This book provides a comprehensive overview of current understanding about the provision of emergency mental health services in an era of community orientated care. Major research findings and theoretical models which will shape future services are described and illustrated by detailed descriptions of successful services both from Europe and North America. A multidisciplinary team of contributors detail the full range of community based services including acute respite care, home based care, day hospitals and family placement schemes, as well as the use of accident and emergency departments and acute in-patient wards. The major factors which influence service development are also explored, including the costs of acute care, the legal framework for emergency mental health work and the views of service users. All those with an interest in or responsibility for mental health will find this insight of value.

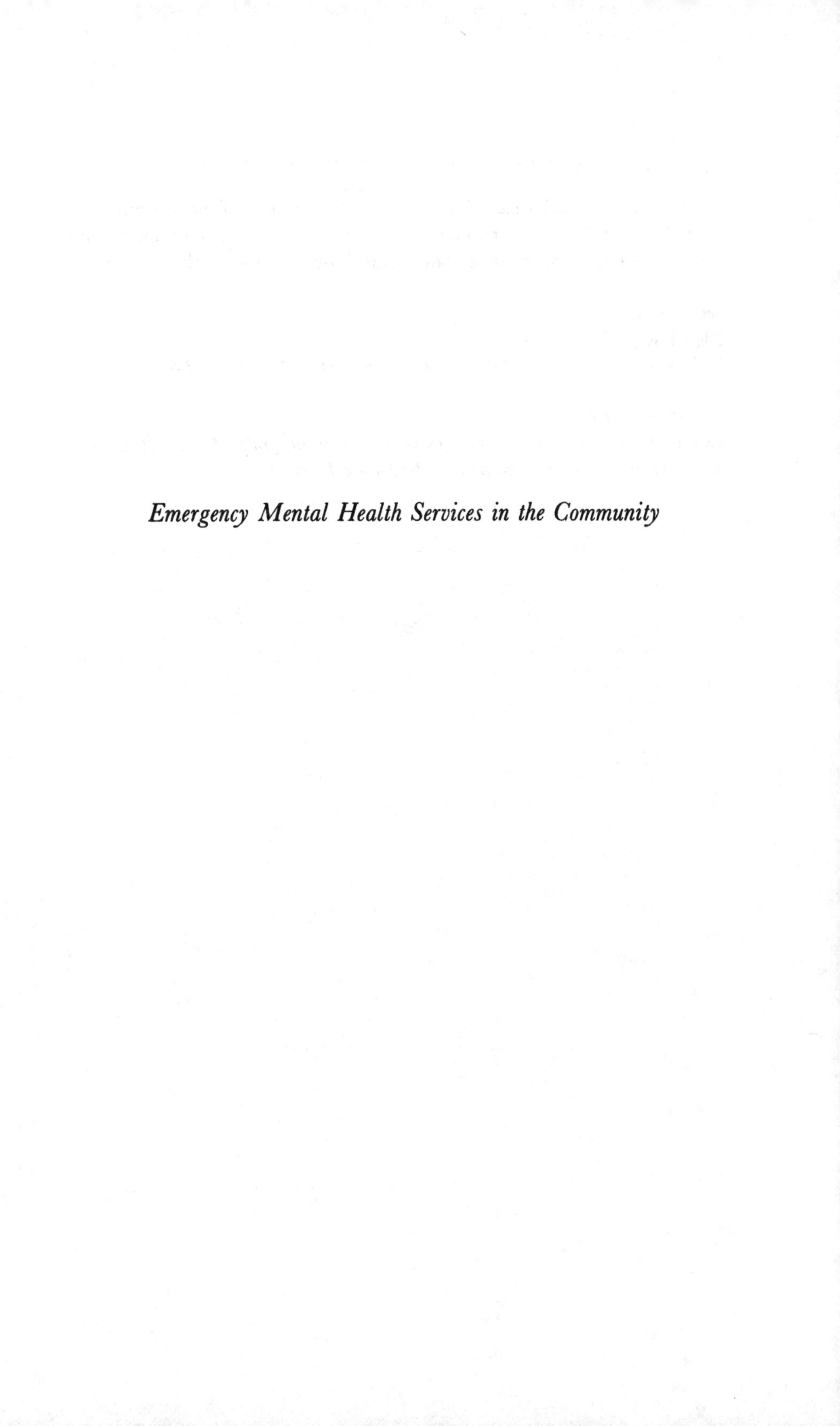

Emergency Mental Health Services in the Community

STUDIES IN SOCIAL AND COMMUNITY PSYCHIATRY

Volumes in this series examine the social dimensions of mental illness as they affect diagnosis and management, and address a range of fundamental issues in the development of community-based mental health services.

Series editor
PETER J. TYRER
Professor of Community Psychiatry, St Mary's Hospital Medical School, London

Also in this series
IAN R. H. FALLOON AND GRAINNE FADDEN *Integrated Mental Health Care*
T. S. BRUGHA *Social Support and Psychiatric Disorder*

Emergency Mental Health Services in the Community

edited by

MICHAEL PHELAN

Institute of Psychiatry

GERALDINE STRATHDEE

Maudsley Hospital

GRAHAM THORNICROFT

Institute of Psychiatry and Maudsley Hospital

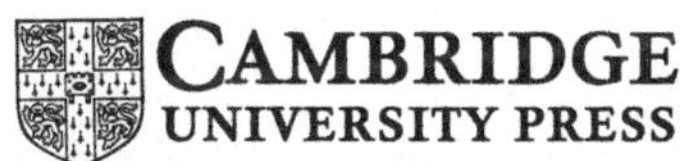

CAMBRIDGE UNIVERSITY PRESS
Cambridge, New York, Melbourne, Madrid, Cape Town, Singapore, São Paulo

Cambridge University Press
The Edinburgh Building, Cambridge CB2 2RU, UK

Published in the United States of America by Cambridge University Press, New York

www.cambridge.org
Information on this title: www.cambridge.org/9780521452519

© Cambridge University Press 1995

This publication is in copyright. Subject to statutory exception
and to the provisions of relevant collective licensing agreements,
no reproduction of any part may take place without
the written permission of Cambridge University Press.

First published 1995
This digitally printed first paperback version 2006

A catalogue record for this publication is available from the British Library

Library of Congress Cataloguing in Publication data
Emergency mental health services in the community / edited by
Michael Phelan, Geraldine Strathdee, Graham Thornicroft
p. cm. – (Studies in social and community psychiatry)
ISBN 0 521 45251 1 (hardback)
1. Psychiatric emergencies. 2. Community mental health services.
I. Phelan, Michael. II. Strathdee, Geraldine. III. Thornicroft,
Graham. IV. Series.
[DNLM: 1. Emergency Services, Psychiatric – organization &
administration. 2. Community Mental Health Services –
organization & administration. WM 30.6 E53 1995]
RC480.6.E436 1995
362.2′04251 – dc20 95–17697 CIP
DNLM/DLC
for Library of Congress

ISBN-13 978-0-521-45251-9 hardback
ISBN-10 0-521-45251-1 hardback

ISBN-13 978-0-521-03455-5 paperback
ISBN-10 0-521-03455-8 paperback

Contents

Contributors

DR HOWARD BADERMAN
University College Hospital, London

CAROLINE BATES
National Union of Teachers Legal and Professional Services, Hamilton House, Mabledon Place, London WC1H 9TX

RUSSELL BENNETT
Mental Health Center of Dane County, 625 West Washington Av., Madison, Wisconsin 53703, USA

PROFESSOR MAX BIRCHWOOD
The Archer Centre, All Saints Hospital, Lodge Road, Winson Green, Birmingham B18 5SD

PROFESSOR LORENZO BURTI
Institute of Psychiatry, University of Verona, Verona, Italy

IAN BYNOE
Institute for Public Policy Research, 30-32 Southampton Street, London WC2E 7RA

YVONNE CHRISTIE
Aveleon Associates, 110 Perry Hill, London SE6 4EY

ALISON COBB
MIND, National Association for Mental Health, Granta House, 15-19 Broadway, London E15 4BQ

PROFESSOR FRANCIS CREED
University of Manchester, Rawnsley Building, Manchester Royal Infirmary, Oxford Road, Manchester M13 9WL

VAL DRURY
The Archer Centre, All Saints Hospital, Lodge Road, Winson Green, Birmingham B18 5SD

ADINA HALPERN
Nightingale Fellow, Commoner in Mental Health Law, Trinity Hall, Cambridge

RACHEL JENKINGS
Department of Health, 133-155 Waterloo Road, London SE1 8UG

DR SONIA JOHNSON
Maudsley Continuing Care Study, Institute of Psychiatry, De Crespigny Park, Denmark Hill, London SE5 8AF

PROFESSOR HEINZ KATSCHNIG
Department of Psychiatry, University of Vienna, Wahringergurter 18-20, A-1090 Wien, Austria

DR DAVID KINGDON
Division of Mental Health, Department of Health, Wellington House, 134-155 Waterloo Road, London SE1 8UG

PAUL MCCRONE
Institute of Psychiatry, De Crespigny Park, Denmark Hill, London SE5 8AF

DR MICHAEL PHELAN
Institute of Psychiatry, De Crespigny Park, Denmark Hill, London SE5 8AF

JAAK RAKFELDT
Yale University, Connecticut Mental Health Center, Office of the Clinical Director, 34 Park Street, New Haven, CT 06519

DR LIZ SAYCE
MIND, National Association for Mental Health, Granta House, 15-19 Broadway, London E15 4BQ

PROFESSOR JAN SCOTT
University Dept of Psychological Medicine, Royal Infirmary, Queen Victoria Road, Newcastle upon Tyne NE1 4LP

DR TOM SENSKY
Department of Psychiatry, Charing Cross & Westminster Medical School, West Middlesex University Hospital, Isleworth, Middlesex TW7 6AF

Mike Slade
Institute of Psychiatry, De Crespigny Park, Denmark Hill, London SE5 8AF

Professor William Sledge
Yale University, Connecticut Mental Health Center, Office of the Clinical Director, 34 Park Street, New Haven, CT 06519, USA

Dr Geraldine Strathdee
Maudsley Hospital, Denmark Hill, London SE5 8AZ

Dr Kim Sutherby
Institute of Psychiatry, De Crespigny Park, Denmark Hill, London SE5 8AF

Dr George Szmukler
Maudsley Hospital, Denmark Hill, London SE5 8AZ

Professor Michele Tansella
Department of Medical Psychology, Institute of Psychiatry, University of Verona, Verona, Italy

Jack Tebes
Yale University, Connecticut Mental Health Center, Office of the Clinical Director, 34 Park Street, New Haven, CT 06519, USA

Dr Graham Thornicroft
Institute of Psychiatry, De Crespigny Park, Denmark Hill, London SE5 8AF

Professor Peter Tyrer
St. Mary's Hospital Medical School, Academic Unit of Psychiatry, St. Charles' Hospital, London W10 6DZ

Ann Watts
Maudsley Hospital, Denmark Hill, London SE5 8AZ

Foreword

Mental illness is a leading cause of distress and disability. Estimates suggest that over a quarter of GP consultations have a mental health component and half of the people seen by social workers have some sort of mental illness.

This authoritative book arose from a study commissioned by the Department of Health and includes contributions from experts who have vast and varied experience of the provision and evaluation of emergency mental health services. It includes both theoretical aspects of the subject and practical examples of mental health care programmes and tells us what patients think of these services. It also highlights that patients want local and accessible community mental health services which provide prompt, appropriate and acceptable help.

Having examined successful models of services in the UK and abroad the authors suggest that no one model can be applied universally. However, it is clear that local agencies must co-ordinate their efforts to ensure that mental health services work together to meet the varying needs of people who suffer from mental illness and the needs of their carers. We can all learn from others' experiences and this book is relevant to anyone responsible for the provision or development or comprehensive, effective and efficient emergency mental health services.

Alan Langlands
NHS Chief Executive

PRINCIPLES AND POLICIES

Introduction

The first section of this book presents the historical background to current thinking about emergency mental health services, the evidence we have about its development, and summarises the evidence on whether such services are indeed effective. Professor Heinz Katschnig bases his findings upon an authoritative review for the World Health Organisation of emergency services throughout Europe, and brings together this vast range of practical experience into themes to guide future service development. Drs Sonia Johnson and Graham Thornicroft fill in the background to this book by detailing the historical roots of current emergency mental health service theories, and by detailing different models of care that have been proposed. It is striking that when users of mental health services express their views, their priorities are often very different from those of professionals. Liz Sayce and colleagues give voice to these priorities, and particularly emphasise that emergency services out of office hours seem guided more by convenience to staff than patients' needs.

For situations in which a patient may not agree to accept mental health treatment and care in an emergency, the provisions of mental health law are commonly applied. Ian Bynoe and colleagues demonstrate that the ethical and clinical dilemmas in such situations need to be framed within mental health legislation that explicitly addresses modern community practices, and that law framed in the era of hospital treatment is now decreasingly relevant. There is increasing recognition that the economics of mental health is an important area of study. Paul McCrone provides an overview of what is known about the costs of emergency mental health care. The common final pathway for people with mental health problems who are in despair is towards suicide attempts, and Drs David Kingdon and Rachel Jenkins clearly set out the national priority within England to reduce suicide rates. They also bring together the evidence that this is a realistic and important goal. For patients not in life-threatening circumstances, initial crisis can be used as a point from which constructive therapeutic relationships can be built, and Prof. Max Birchwood and Val Drury show that the body of evidence for these early interventions is now becoming powerful and persuasive. In the last chapter of this section, Drs Kim Sutherby and George Szmukler describe the principles and practical implications of conducting emergency assessments in the community.

1

The scope and limitations of emergency mental health services in the community

Heinz Katschnig

Introduction

When psychiatric care was based in large psychiatric hospitals there was a limited professional response to what would nowadays be called, a psychiatric emergency – i.e., disturbed patients who, posing a risk to themselves or to others, were taken to hospital and admitted. These hospitals were often many miles from where the patients lived, and as admissions were long-term, patients were isolated from their relatives and other social supports. Emergency care was passive and curative.

The advent of community psychiatry has changed this. In contrast to the traditional waiting attitude of the psychiatric hospital, community psychiatry is concerned with actively reaching out into the community and providing local and flexible services which meet the differing needs of those requiring help. The philosophy of community psychiatry is to be active and preventive, instead of passive and curative. However, to provide appropriate early intervention in emergency situations is clearly a difficult and complex task.

Isolated attempts to provide non-hospital based help to those in crisis are not new. For instance, in New York a telephone hotline had been established at the beginning of the twentieth century by Warren, an Anglican clergyman, in order to prevent suicides (Allen, 1984), and in Amsterdam during the 1930s a mobile psychiatric emergency service was set up with the aim of preventing hospitalisation and thus reduce the costs of care for the city (Querido, 1968). However, it is only recently that the importance of such services has been widely recognised and that attempts to provide comprehensive emergency care have become more widespread.

Despite the fact that the need for efficient and high quality psychiatric emergency services has been demonstrated, there is still a long way to go before they are provided universally. After 30 years of community psychiatry there is, in most Western countries, consensus about the standards required for psychiatric rehabilitation, and how such services can best be organised. But there is great uncertainty about how best to organise community psychiatric emergency services. It seems that it is easier to organise the return of psychiatric patients into the community – despite the frequent problems of fragmented legal and financial responsibilities and public rejection of psychiatric patients – than the entry from the community into psychiatry of those needing urgent psychiatric help.

All too often, a psychiatric emergency still results in a rough entry into psychiatric care for patients. There appear to be four main reasons why it is difficult to ensure the smooth transition that everyone would want:

1 The uncertainty – which cannot be reduced because of pressure of time – about the nature of the specific problem which has to be dealt with.
2 The geographical distance between those needing and those providing help.
3 The necessity for immediate action despite the geographical distance and the lack of information (e.g. making far-reaching decisions about admitting a person against his will to a psychiatric hospital or leaving him in the community with the risk of harm to self or to others).
4 The clash of different concepts held by those afflicted, their carers and the mental health staff (who often disagree among themselves) about what constitutes a psychiatric emergency and what action should be taken, as opposed to psychiatric rehabilitation, where the problem is usually already defined as being a psychiatric one.

The historical roots of emergency mental health services in the community

In a review, carried out in the 1980s (Katschnig *et al.*, 1993), of 32 psychiatric emergency and crisis intervention services in 19 European countries some patterns were detectable but no two services closely resembled each other. Most services had been created out of local initiatives because of dissatisfaction with existing emergency provision. In most of the countries visited no systematic attempts had been made to provide good psychiatric emergency care on a nation-wide basis.

This variation is understandable when the different origins and reasons behind the establishment of such services are considered. At least four factors appear to have shaped service development:

- Prevention of hospitalisation.
- Prevention of suicide.
- Crisis intervention theory.
- The necessity of coping with de-institutionalisation.

'Prevention of hospitalisation' was a core concept in the early days of community psychiatry. The United States 'Community Mental Health Centre Programme' of the Kennedy administration included an emergency component with the explicit aim of preventing hospitalisation. Today there is no convincing evidence that the number of psychiatric hospital admissions is necessarily reduced by community psychiatric services. Whenever there is a fall in the number of in-patient beds in use, it is due to a decrease in the average length of stay, and not to a reduction in the numbers of admissions. There is even some evidence that the total number of admissions, especially of re-admissions, increases when community psychiatric services are established. This may be partly due to the fact that, while these services may prevent some hospitalisations, they may simultaneously recruit new patients, who would otherwise have not received the care they needed.

The 'suicide prevention' movement has its roots not in the professional mental health field but in lay activities, frequently associated with religious institutions. In the UK, the 'Samaritans' are a typical example. It is doubtful whether specialised suicide prevention centres have contributed to any substantial reduction in suicide rates (Reimer, 1986). From an analysis of the data on callers to telephone hotlines it is also evident that very few are, in fact, suicidal. Today, there is less isolated emphasis on suicide prevention, and instead it is viewed as an important aim for all mental health services.

'Crisis intervention theory' has been one of the prime movers behind the setting up of specialised crisis intervention services in Europe. The essential ingredient of crisis theory is the notion that, as in the non-developmental crises of a healthy personality, there is always the chance of growth, and that a well managed crisis may lead to better functioning in the future (Lindeman, 1944; Caplan, 1964; Jacobson, 1980). Crisis intervention centres are meant to provide this type of assistance using specific crisis intervention techniques, but few users of these services correspond to this concept. Such crises, which by definition do not involve a diagnosable psychiatric illness, are seen as brief non-specific states, characterised by distress, worry and tension, often with short lived feelings of hopelessness, helplessness, sadness and futility, and are said to occur in previously stable individuals free from psychiatric illness, coming on suddenly as a result of severe stress. 'Pure' instances of crisis of this type are rare in practice, since most patients who turn up in crisis intervention centres have chronic domestic, social and relationship problems and/or personality disorders.

Finally, an important motive for setting up psychiatric emergency services comes from the consequences of 'de-institutionalisation'. It has already been stated that the number of re-admissions increases whenever psychiatric hospital beds are dramatically reduced, and a parallel increase in the number of patients turning up in emergency services is observed (Kaskey & Ianzito, 1984).

In Europe, the provision of psychiatric emergency care in the community is not only patchy, but is also confusing, since services – depending on their historical roots – often have a specific ideology which is not easily understood by clients. The use of the terms 'crisis intervention' and 'emergency psychiatry' are often confused and used interchangeably in the descriptions and names of services. To the patient and his family, fine distinctions between problems and symptoms, or reactions and illnesses are of little interest; they feel unwell and know they need help.

Who needs psychiatric emergency care?

In the fourth edition of the *Handbook of Psychiatric Emergencies* by Slaby (1994) more than 250 psychiatric emergency conditions are described. A selected list of just some of these conditions highlights the difficulty in providing psychiatric emergency services: abdominal pain of psychogenic origin, acute psychosis, alcohol withdrawal, anxiety, carbamazepine-induced disorders, bereavement, encephalitis, erotomania, gambling addiction, headache, homelessness, hypoglycaemia, lead toxicity, marital crises, mutism, opiate dependence, phencyclidine intoxication, post-cardiotomy delirium, rape, self mutilation, steroid-induced disorder and suicide attempts.

Apart from the overriding necessity to prevent harm towards self or others, there are clear clinical priorities when dealing with these conditions, for instance an organic aetiology must be excluded before a diagnosis of a functional psychosis can be considered. Unfortunately, the presenting psychopathological picture, including the circumstances, often give little hint to the aetiology and may even be misleading. For example, acute schizophrenic states are often precipitated by life events, seducing the uninitiated into believing in a simple stress reaction; anxiety states can be the consequence of traumatic experiences but they can be the result also of hyperthyroidism; and acute psychosocial crises are often masked by psycho-organic symptoms when, for instance, alcohol is used as a means of coping or suicide is attempted with tricyclic antidepressants. It is often impossible, even for those skilled in psychiatric emergency work, to solve the puzzle on the spot. Fortunately, it is sufficient in many cases to just consider the presence of an organic or 'endogenous' aetiology and to manage safely the situation by appropriate referral.

In order to clarify the situation, it is suggested that three types of patients requiring emergency psychiatric care are distinguished and considered when planning services:

1 Those in acute psychosocial crises (mainly because of personal losses; often, however, with a background of long-standing psychosocial problems and of personality disorders).
2 Those with acute psychoses of organic or endogenous origin not yet known to psychiatric services.
3 Those with a chronic mental illness, living in the community, who are overtaxed by the stresses of normal community life – a population of emergency service users which is a result, in part, of the reduction in the number of long-term hospital patients.

Obviously many patients do not fit neatly into any of these categories, and others have features of all three. However, it is clear that a wide range of services and skills are required if these three groups are to be adequately cared for. Individuals in psychosocial crisis may benefit from crisis intervention techniques (but, if suicidal, may also require compulsory admission). Organic and endogenous acute psychoses usually need complex psychiatric management including psychotropic medication and, at times, hospital admission, whereas patients with chronic mental illness living in the community may need a combination of both.

It is also important to accept that there is a sub-population of patients who use emergency services repeatedly, often because their needs are not being met elsewhere. They have been called 'chronic crisis patients' (Bassuk & Gerson, 1980) and 'emergency room repeaters' (Walker, 1983). Groves (1978) has categorised some of these patients and in doing so has highlighted the negative feelings expressed by staff towards them: 'dependent clingers', who use flattery and childlike behaviour to seduce the doctor into giving endless medical attention and reassurance; 'entitled demanders', who are often well-educated and articulate, know their rights to health care and expect to have their questions answered and needs met; 'manipulative help rejecters', who insist that no doctor or medicine has ever helped them, yet keep appearing to follow doctors' orders; and finally, 'self-destructive deniers', who by their behaviour take no responsibility for themselves, forcing others to be responsible for them and are repeatedly brought to an emergency service in a moribund state.

The organisation and range of services

There are two main components to the quality of psychiatric emergency care in the community: **accessibility** and the provision of **comprehensive assessment and management**. Accessibility is essential if help is to be provided quickly, and undue suffering and complications, such as self-harm, are to be reduced. It also includes several components: psychological visibility and acceptance of the service by the general public, availability around the clock, immediate availability and, last but not least, financial accessibility. The components of actual service provision include: a thorough evaluation of the person concerned, including such diverse aspects as the motives behind calling the emergency service (in whose interest was it?), a medical examination (requiring medical skills and access to a medical infrastructure), the necessary medical, psychosocial and legal interventions and at times the control of violent behaviour.

There will always be tension when trying to achieve both components. Permanent and quick accessibility cannot be married with a comprehensive and competent assessment and management of the emergency condition on the spot. One aspect can only be maximised at the expense of the other. For both components of quality of care, the **size of the catchment area** and the **types of available services** are of crucial importance.

Size of the catchment area must be considered in terms of the **geographical size** and the number of people living in the area – a geographically small urban catchment area may well have more inhabitants than a large but thinly populated rural area. The geographical size largely determines quick accessibility of a service, if a face-to-face contact is regarded to be necessary. Where distances are short, those needing help and those providing it, can come together quickly. Also, a mobile service can manage a series of emergencies more easily in a small catchment area. If a person needs help, he/she and their family will more readily accept it if they do not have to travel far. For emergency psychiatry a geographically small catchment area has the same advantages of high accessibility as it has for community psychiatry in general.

The **size of the population** covered by a service is equally as important as geographical size. A population of 50,000 or 80,000 (the typical sector size in France and Italy) will allow staff to get to know many of the patients living in the community, which is clearly helpful when an emergency arises. However, a small population may have the disadvantage that psychiatric emergencies are relatively rare, and that given the broad spectrum of conditions which can present as emergencies, those providing emergency care may not gain sufficient experience in the required diagnostic and management skills.

This dilemma is illustrated by the services in Paris where two types of sector size have co-existed since the 1980s. In 1982, a centralised psychiatric emergency service, the *Centre Psychiatrique d'Orientation et d'Accueil* (CPOA), for the whole city of four million inhabitants, saw around 40 emergencies in 24 hours, while an experimental sectorised service with around-the-clock coverage of 30,000 inhabitants saw 500 patients during a whole year, of whom most were long-term users. It is simply impossible, therefore, for the staff of the sectorised team to become as experienced in assessing psychiatric emergencies as the staff of the centralised services.

It is clear to all those involved in planning emergency community mental health services that it will not always be possible to provide high quality, around-the-clock coverage for individual small-sized catchment areas. It would appear sensible for services with small catchment areas to combine efforts when providing cover at night and at weekends. In Paris, apart from the experimental sector already mentioned, there is co-operation between the 38 sectorised community mental health centres (mostly only open during the day and on weekdays) and the CPOA. In the last 10 years several of these sectorised services have started to work 24-hours, seven-days a week. Also, more and more psychiatrists have been allocated to general hospitals. This is reflected in fewer patients being seen at the centralised CPOA, and a higher proportion of these patients are homeless and non-nationals than previously. In Triest an interesting variant of this model has been working successfully for many years. Doctors from the seven community mental health centres, which are open from 8 a.m. to 8 p.m. and cover 280,000 inhabitants, work a night rota on the psychiatric emergency ward of the general hospital which covers the whole catchment area. This ward receives on average seven emergencies in 24 hours.

In addition to geographical and population size, the types of services and the settings in which they are delivered will have a strong influence on the quality of care. Throughout this book examples are provided of the range of emergency services that have been established. There are four broad categories: telephone services, mobile services, out-patient and day-hospital services and services with overnight-stay facilities.

Telephone services

There is an important role for telephone lines in any emergency service. They provide an easily accessible and highly acceptable source of support for those in crisis. Traditionally, in Western Europe, most telephone services are staffed by volunteers, independent from formal psychiatric services, and provide anonymity and security to callers. Alongside these, the provision of 24-hour telephone lines by local community psychiatric services appears to be increasing. Patients and their carers are grateful to have someone they can contact at anytime, and problems can often be sufficiently resolved so that staff and patient can avoid having to make immediate face-to-face contact. This has advantages in rural areas where distances are great, and at night in inner city areas where home visiting may be dangerous for staff. However, a telephone call will only provide a limited amount of information about a caller's condition and surroundings, and the possibilities for intervention are extremely restricted.

Mobile services

Teams which provide acute care in patients' homes can be an important component of an emergency service. The feasibility and effectiveness of such teams are discussed in detail in subsequent chapters. The opportunity of seeing someone in their normal surroundings offers enormous advantages for staff trying to make a full assessment, and the maintenance of normal social support during times of crisis will often be very beneficial to the patient. However, such services may at times place an excessive burden on carers, and may be regarded as an unwanted intrusion by some. Also, there will always be some situations which cannot, or should not, be managed without transferring the patient elsewhere.

Out-patient and day hospital services

Although out-patient clinics are usually viewed as a non-emergency service they can play a role in the provision of emergency care, if time is allocated for urgent cases to be seen. Day hospitals have tended to be seen as primarily providing long-term care, but Professor Francis Creed (Chapter 15) outlines the effective role that they can play for those in crisis. Other out-patient services, such as specialised emergency clinics and Accident and Emergency departments in general hospitals will be dealt with elsewhere in this book, and again are an important component. Overall the acceptability of such services will depend on their location, with those based in psychiatric hospitals being less acceptable than stand-alone services, especially when they have neutral names such as 'crisis intervention centre' or 'walk-in clinic'. All out-patient services offer staff the opportunity of face-to-face contact, and usually there will be access to the medical investigation services.

Services with overnight stay facilities

The commonest overnight facility for those in crisis remains the hospital ward, and legal procedures for compulsory admission are often required. The development of alternatives to hospital admission are seen as a priority by those who use services (see Chapter 3), but progress has been slow. The descriptions in this book of some successful alternatives may encourage their development, and allow fuller evaluation of their effectiveness. In some European cities, so-called ‘crisis admission wards’ have been set up within a non-psychiatric setting, with the aim of helping the patient overcome his/her crisis within a couple of days and thus avoid admission to a psychiatric hospital. Such wards usually have a multidisciplinary team and provide a high quality of care. However, it is often not possible to resolve the emergency situation within a couple of days, and many patients have to be referred to psychiatric in-patient units.

Staff problems related to psychiatric emergency work

The rapid turnover of patients, many in great distress, inevitably puts a heavy burden on the staff of an emergency service. Particularly stressful aspects of the work that staff complain of are:

- having to break up relationships with patients, and their families, after a brief period of intense involvement;
- having frequent encounters with severely distressed, aggressive, and at times dangerous patients;
- a need to make rapid decisions, often based on limited information;
- frequent complaints from other agencies that have taken over the care of patients, and who have had more time to do a comprehensive assessment;
- practical problems such as difficult hours of work and occasional shortage of sleep.

Concepts such as ‘burn-out syndrome’ and ‘overload’ are frequent topics of discussion in these units. A general burn-out syndrome was first described by Freudenberger (1974), and other authors (e.g., Aguilera & Messick, 1982) provide a detailed description of the stages of this syndrome (enthusiasm, stagnation, frustration, apathy, hopelessness), which occurs in staff working for emergency services.

Strategies to minimise stress, and avoid its harmful effects upon staff, have been discussed by Slaby (1994) and Kaskey & Ianzito (1984). A measure which is easy to recommend, but may be difficult to achieve, is good selection of staff. In addition, the duties of the emergency team should be arranged so that staff see a wide variety of patients; it is, for example frustrating, and at times distressing, to work only with parasuicide patients.

Supervision of all team members, particularly the junior members, by experienced workers of all the disciplines concerned must be a high priority. Continuing education of the team members by means of seminars and educative case discussions should always be a part of the overall programme of a unit.

The question of whether or not the members of a crisis and emergency team should keep on a number of patients for after-care is largely an individual decision. Some crisis workers find that after-care work is particularly satisfying, whereas others prefer the rapid turnover without the implications of the development of a long-lasting relationship with the patient.

One of the most obvious precautions against the development of excessive stress and exhaustion is the provision of enough staff, particularly at night and at weekends, on those units where a 24-hour cover is involved. However, this is often the most difficult to achieve.

The multidisciplinary team, which is a particular feature of emergency and crisis centres, has been described by many authors. It has a particular style of working, characterised by the sharing of responsibility and blurring of professional roles (Cooper, 1979). It is likely that this style was evolved as a response to the varieties of stress already mentioned, since the sharing of responsibilities and decisions among the members of the team obviously helps to minimise both the stress and workload. Such sharing is on the whole beneficial, but there are occasions when it is clearly stressful for the team if a specific person cannot be made responsible for mistakes or wrong decisions.

Despite an overall beneficial effect, multidisciplinary team work may result in problems, because of overt disagreement or latent conflict between staff members about their different roles. Sometimes it is clear that staff are using team meetings to work through their own conflicts with other members, or even to try and resolve their own emotional problems. This can be indicated by the increasing frequency and duration of team meetings, and by the meetings being focused on the organisation and relationships between staff members, rather than patient management.

Conclusions

This chapter has attempted to provide a brief overview of the historical background of the development of emergency psychiatric services, and to introduce some of the major issues facing those who are responsible for providing such services both today and in the future. With wide variation in the organisation of health and social services available in each of the European countries it is not possible, and would anyway be inappropriate, to give precise guidelines about how emergency mental health services should be organised in different settings. However, based on past experience it is possible to give some tentative suggestions about the direction in which future developments should progress.

The move to providing services close to where people live, whether this involves admission to a local hospital or actual care in the home, should continue. More attention needs to be given to the specific requirements of local communities, and greater recognition of specific cultural and other special needs. There is increasing evidence that rates of psychiatric disorder are closely correlated to levels of deprivation, and the allocation of resources should be closely matched to the social characteristics of the area served.

The wide range of problems and disorders presenting to services requires an equally diverse mix of skills and responses from staff. Multidisciplinary working and greater involvement of the non-medical professions will help to broaden the expertise available. However, there are clear advantages in maintaining a close integration with primary and secondary general health care services, rather than establishing them as separate, specialised psychiatric emergency/ crisis intervention services. General health services are accessible to the public around-the-clock, both in large cities and rural areas. General hospitals are usually within easy reach of the population, and primary care physicians may visit patients at home. Another reason for integration is the frequent presence of either physical causes (e.g., intoxication, brain disease, metabolic disorder) or physical concomitants (e.g., overdose, drunkenness) in psychiatric emergencies, and the necessity for medical expertise, especially during the initial assessment and management. Finally, general medical services have the advantage of having fewer stigmas attached to them, and for this reason are more acceptable to many people.

While it may be advisable to graft emergency psychiatric services on to existing general health services, there is still a need for specialisation within such an integrated setting. Emergency psychiatry is not simply general psychiatry in an acute setting. Interventions have to be carried out immediately, without time for detailed treatment planning; information available about the immediate history and background of the condition is frequently scanty when action has to be taken; available resources for diagnosis and management are limited; and, finally, a potentially omniscient emergency worker is required, since any psychiatric condition – organic, functional or purely psychogenic – can present itself as an emergency. Working under such circumstances is quite different from ordinary psychiatric duties.

References

Allen, N. (1984). Suicide prevention. In *Suicide. Assessment and Intervention*, 2nd edn. ed. C. Loing Hatton, S. McBride Valente, Norwalk, Connecticut, Appleton-Century-Crofts.

Aguilera, D. C. & Messick, J. M. (1982). *Crisis Intervention. Theory and Methodology*, 4th edn. St. Louis, CV Mosby.

Bassuk, E. & Gerson, S. (1980). Chronic crisis patients. A discrete clinical group. *American Journal of Psychiatry*, **137**, 1513–17.

Caplan, G. (1964). *Principles of Preventive Psychiatry*. New York, Basic Books.

Cooper, J. E. (1979). Crisis admission units and emergency psychiatric services. *Public Health in Europe*, No. 2. Copenhagen, World Health Organization.

Freudenberger, H.J. (1974). Staff burnout. *Journal of Social Issues*, **30**, 159–65.

Groves, J. (1978). Taking care of the hateful patient. *New England Journal of Medicine*, **298**, 883–7.

Jacobson, G. F. (Ed.) (1980). Crisis intervention in the 1980s. *New Directions for Mental Health Services*, No. 6. San Francisco, Jossey Bass.

Kaskey, G. B. & Ianzito, B. M. (1984). Development of an emergency psychiatric treatment unit. *Hospital Community Psychiatry*, **35**, 1220–2.

Katschnig, H., Konieczna, T. & Cooper, J. E. (1993). *Emergency Psychiatric and Crisis Intervention Services in Europe*. A report based on visits to services in seventeen countries. Copenhagen, World Health Organization.

Lindeman, E. (1944). Symptomatology and management of acute grief. *American Journal of Psychiatry*, **101**, 141–8.

Querido, A. (1968). The shaping of community mental health care. *British Journal of Psychiatry*, **114**, 293–302.

Reimer, C. (1986). Praevention und Therapie der Suizidalitaet. In *Psychiatrie der Gegenwart* 2. *Krisenintervention Suizid Konsiliarpsychiatrie*, ed. K. P. Kisker, H. Lauter, J.-E. Meyer, C. Mueller & E. Stroemgren. Berlin, Springer-Verlag.

Slaby, A. E. (Ed.) (1994). *Handbook of Psychiatric Emergencies*. Norwalk, Connecticut, Appleton & Lange.

Walker, J. I. (1983). *Psychiatric Emergencies. Intervention and Resolution*. Philadelphia, J. P. Lippincott.

2

Service models in emergency psychiatry: an international review

SONIA JOHNSON AND GRAHAM THORNICROFT

Introduction

Services for the assessment and management of psychiatric emergencies have been of central importance during deinstitutionalisation and the continuing development of community care. However, discussion and evaluation of this aspect of care have lagged behind that of rehabilitation. The literature in this area is limited and mainly consists of descriptions and, more rarely, evaluations of small model services. There are few general surveys of services for psychiatric emergency care, and very few evaluative studies have taken place outside small experimental services. However, by summarising the various contributions which have been made in this chapter, we aim to construct a general overview of the range of service models, many of which are discussed in more detail in subsequent chapters.

Before reviewing this area, it is important to address the question: what counts as a 'real' psychiatric emergency? In particular, should psychosocial crises be distinguished from deteriorations in mental state in those whom psychiatrists would regard as severely mentally ill? In practice, services vary greatly in what they regard as 'real' psychiatric emergencies, and consequently in the situations they regard as proper priorities for their interventions. In this review we have included services which serve each of these patient groups. Our discussion is, however, confined to research about those emergency services which, if not based on a purely 'medical model', do involve participation by psychiatrists.

There are two main paths along which emergency services may develop (Katschnig & Konieczna, 1990). The first, which is the basis for most of the earlier innovative services, is the provision of centralised, specialised emergency psychiatric services, staffed by people exclusively responsible for emergency work and usually serving large catchment areas. The second, which appears to have overtaken the first in popularity in the last 20 years, is the development of decentralised, locally based services, where emergency intervention is not the responsibility of distinct staff or separately organised from the rest of patient care, but rather forms an integrated part of the comprehensive service offered to the local population. Products of the first 'specialised' tendency in the evolution of services include the specialist psychiatric emergency clinic, brief treatment wards in hospital, deliberate self-harm teams, crisis intervention services and home treatment teams. The second tendency has aimed for an integrated organisation of all services, including emergency intervention, at a local, sector level, often with a community mental health centre providing the base for comprehensive service delivery.

In this chapter, we will begin by discussing the small number of general surveys of overall patterns of emergency psychiatric services which have been published, and then review those papers which focus on a particular form of emergency service. This literature has been divided into two broad categories according to the distinction outlined above between the specialised/centralised and the decentralised/integrated. The two modes of working are not of course entirely distinct. For example, sector teams may do work in patients' homes resembling that of specialised crisis intervention teams and home treatment teams, and the community mental health centre, like the emergency clinic, will often provide a walk-in facility. However, the sector team and the community mental health centre staff will generally have responsibilities other than emergency intervention, and they may continue to work with the same patients both through crises and through periods of relative stability.

Comparative studies of emergency services

Few discussions of general patterns in emergency care have been published, and those which are available tend to focus on qualitative comparisons between a few major centres. One exception is an early review of the status of psychiatric services throughout the United States (Blanes *et al.*, 1967), which includes the results of a national survey. This showed that, while a few centres had innovative services such as multidisciplinary walk-in emergency clinics, the great majority of hospitals relied on a single duty psychiatric resident, whose time was rarely committed exclusively to emergency work. This useful paper thus demonstrates that the innovative services to which much of the literature was devoted were quite unrepresentative of most emergency work at that time.

Wellin *et al.* (1987) identify three lines of development in the North American emergency services. During the 1920s, psychiatric residents began to provide makeshift emergency services within the emergency wards of general hospitals. In the 1930s, emergency services were developed for patients released from large psychiatric hospitals. Then, beginning in the 1950s, community mental health centres began to provide facilities for emergency care. It is suggested that these lines have now converged, with co-operative arrangements between various agencies and a marked tendency for the general hospital to become the main provider of emergency mental health care.

One general survey of emergency psychiatric provision throughout England and Wales has been reported. Johnson and Thornicroft (1991) found a strong trend towards a decentralised, sectorised model for psychiatric emergency provision during the day: 81% of health districts had been sectorised by 1991, and sector teams usually provided the main daytime emergency service. Junior psychiatric staff were most often involved in emergency assessment, although some multidisciplinary assessments were being used in around half the districts. Centralised and specialised forms of emergency service, such as emergency clinics, crisis and respite houses, short-stay evaluation and brief treatment wards and crisis intervention teams were uncommon. Urgent admission to a day hospital was, however, available in the majority of districts, and community mental health centres or day hospitals were used for some daytime emergency assessments in more than half the districts.

In Europe, two major studies undertaken under the auspices of the World Health Organization have surveyed emergency psychiatric service provision. Cooper (1979) visited 15 centres in eight countries, which varied in degree of adherence to a brief treatment, crisis intervention model. Cooper noted that this model often appeared to be operating with some success, but that disappointment was widespread in the degree to which patients were not previously well adjusted people coming forward in crisis, but rather people with many long-standing social and psychological difficulties.

Katschnig and Konieczna (1990) provide a supplement to this report, with a further survey undertaken between 1982 and 1985. They discuss a range of service types, including traditional psychiatric acute wards, psychosocial crisis intervention services, telephone hotlines and mobile services. They draw attention to a number of important questions for the providers of emergency services. In particular, difficulties may result from the same professional having to cope with quite disparate groups of patients, including people in acute psychosocial crisis, often on a background of personality disorder and chaotic lifestyle, people with acute mental illnesses, and those with chronic psychotic illnesses who may be at risk of decompensating in the face of quite minor psychosocial stressors. The provision of services which are multidisciplinary may provide more flexibility in responding to a variety of types of patient. These reviews provide the most enlightening insight available into the range of modes of organisation of psychiatric emergency care operating in Europe. The centres visited are, however, predominantly centres of excellence, with relatively well funded and highly developed emergency services, so that considerable scope remains for more precise delineation and evaluation of the range of services operating outside these centres.

Centralised emergency psychiatry: service models

The emergency clinic

The emergency clinic features prominently in the literature of the United States from the 1950s, and was the first innovative form of emergency service to be extensively described. Early examples are described by Coleman and Zwerling (1959), who established the first service in the United States of this type at the Bronx Municipal Hospital Centre. Similar clinics are described by Bellak (1960), Normand *et al.* (1963) and Atkins (1967).

Early emergency clinic work was closely linked to two theoretical schools. Firstly, the approach of ego psychology provided a psycho-dynamic view of the genesis of psychosis, and suggested it might be prevented by a brief psychotherapeutic intervention aimed at restoring the defence mechanisms which had previously been effective in maintaining ego integrity. Secondly, crisis intervention theory was also highly influential at this time (Caplan, 1961, 1964; review in Hobbs, 1984).

Short interventions in the United States emergency clinics of the 1960s consisted of up to about five arranged repeat attendances at the emergency clinic, aimed at preventing decompensation and promoting growth by bringing about a healthy resolution of the crisis. Initially, there was optimism about the efficacy and the scope for wide application of this model. For example, Bellak viewed brief psychotherapy as 'on the spot treatment for troubled feelings and the vexing ordinary problems of everyday life', and believed that in a few sessions at the time of crisis, 'a quick and better restructuration of patient and situation' could be achieved. He proposed that this form of intervention should not be confined to medical settings, but should be taught to teachers, lawyers, chaplains and parents, in order to solve the problems of a world of 'lonely crowds'. These clinics usually operated on a walk-in basis, and were often based in general rather than psychiatric hospitals. The move of the psychiatric acute units to the general hospital, and the setting up of out-patient clinics in the general hospital, were at that time perceived as cornerstones for a more accessible, community-based form of psychiatric care. These services were also innovative in being multidisciplinary, rather than based exclusively on medical intervention.

During the 1970s the crisis intervention model appears to have declined in importance in the United States (Goldfinger & Lipton, 1985; Farberow, 1968), as interest in more biomedical models of mental illness re-emerged. Disillusionment resulted from the realisation that the population attracted and treated by this form of service were not an otherwise healthy group requiring brief preventive intervention in severe social crisis as originally envisaged, but were often 'chronic crisis patients' – recurrent, disorganised attenders of the emergency services (Bassuk & Gerson, 1980, Bassuk, 1985). 'Chronic crisis patients' are described as having insecure relationships and disrupted employment histories, with highly impulsive behaviour and immature and dependent personalities. Some have primary diagnoses of personality disorder or chronic neurosis; others are young people with psychotic illnesses who have never been institutionalised and have not maintained stable contact with any other services. These patients provoke hostility and disillusionment among emergency staff, and present recurrently to the emergency services when in crisis, rather than engaging in any consistent treatment

(Chafetz *et al.*, 1966; Farberow, 1968; Gomez, 1983; Bassuk, 1985; Perez *et al.*, 1986).

Paradoxically, whilst specialist emergency clinics of this type went into decline in the United States in the 1970s and 1980s, a number of similar model services, providing walk-in facilities and broadly based on crisis intervention theory, were developing in Europe, particularly in the Netherlands and in the German speaking countries. Cooper's (1979) survey of European emergency services describes a number of such services, including clinics in Utrecht, the Netherlands and in Stockholm, Sweden. Häfner-Ranabauer *et al.* (1987) and Schöny (1983) describe walk-in crisis intervention services in Mannheim, Germany and in Linz, Austria.

Emergency clinics based on a more 'biomedical' model have also been established. A number of British papers have been devoted to the Emergency Clinic at the Maudsley Hospital (Brothwood, 1965; Mindham *et al.*, 1973; Lim, 1983; Haw *et al.*, 1987). When the clinic was first established in the 1950s, there was very little facility for emergency work at the large mental hospitals, and patients were screened at the clinic, prior to being admitted to various London hospitals. Since then a 24-hour emergency service has been offered, with repeat appointments for brief interventions until routine out-patient follow-up is established. This model has not, however, become widespread in the UK; in contrast to the United States, British services have generally aimed to integrate emergency services into the comprehensive work of hospitals and clinics rather than to develop distinct emergency services (Morrice, 1968). Smithies (1986) describes the setting up of an emergency clinic in Southampton and the subsequent decision to close it and to develop a decentralised sectorised service in its place. Interestingly, although problems arose with poorer assessment facilities on the wards, this transition was accompanied by a fall in emergency admission rate from 24 to 14% of patients assessed.

Psychiatry in the general hospital casualty department

Various groups of patients may need urgent psychiatric attention in the general hospital casualty department (i.e. accident and emergency in the UK; emergency room in the United States). Firstly, there has been an overall increase over the last 30 years in numbers of patients presenting in the casualty department after self-poisoning (Hawton

& Catalan, 1987). Secondly, patients with primarily psychiatric complaints may present themselves here, or, as in some areas, general practitioners (GPs) and other professionals in the community may be directed to send their referrals for urgent psychiatric assessment to the casualty department. Finally, it is well documented that psychiatric morbidity is high among patients seen by casualty officers, even where their presenting complaints are ostensibly physical (Bell *et al* 1990).

Psychiatric provision in casualty for people who present to casualty officers with psychiatric problems varies greatly in extent. In the United States model services of the 1960s, a multidisciplinary crisis intervention model similar to that used in the psychiatric emergency clinics was in use in the general emergency room (Frankel *et al.*, 1966; Blanes *et al.*, 1967; Spitz, 1976). Innovative services in the UK have used a variety of professionals other than psychiatrists to deliver brief interventions following self-harm: pioneers in the development of multidisciplinary self-harm services have included the Regional Poisoning Unit in Edinburgh and the Barnes Unit in Oxford (Kennedy, 1972; Chowdhury *et al.*, 1973; Hawton *et al.*, 1981; Hawton *et al.*, 1987). One of very few innovative casualty department services not primarily targeting deliberate self-harm is described by Atha *et al.* (1992). They developed a programme in which brief cognitive interventions were offered by a community psychiatric nurse to attenders in the casualty department, including those who attend with apparently physical problems, but on screening show evidence of psychological distress.

Hopkin (1985), Goldfinger and Lipton (1985), Hillard (1994) and Wellin *et al.* (1987) have documented an increasing tendency in the United States for the general hospital emergency room to be used as the primary site for emergency intervention, and in the UK the accident and emergency department retains a central place, particularly in night-time emergency services (Johnson & Thornicroft, 1991). However, a number of criticisms may be made of many casualty department emergency services: physical facilities are often poor, safety measures may be inadequate; there may not be adequate mechanisms for ensuring continuity of care and engagement with other services after initial attendance; and training and supervision both of casualty staff and of psychiatric staff are often poor. The psychiatric work of the casualty department and the difficulties which arise in it are discussed further by Johnson and Baderman in Chapter 11.

The emergency ward

A third form of hospital-based specialist emergency service has been the provision of beds designated specifically for brief intervention and assessment. These are of two broad types. Firstly, some North American work has described the benefits of evaluation areas or diversion beds, in which assessment may be continued for up to 24 hours and alternatives to hospitalisation sought before a decision is made about further treatment. Hughes (1993) notes the particular benefits of diversion beds for intoxicated suicidal patients, who cannot adequately be assessed until sober. Gillig *et al.* (1989) compared hospitalisation rates in two similar university hospitals, one with a psychiatric holding area for extended assessments, the other without such a facility. They found a significantly lower rate of hospitalisation, not accounted for by demographic or diagnostic differences, in the hospital with this facility. The 'guesting' system at the Maudsley, where patients were accommodated overnight on wards, but were not formally admitted and remained the responsibility of the emergency clinic staff, was a similar type of service, and was a useful means of avoiding some full admissions (Lim, 1983).

The second form of emergency bed provision, decribed extensively in the American literature, is the brief-treatment bed, designated for intensive multidisciplinary treatment, with discharge usually planned within one week (Guido & Payne, 1967; Herz *et al.*, 1977; Comstock, 1983). Good results have been reported, with a swifter return to normal roles, no added burden on family and no loss of treatment compliance for patients treated by brief hospitalisation in comparison with conventional admission. Some European services, for example those in Bern and Munich, make similar use of beds, providing brief intensive treatment which is based on a crisis intervention model (Feuerlein, 1983; Hülsmeier & Ciompi, 1984; Maier, 1987).

The acute day hospital

The day hospital was one of the earliest established facilities which aimed to provide acute intervention without admission. The first attempts to set up acute day hospitals seem to have been in the former USSR in the 1930s (Shepherd, 1991), and they are now in use in North America and many European countries. Their growth may have been slowed recently by the advent of the community mental health centre. In Britain, the day hospital was initially envisaged as a specialist acute service, complemented by separate provision of continuing care and rehabilitation for the chronically ill at local authority day centres. A number of studies have suggested that the efficacy of the day hospital in caring for a substantial proportion of the acutely mentally ill without in-patient admission is high (Creed *et al.*, 1989). Day hospitals have increased rapidly in numbers, although government targets have not yet been fully met. However, considerable doubts have been raised about the degree to which day hospitals may have deviated from their intended function of providing acute care and taken on the function of giving long-term support to the chronically ill (Pryce, 1982; McGrath & Tantam, 1987).

Crisis intervention and home treatment teams

The specialist services of crisis intervention teams provide initial multidisciplinary assessment and, if possible, treatment, in the patients' homes. In home treatment teams, the central aim is to provide intensive treatment for the severely mentally ill at home, although initial assessment may take place in various settings. The earliest such service was established in Amsterdam in the 1930s, where a social worker and a psychiatrist visited all patients at home who had been referred for admission, with the aim of avoiding hospitalisation (Querido, 1965).

In the 1980s, multidisciplinary home assessment services became an important form of innovative provision in the United States. 'Mobile assessment units' were reported to reduce hospital admissions and make possible a 'systems theory' approach, which takes into account the patient's family and support network, as well as other agencies already involved (Bengelsdorf & Alden, 1987; Gillig *et al.*, 1990; Zealberg *et al.*, 1993). Bengelsdorf *et al.* (1993) report that despite the relatively high cost of such services, savings due to admission diversion appear to make them cost effective. In the UK, the evolution of such services seems to have been slower, perhaps partly because the primary health care system already allows for home visiting by GPs, and, at their request, domiciliary visits by consultant psychiatrists. However, the use of extensive home visiting and multidisciplinary assessment has long been a feature of the highly developed community services at Dingleton in Scotland. More recently, descriptions have been published of crisis intervention teams carrying out multidisciplinary home assessments in the London areas of Barnet (Ratna, 1982; Katschnig & Konieczna, 1990), Lewisham (Tufnell *et al.*, 1985; Wood, 1991) and Tower Hamlets (British Medical Journal, 1981).

In a few centres, extensive home treatment programmes have been developed for emergency care, although initial assessment for entry to these programmes has not necessarily taken place in the home. The most prominent model service is the home treatment programme for the severely mentally ill operating in Madison, Wisconsin, USA (Stein & Test, 1980). In this programme, a group of chronically ill patients presenting to the admissions office in crisis were treated in their homes. They were trained in community living skills and an 'assertive case management' approach was adopted both during and after the crisis, with great efforts to maintain contact and treatment. Results suggested that the effect of this approach was to reduce in-patient days, unemployment and symptoms, and to improve overall satisfaction with life, compared with a matched control group treated by conventional hospitalisation. Since the publication of this work, many other United States and Australian centres have used this approach, generally with similar or better outcomes for home treatment compared with conventional hospital care (Soreff, 1983; Hoult, 1986; Bush *et al.*, 1990).

In recent UK literature, a number of services have been described which aim to provide similar intensive treatment for the severely mentally ill without in-patient admission. Sparkbrook, in South Birmingham has a home treatment programme operating (Dean, 1993), where daily visits by a nurse and a doctor can be provided, nursing assistants are available to spend several hours a day in the patients' home, medication is dispensed daily, and a nurse can be contacted by patients and families 24-hours a day. Evaluation of this service suggested that the home treatment programme led to a generally similar outcome on clinical outcome measures, with greater satisfaction among relatives and greater success in maintaining contact with patients after one year. The Daily Living Programme at the Maudsley Hospital (Marks *et al.*, 1988, Muijen *et al.*, 1991; Marks *et al.*, 1994) is a UK randomised controlled trial of the efficacy of home treatment for patients with serious mental illness presenting to an emergency clinic. This has shown an initially superior clinical and social outcome and improved satisfaction for home-based care in the first 20 months of the study, although, perhaps because of low morale among staff, these gains largely disappeared in a later phase. Tufnell *et al.* (1985) describe the efforts of the Lewisham Crisis Intervention Team to continue treatment at home after home assessment, in co-operation with GPs. They have successfully managed 45% of those assessed at home in the community (31% were admitted to hospital, the rest referred to out-patients clinics or psychotherapists). They note that work on crisis interventions at home has tended to focus relatively little on the seriously mentally ill, and that treating this group requires easily accessible helpers who can provide long, frequent visits, so that they need to be free from the traditional hospital workload. Merson *et al.* (1992) describe a randomised controlled trial with patients presenting in an emergency in Paddington, London, where those assigned to a community-based 'early intervention team' showed significantly greater patient satisfaction and symptomatic improvement than controls assigned to conventional hospital-based services, as well as an eight-fold reduction in in-patient days.

Emergency residential care outside hospital

The literature on emergency residential facilities outside hospital is predominantly from the United States and tends to describe single model programmes. Stroul (1988) provides a helpful review of this literature on such services and the results of a survey of 40 residential crisis facilities. She finds that the commonest form of care of this type is the provision of short-term housing and support in the homes of carefully selected families. Other crisis facilities take the form of crisis housing or hostels for groups. These approaches to the management of emergencies emphasise a rapid return to normal functioning and normal roles. Stroul suggests that residential crisis programmes provide an effective means of stabilising a high proportion of the long-term severely mentally ill in relapse. In addition, people presenting in acute crisis who do not have a long history of admissions can be managed in these crisis facilities without leading them to become reliant on hospital admission as a means of coping with crises. However, she also emphasises that these programmes only function effectively if adequate longer term community based treatment is available following the crisis, and if adequate professional support is available for families providing crisis housing. Wiesman (1985), in his account of the varying types of crisis housing provided by the San Francisco Mental Health Services, emphasises the importance of having a range of types of crisis housing available, so that appropriate levels of support and supervision can be provided to meet the varying needs of a wide range of patients.

Decentralised emergency psychiatry: service models

Two prominent and allied developments in community psychiatry have brought about a move away from the development of specialist emergency services with staff devoted exclusively to emergency assessment and intervention. These movements are sectorisation and the related development of community mental health centres.

Sectorisation

The establishment of small catchment areas, with teams or consultants taking responsibility for single small geographical zones, has been a fundamental element in the planning of community services in several countries. *La politique du secteur* has been central in French mental health policy since 1960, although France has continued to have very large numbers of mental hospital beds, and it is doubtful how extensive the provision of sector based services really is (Barres, 1987; Bennett, 1991). In the United States, sectorisation occurred together with the development of the community mental health centres, although other services, such as the mental hospital system, were not concurrently sectorised in most areas. Planning of services in all or parts of Denmark, Norway, Finland, West Germany, Austria, Spain, Italy and Sweden has also been based on a sectorisation principle in recent years, the process of establishing sectorised services having generally reached very different stages in different areas of each country (Lindholm, 1983; Freeman *et al.*, 1985; Bennett, 1991). The former Yugoslavia appears to have had a comparatively old and highly evolved sectorised service, which made extensive use of day hospitals (WHO, 1988).

Unfortunately, few detailed evaluations of the effects of sectorisation seem to have been published. Lindholm (1983) provides a thorough and well controlled evaluation of the implementation of sector based services in Stockholm, and does suggest some benefits in sectorisd service organisation.

The UK situation is somewhat different from that of many other countries, in that district health authorities have been the basic unit in planning and service provision, so that a degree of sectorisation is already in place. However, districts are larger than the sectors used in most countries where implementation of sectorisation has been attempted, as sector sizes not exceeding around 100,000 have usually been planned. Further division of districts into smaller units is generally necessary if services for each sector are to be provided by a single multidisciplinary team. There has been little evaluation of this process in the UK. A longitudinal study in Nottingham, examined the effects of giving responsibility for emergency admissions to sector teams (Tyrer *et al.*, 1989). Following sectorisation, there was a significant fall in both the number and the average duration of admissions in Nottingham compared to the rest of the country. This finding was attributed to good continuity of care between the hospital and sectorised community services.

The community mental health centre

Sectorised services may continue to have their main base in the hospital, with different teams within a single hospital serving different sectors. However, in order to develop a service which is genuinely accessible to the community it serves, and which appears approachable to patients, sectorised services have often moved their base to a centre within the locality served. Centres of this type have been given a number of names, but have often been called community mental health centres (CMHCs), after the centres established by the United States federal initiative of the 1960s, or 'mental health resource centres'.

The United States community mental health centre movement, funded by the federal government from 1963 until 1981, aimed to sectorise the whole country and to establish within each sector centres providing all mental health services needed by their local community, including emergency care. Since the end of federal funding, some of these centres have continued to operate, and some new centres have been established. As with the use of crisis intervention theory, CMHCs have expanded in Europe whilst declining in the United

States. In Italy, for example, the *Servizi Psichiatrici di Diagnosi e Cura*, established following the decision to close the mental hospitals, aim to provide all services necessary in each community. In many areas, they are in fact based within general hospitals (Morosini *et al.*, 1985). However, descriptions of the model services established in highly developed centres such as Trieste and Verona do suggest that small neighbourhood-based centres with a few beds at their disposal are providing comprehensive services with some success (Dell'Acqua & Dezza, 1985; Zimmermann-Tansella *et al.*, 1985: Tansella, 1991). In Madrid, each of the 20 sectorised barrios has a 'health promotion centre'. An attempt is being made to avoid overloading these centres by assigning responsibility for people discharged from hospital to other agencies, so that they take new referrals only (Dowell *et al.*, 1987). In a few sector-based centres in France, such as those in the 7th and 13th arrondissements of Paris, mobile teams provide emergency services with some success (Gittelman *et al.*, 1973). Social psychiatric services in West Germany, based at public health departments, have also often aimed to provide a comprehensive range of community services, although they have been criticised for failing to assign a sufficiently high priority to emergency care (Härlin, 1987).

In Britain, the establishment of CMHCs also appears to be proceeding apace (Sayce, 1991). At the end of 1989, almost three-quarters of a sample of districts had or planned at least one CMHC, although they are not necessarily sector-based; in some places a single centre has been established to serve a whole district.

Emergency services in a sectorised system

One of the remits of sector teams and of CMHC staff is very often the provision of emergency services. This has some notable advantages: continuity of care is more likely to be a feature of services and CMHCs can offer emergency services to which self-referrals may be made and which are locally accessible. Sector teams may also be in a good position to undertake crisis intervention work with patients in their own homes.

There are, however, some important problems with this form of decentralised, undifferentiated service, as Katschnig and Konieczna (1990) have argued. Firstly, it is uncommon for sectorised emergency care to continue to operate outside working hours, perhaps because small sectors will not generally have enough emergencies for the retention of staff at night for a single sector alone to be cost effective (Johnson & Thornicroft, 1993). Secondly, generic staff do not gain experience as rapidly as staff in a specialist service. Thirdly, a variety of types of work and of patient groups compete for their time and attention. A particular problem in the United States was that CMHCs did not always appear to be treating the most severely ill patients. They often had very broad objectives, aiming to promote high standards of mental health in the whole community, and sometimes provided more services for 'the worried well' and the 'healthy but unhappy' than for those with severe and chronic mental illnesses (Bachrach, 1991). The provision of emergency services appears in any case to be a role which has gradually declined in CMHCs in the United States (Hillard, 1994). Solomon and Gordon (1986) note that at the time when their provision was still a statutory responsibility for the CMHCs, it was frequent for them to contract general hospital emergency wards to provide them, and more recently Scherl and Schmetzer (1989) observe that general budget cuts seem to be causing a decline in the proportion of CMHCs providing emergency services.

Sayce *et al.* (1991) point to some risk of similar difficulties arising in the UK, as many of the first CMHCs did not specifically prioritise emergency work or the care of the severely mentally ill. However, they also see some evidence of a recent reversal of this trend, with clearer boundaries and more explicit priorities set. Hutton (1985), studying self-referrals to a CMHC with a walk-in service in Lewes, Sussex, observed that few of the people seen appeared to be acutely mentally ill, and that over three years none required admission at the time of self-referral. At another early service of this type, the Lewisham Mental Health Assessment Centre, London a dearth of referrals of the acutely and severely ill was similarly noted (Tufnell *et al.*, 1985; Boardman *et al.*, 1988; Wood, 1991).

Six CMHCs with varying histories were visited by Patmore and Weaver (1991), who conclude that there is great variation in the degree to which these centres serve the seriously mentally ill, and that they are more likely to do so if the workloads of community psychiatric nurses already employed in their catchment areas are included in their initial client group. Their descriptions of the centres' services suggest that emergency work is not currently a central element in most CMHCs.

One possible way of resolving some of the difficulties of emergency care in a decentralised system is to establish a centralised out-of-hours emergency system, alongside a sectorised system for managing emergencies during office hours. Arrangements of this type operate in Verona and in Trieste (Dell'Acqua & Dezza, 1985), where an eight-bed emergency ward operates at night, with a maximum stay of 24 hours, and with referral back to district centres the following day. A second, more radical, way in which cost effective 24-hour sectorised emergency services may be feasible would be if they operated as intensive home treatment services, providing high levels of support for the severely mentally ill in the community, so that substantial numbers of staff could be moved out of the hospital in-patient unit into the community.

Methodological issues

The literature on the provision of emergency services describes a range of ways to organise emergency assessment and treatment. Unfortunately, although the services described are often innovative and interesting, the usefulness of much of this work is severely limited by its methodological weakness. The main focus has been on descriptions and, more rarely, evaluations, of individual model services. From the point of view of experimental design, it is uncommon to find randomised controlled trials, and indeed many of the studies make no attempt to find a control group of any type. The usefulness of evaluations of services is also limited by small study sizes.

Certain characteristics of model services also limit the usefulness of a literature focusing almost exclusively on them. They may emerge particularly well from evaluation simply because, as innovative services, they often attract extra resources and highly skilled and committed staff. A criticism often levelled against them is that they may function well for a limited period, fuelled by charismatic leaders and energetic and committed staff, but that staff are highly susceptible to 'burn-out' and are unable to sustain this initial momentum. They also may be operating with a more carefully selected patient group than would be feasible in most services: experimental services often have rigorous exclusion criteria for admission to the study.

A further difficulty arises if one considers replication of these studies. Descriptions of the exact forms of intervention used, for example in the work of 'crisis intervention services' are often too vague to allow replication, and the characteristics of the patient groups are not well described or defined. In particular, with services such as CMHC emergency services or crisis houses, it is not clear how far the services are targeting the severely mentally ill in their provisions. Clear operational definitions of psychiatric emergencies are also rare.

Economic data, showing the cost-effectiveness of different types of service are also found only rarely, and such information is a further important requirement for service planning.

Conclusion

Literature on psychiatric emergency services, especially that of the 1960s and 1970s, provides descriptions of a wide variety of models specialising in emergency interventions, for example, psychiatric emergency clinics, acute day hospitals and crisis intervention teams. More recently, specialist services of these types seem to have lost favour, with the development of sectorisation and CMHCs, where emergency care is provided alongside other generic services by a single team.

Whilst descriptions of individual model services are relatively abundant they are not necessarily typical, and evaluation is often surprisingly scanty. Fashion, rather than evaluative data dictates service planning. CMHC emergency services, sectorised care and crisis houses, amongst others, emerge as interesting and promising models of emergency care, which may well have an important place in the provision of comprehensive community psychiatric services. However, the empirical case for these forms of care remains largely unproved.

The literature is also notably silent on how psychiatric emergencies are managed outside major centres of excellence. As noted by Blanes *et al.* (1967), innovative research programmes may be far from typical, and if service planning is to be effective, more information is needed about the extent and adequacy of provision and the favoured directions for service development outside model programmes. The roles in the management of psychiatric emergencies not only of psychiatrists, but also of GPs, social workers and community nurses need to be studied.

This overview of work on emergency services in psychiatry indicates a need both for rigorous evaluation of individual services and for accurate surveys showing the current broad national pattern of services. Central questions for psychiatric research which remain unanswered are: why do psychiatric emergencies arise, how are they related to the way in which psychiatric services are organised, and can relapse prevention and early intervention reduce the frequency and urgency of emergencies?

References

Atha, C., Salkovskis, P. M. & Storer, D. (1992). Cognitive-behavioural problem solving in the treatment of patients attending a medical emergency department: a controlled trial. *Journal of Psychosomatic Research*, **36**, 299–307.

Atkins, R. W. (1967). Psychiatric emergency service: implications for the patient, the physician, the family, the community and the hospital. *Archives of General Psychiatry*, **17**, 176–82.

Bachrach, L. (1991). Community mental health centres in the USA. In *Community Psychiatry: The Principles*, ed. D. H. Bennett & H. L. Freeman. Edinburgh, Churchill Livingstone.

Barres, M. (1987). Sectorisation and overcapacity in France. *International Journal of Social Psychiatry*, **33**, 140–3.

Bassuk, E. L. (1985). Psychiatric emergency services: can they cope as last resort facilities? *New Directions for Mental Health Services*, **28**, 11–20.

Bassuk, E. & Gerson, S. (1980). Chronic crisis patients: a discrete clinical group. *American Journal of Psychiatry*, **137**, 1513–17.

Bell, G., Hindley, N., Rajiyah, G. & Rosser, R. (1990). Screening for psychiatric morbidity in an accident and emergency department. *Archives of Emergency Medicine*, **7**, 155–62.

Bellak, L. (1960). A general hospital as a focus of community psychiatry: a trouble shooting clinic combines important functions as part of a hospital's emergency service. *Journal of the American Medical Association*, **174**, 2214–17.

Bengelsdorf, H. & Alden, D. C. (1987). A mobile crisis unit in the emergency room. *Hospital and Community Psychiatry*, **38**, 662–5.

Bengelsdorf, H., Church, J. O., Kaye, R. A., Orlowski, B. & Alden, D. C. (1993). The cost effectiveness of crisis intervention: admission diversion savings can offset the high cost of service. *Journal of Nervous and Mental Disease*, **181**, 757–62.

Bennett, D. H. (1991). The international perspective. In *Community Psychiatry: The Principles*, ed. D. H. Bennett & H. L. Freeman. Edinburgh, Churchill Livingstone.

Blanes, H. T., Muller, J. & Chafetz, M. E. (1967). Acute psychiatric services in the general hospital: current status of emergency psychiatric services. *American Journal of Psychiatry Supplement*, **124**, 37–45.
Boardman, A. P., Bouras, N. & Craig, T. K. J. (1988). General practitioner referrals to an ambulatory psychiatric service: the effects of establishing an ease of access service. *International Journal of Social Psychiatry*, **34**, 172–83.
British Medical Journal Leader (1981). Crises and interventions. *British Medical Journal*, **282**, 1737–8.
Brothwood, J. (1965). The work of a psychiatric emergency clinic. *British Journal of Psychiatry*, **111**, 631–4.
Bush, C. T., Langford, M. W., Rosen, P. & Gott, W. (1990). Operation Outreach: intensive case management for severely psychiatrically disabled adults. *Hospital and Community Psychiatry*, **41**, 647–9.
Caplan, G. (1961). *An Approach to Community Mental Health*. New York, Grune and Stratton.
Caplan, G. (1964). *Principles of Preventive Psychology*. New York, Basic Books.
Chafetz, M. E., Blanes, H. T. & Muller, J. J. (1966). Acute psychiatric services in the general hospital: 1. Implications for psychiatry in emergency admissions. *American Journal of Psychiatry*, **123**, 664–70.
Chowdhury, N., Hicks, R. C. & Kreitman, N. (1973). Evaluation of an aftercare service for parasuicide (attempted suicide) patients. *Social Psychiatry*, **36**, 67–81.
Coleman, M. D. & Zwerling, I. (1959). The psychiatric emergency clinic: a flexible way of meeting community mental health needs. *American Journal of Psychiatry*, **115**, 980–4.
Comstock, B. S. (1983). Psychiatric emergency care. *Psychiatric Clinics of North America*, **6**, 305–16.
Cooper, J. E. (1979). Crisis admission units and emergency psychiatric services. *Public Health in Europe* No. 2. Copenhagen, World Health Organization.
Creed, F., Black, D. & Anthony, P. 1989). Day hospital and community treatment for acute psychiatric illness: a critical appraisal. *British Journal of Psychiatry*, **154**, 300–10.
Dean, C., Phillips, J., Gadd, E. M., Joseph, M. & England, S. (1993). Comparison of community based service with hospital based service for people with acute severe psychiatric illness. *British Medical Journal*, **307**, 473–6.
Dell'Acqua, G. & Dezza, M. G. C. (1985). The end of the mental hospital: a review of the psychiatric experience in Trieste. *Acta Psychiatrica Scandinavica, Supplement*, **316**, 45–69.
Dowell, D. A., Poveda de Augustin, J. M. & Lowenthal, A. (1987). Changing mental health services in Madrid. *Hospital and Community Psychiatry*, **36**, 68–72.
Farberow, N. (1968). Crisis prevention. *International Journal of Psychiatry*, **6**, 371–9.
Feuerlein, W. (1983). Kriseninterventionstechniken und Organisation der

Krisenintervention. Eine station für Notfallpsychiatrie und Krisenintervention – Konzepte, Struktur und erste Erfahrungen. *Wiener Klinische Wochenschrift Supp.*, **1445**, 13–17.
Frankel, F. H., Chafetz, M. E. & Blanes, H. T. (1966). Treatment of psychosocial crises in the emergency service of a general hospital. *Journal of the American Medical Association*, **195**, 626.
Freeman, H. L., Fryers, T. & Henderson, J. H. (1985). Mental health services in Europe 10 years on. *Public Health in Europe* No. 25. Copenhagen, World Health Organization.
Gillig, P., Dumain, M. & Hillard, J. R. (1990). Whom do mobile crisis services serve? *Hospital and Community Psychiatry*, **38**, 662–5.
Gillig, P., Hillard, J. R. & Bell, J. (1989). The psychiatric service holding area: effects on utilisation of resources. *American Journal of Psychiatry*, **146**, 369–72.
Gittelman, M., Dubius, J. & Gillet, M. (1973). Recent developments in French public mental health. *Psychiatric Quarterly*, **47**, 509–20.
Goldfinger, S. M. & Lipton, F. R. (1985). Emergency psychiatry at the crossroads. *New Directions for Mental Health Services*, **28**, 107–10.
Gomez, R. (1983). Demographic and non-demographic characteristics of psychiatric emergency patients. *Psychiatric Clinics of North America*, **6**, 213–23.
Guido, J. A. Payne, D. H. (1973). 72-hour psychiatric detention: clinical observation and treatment in a county general hospital. *Archives of General Psychiatry*, **16**, 233–8.
Häfner-Ranabauer, W. & Günzler, G. (1987). Entwicklung und Funktion des psychiatrischen Krisen- und Notfallsdiensts in Mannheim. *Fortschritte Neurologie Psychiatrie*, **52**, 83–90.
Härlin, C. (1987). Community care in West Germany: concept and reality. *International Journal of Social Psychiatry*, **33**, 105–10.
Haw, C., Lankily, C. & Vickers, S. (1987). Patients at a psychiatric walk in clinic. *Bulletin of the Royal College of Psychiatrists*, **10**, 329–32.
Hawton, K. Bancroft, J., Catalan, J., Kingston, B., Stedeford, A. & Welch, N. (1981). Domiciliary and out-patient treatment of self-poisoning patients by medical and non-medical staff. *Psychological Medicine*, **11**, 169–77.
Hawton, K. & Catalan, J. (1987). *Attempted Suicide: A Practical Guide to its Management*, 2nd edn. Oxford, Oxford University Press.
Hawton, K., McKeown, S., Day, A., Martin, P., O'Connor, M. & Yule, J. (1987). Evaluation of out-patient counselling compared with general practitioner care following overdoses. *Psychological Medicine*, **17**, 751–61.
Herz, M. I., Endicott, J. & Spitzer, R. L. (1977). Brief hospitalization: a two-year follow up. *American Journal of Psychiatry*, **134**, 502–7.
Hillard, J. R. (1994). The past and future of emergency psychiatry in the US. *Hospital and Community Psychiatry*, **45**, 541–3.
Hobbs, M. (1984). Crisis intervention in theory and practice: a selective review. *British Journal of Medical Psychology*, **57**, 23–34.
Hopkin, J. T. (1985). Psychiatry and medicine in the emergency room. *New*

Directions for Mental Health Services, **28**, 47–53.
Hoult, J. (1986). Community care of the acutely mentally ill. *British Journal of Psychiatry*, **149**, 337–44.
Hülsmeier, H. & Ciompi, L. (1984). Stationäre sozialpsychiatrie: Krisenintervention am Beispiel der Kriseninterventionsstation der sozialpsychiatrischen Universitätsklinik Bern. *Psychiatrische Praxis*, **11**, 67–73.
Hughes, D. H. (1993). Trends and treatment models in emergency psychiatry. *Hospital and Community Psychiatry*, **44**, 927–8.
Hutton, F. (1985). Self referrals to a Community Mental Health Centre: a three year study. *British Journal of Psychiatry*, **1417**, 540–4.
Johnson, S. & Thornicroft, G. (1991). *Emergency Psychiatric Services in England and Wales*. Report to the Department of Health. London, PRiSM, Institute of Psychiatry.
Johnson, S. & Thornicroft, G. (1993). The sectorisation of psychiatric services in England and Wales. *Social Psychiatry and Psychiatric Epidemiology*, **28**, 45–7.
Katschnig, H. & Konieczna, T. (1990). Innovative approaches to delivery of emergency services in Europe. In *Mental Health Care Delivery*, ed. I. M. Marks & R. A. Scott. Cambridge, Cambridge University Press.
Kennedy, P. (1972). Efficacy of a regional poisoning treatment centre in preventing further suicidal behaviour. *British Medical Journal*, **4**, 255–7.
Lim, M. H. (1983). A psychiatric emergency clinic: a study of attendances over six months. *British Journal of Psychiatry*, **143**, 460–6.
Lindholm, H. (1983). Sectorised psychiatry. *Acta Psychiatrica Scandinavica, Supp.*, **67**, 1–69.
Maier, C. (1987). Stationäre Krisenintervention: Behandlungskonzept und therapeutischer Alltag. *Schweizer Archiv für Neurologie und Psychiatrie*, **138**, 35–43.
Marks, I., Connolly, J. & Muijen, M. (1988). The Maudsley Daily Living Programme. *Bulletin of the Royal College of Psychiatrists*, **12**, 22–4.
Marks, I., Connolly, J., Muijen, M., Audini, B., McNamee, G. & Lawrence, R. E. (1994). Home-based versus hospital-based care for people with serious mental illness. *British Journal of Psychiatry*, **165**, 179–94.
McGrath, G. & Tantam, D. (1987). Long-stay patients in a psychiatric day hospital: a case note review. *British Journal of Psychiatry*, **150**, 836–41.
Merson, S. Tyrer, P., Onyett, S., Lack, S., Birkett, P., Lynch, S. & Johnson, T. (1992). Early intervention in psychiatric emergencies: a controlled clinical trial. *Lancet*, **339**, 1311–13.
Mindham, R. H. S., Kelly, M. J. & Birley, J. L. T. (1973). A psychiatric casualty department. *Lancet*, pp. 1169–71.
Morosini, P. L., Repetto, F., De Salvia, D. & Cecere, F. (1985). Psychiatric hospitalisation in Italy before and after 1978. *Acta Psychiatrica Scandinavica, Supp.*, **316**, 27–43.
Morrice, J. K. (1968). Emergency psychiatry. *British Journal of Psychiatry*, **114**, 485–91.

Muijen, M., Marks, I. M. & Connolly, J. (1991). The Daily Living Programme: a controlled study of community care for the severely ill in Camberwell. In *The Closure of the Mental Hospitals*, ed. P. Hall & I. P. Brockington. London, Gaskell.

Normand, W., Fensterheim, H., Tannebaum, G. & Sager, C. J. (1963). The acceptance of a walk-in clinic in a highly deprived community. *American Journal of Psychiatry*, **120**, 533–9.

Patmore, C. & Weaver, T. (1991). *Community mental health teams: Lessons for planners and managers*. London, Good Practices in Mental Health.

Perez, E., Minoletti, A., Blonin, J. & Blonin, A. (1986). Repeated users of a psychiatric emergency service in a Canadian General Hospital. *Psychiatric Quarterly*, **58**, 189–201.

Pryce, I. G. (1982). An expanding 'stage army' of long-stay psychiatric day patients. *British Journal of Psychiatry*, **142**, 595–601.

Querido, A. (1965). Early diagnosis and treatment services. In *The Elements of a Community Mental Health Programme*. New York, Milbank Memorial Fund.

Ratna, L. (1982). Crisis intervention in psychogeriatrics: a two-year follow-up study. *British Journal of Psychiatry*, **141**, 296–301.

Sayce, L., Craig, T. K. J. & Boardman, A. P. (1991). The development of Community Mental Health Centres in the United Kingdom. *Social Psychiatry and Psychiatric Epidemiology*, **26**, 14–20.

Scherl, E. K. & Schmetzer, A. D. (1989). CMHC emergency services in the 1980s. *Community Mental Health Journal*, **25**, 267–75.

Schöny, W. (1983). Organisation ambulanter Krisenintervention. *Wiener Klinische Wochenschrift, Supp.*, **145**, 17–19.

Shepherd, G. (1991). Day treatment and care. In *Community Psychiatry: The Principles*, D. H. Bennett, & H. L. Freeman. Edinburgh, Churchill Livingstone.

Smithies, J. M. A. (1986). A psychiatric emergency clinic. *Bulletin of the Royal College of Psychiatrists*, **10**, 357–9.

Solomon, P. & Gordon, B. (1986). The psychiatric emergency room and follow up services in the community. *Psychiatric Quarterly*, **58**, 119–27.

Soreff, S. M. (1983). New directions and added dimensions in home psychiatric treatment. *American Journal of Psychiatry*, **140**, 1213–16.

Spitz, L. (1976). The evolution of a psychiatric emergency service in a medical emergency room setting. *Comprehensive Psychiatry*, **1**, 99–113.

Stein, L. I. & Test, M. A. (1980). Alternatives to mental hospital treatment. *Archives of General Psychiatry*, **37**, 392–7.

Stroul, B. A. (1988). Residential crisis services: a review. *Hospital and Community Psychiatry*, **39**, 1095–9.

Tansella, M., Balestieri, M., Meneghelli, G. & Micciolo, R. (1991). Trends in the provision of psychiatric care 1979–1988. *Psychological Medicine Monograph Supplement*, **19**, 5–16.

Tufnell, G., Bouras, N., Watson, J. P. & Brough, D. I. (1985). Home assessment and treatment in community psychiatric service. *Acta Psychiatrica Scandinavica*, **72**, 20–8.

Tyrer, P., Turner, R. & Johnson, A. L. (1989). Integrated hospital and community psychiatric services and use of inpatient beds. *British Medical Journal*, **299**, 298–300.

Wellin, E., Slesinger, D. P. & Hollister, C. D. (1987). Psychiatric emergency services: evolution, adaptation and proliferation. *Social Sciences and Medicine*, **24**, 475–82.

Wiesman, G. (1985). Crisis houses and lodges: residential treatment of acutely disturbed chronic patients. *Psychiatric Annals*, **15**, 642–7.

Wood, S. (1991). Home treatment and crisis intervention in Lewisham. In *The Closure of the Mental Hospitals*, eds. P. Hall & I. P. Brockington. London, Gaskell.

World Health Organization Regional Office for Europe (1988). *Mental health services in Southern countries of Europe*. Report on WHO meeting Madrid, 25–29th May, 1986. WHO Euro reports and statistics, 107. Copenhagen, World Health Organization.

Zealberg, J. J., Santos, A. B. & Fisher, R. K. (1993). Benefits of mobile crisis programs. *Hospital and Community Psychiatry*, **44**, 16–17.

Zimmermann-Tansella, C., Burti, L., Faccincani, C., Garzotto, N., Siciliani, O. & Tansella, M. (1985). Bringing into action the psychiatric reforms in South Verona: a five year experience. *Acta Psychiatrica Scandinavica, Supp.*, **316**, 71–85.

3

Users' perspective on emergency needs

LIZ SAYCE, YVONNE CHRISTIE, MIKE SLADE AND ALISON COBB

A growing call for crisis services

In this chapter we will attempt to give a representative picture of the views of mental health service users, on current acute mental health services and outline suggestions for improvement. As we are all based in Britain, our account will inevitably focus on the current British situation, but it is our belief that this mirrors the situation in many other countries Wherever user groups have emerged, they have consistently and independently come up with the demand for a better response to people experiencing a mental health crisis. There are a number of common complaints. Sometimes the system offers next to nothing:

> I have padded through the streets at 2 a.m. before now, seeking help from the nearest police station. It would have been nice to think I could have rung up a caring person in a crisis house.
>
> *(User contacting MIND.)*

Sometimes it offers admission to the acute unit of a district general hospital, which may be experienced as bewildering or unhelpful:

> I was taken to a psychiatric unit which is part of a large general hospital. My clothes and personal belongings were taken away from me. I had no idea why I needed to be placed somewhere where contact with my family and friends disappeared so suddenly when I needed it most.
>
> *(Beeforth* et al., *1990.)*

Sometimes it involves the use of legal powers or other forms of control. Users have described how frightening it can be to be taken to a police station, and to be forcibly medicated or placed in seclusion:

> I found the imposition of a major tranquilliser, administered against my will in injection form on a number of occasions, very destructive to my self-confidence and integrity as a person. There are clear similarities between the experience and accounts I've read of rape – the shame and feeling 'I must have been to blame'.
>
> *(Cobb, 1993.)*

> Why do people in the psychiatric system feel they are being punished?
>
> *(Campbell, 1988 quoted in Sargeant, 1988.)*

In 1975 the British government advocated the development of hospital acute units and an accompanying range of community supports, but as Professor Elaine Murphy (Murphy *et al.*, 1991) put it:

> The first of these themes has become a major symphonic work whilst the second, the community support, has been scarcely audible.

When the Minister for Health was asked in 1991 how many crisis centres 'for the mentally ill' were available, he gave the stock answer – with all its implications of low priority – 'this information is not collected centrally'. Whilst almost every health authority had or planned at least one acute unit in a district general hospital (DoH, pers. comm.), recent surveys of health authorities found only a limited non-hospital emergency service outside office hours (Johnson & Thornicroft, 1991), with only 7 out of 82 local authorities offering a 'crisis team' service (Huxley, 1993).

The 'symphony' (if so it can be called) of the acute unit has taken most of the resources. Britain still spends 77% of its National Health Service (NHS) mental health budget (over £2 billion in 1991) on hospital and medication costs, and only 23% (about £0.6 billion) on general practitioner (GP) services, community psychiatric nursing, day hospitals and all other community health responses. Meanwhile social services mental health spending is a mere £0.2 billion (Mental Health Foundation, 1993). This is partly because of the running costs of the 90 remaining large psychiatric hospitals, but it is also because the money has in effect been transferred from one institution – the Victorian asylum – to another, the acute unit. This has enabled the Government's Task Force to announce proudly that numbers of beds have not reduced over the last 10 years (if one includes private hospital and nursing home beds) (Davidge *et al.*, 1993). This is not a popular claim with the hundreds of thousands of people waiting for decent services in the community.

What this means in human terms is that many people are in hospital whose admission could have been avoided. Professional staff in one survey (Health Advisory Service, 1991) believed that 50% of admissions could have been prevented, if they had had access to alternatives such as a crisis intervention team, a crisis house and a day hospital. Another study (Barbour *et al.*, 1991) found that 87% of users and carers could identify at least 50 people who could benefit from a 24-hour non-hospital crisis centre, compared with only 18% of statutory sector staff.

Until the 1980s the call for new forms of response to crisis went largely unheard. Despite a small number of UK non-hospital crisis services – the Laingian Arbours centre set up in 1973, the Coventry crisis service, the Barnet, London, crisis intervention team – and despite a minority interest in international user literature on alternatives (e.g. Judi Chamberlin, 1988), most professionals and policy makers ignored non-hospital crisis approaches. Occasionally such approaches roused enough interest to merit a brief attack on the 'unworkable' idea of crisis services, from an orthodoxy stating that non-traditional services would simply see a new clientele and would do nothing to prevent hospitalisation for those who 'really needed it':

> crisis intervention is seen by many as an impractical approach to mental health care practised by a small minority of isolated enthusiasts.
>
> *(Johnstone* et al., *1991.)*

During the 1980s the case for change began to be articulated strongly, at a national level, and people began to listen. Crisis houses and crisis cards – carried like kidney donor cards and outlining the response people do, and do not, want when in crisis – became integral to debates about mental health. This was related to the rapid growth of user groups – UK Advocacy Network knew of over 100 user groups by the early 1990s – which began to unite in powerful national networks. Survivors Speak Out and MINDLINK (both formed in 1987) and the UK Advocacy Network (1992) all identified crisis services as priorities across the country and placed the issue high on their agendas. User influence in voluntary organisations like MIND ensured that alternative crisis services were also included in their policy thinking and lobbying – MIND's policies call for a range of different responses to crisis including crisis houses, non-hospital crisis teams and respect for crisis cards (MIND's Policy Pack, 1993). A growing user literature has also repeatedly called for awareness of problems, such as lack of safety in acute units (e.g. Camden Consortium/GPMH, 1988), and for a major investment in alternatives:

> Resources for community services should be redirected to develop services that users want. We need to develop crisis intervention houses, where one can go 24 hours a day seven days a week to get support so often needed at such times.
>
> (*Beeforth* et al., *1990)*

The case of Christopher Clunis, who killed Jonathan Zito in 1992, shows graphically what can go wrong when there are almost no resources in community care. Mr Clunis went in and out of acute hospital wards – but when he was out, there was no planning of his care, no regular contact by any professional and a 'lack of clear and co-ordinated response to a psychiatric crisis' (Ritchie *et al.*, 1994). Unfortunately some commentators draw the erroneous conclusion that what is needed is more acute beds. The beds are indeed full, especially in London. However, a third to a half of patients in London acute wards are typically not discharged only because they are homeless, and in any case a high proportion – 50% according to one study (Health Advisory Service, 1991) – would never have been admitted if there had been other crisis services. The conclusion is inescapable: provide support in the community and pressure on acute beds will diminish.

By 1994 the issues had hit official and professional debates in a major way. The House of Commons Health Committee, following evidence from Survivors Speak Out and MIND, called for an examination of the possibility of giving crisis cards a legal status (House of Commons Health Committee, 1993). The Government's Mental Health Task Force decided to produce a video on alternatives to hospital admission. The *British Medical Journal* published articles on the success in Birmingham of 'home treatment'. The British Medical Association called for 24-hour crisis services as a national community care standard (British Medical Association, 1994). The National Association of Health Authorities and Trusts and the Association of Directors of Social Services joined with MIND in a national conference promoting different models of crisis service (April 1994). The Ritchie Report (Ritchie *et al.*, 1994) into the care and the treatment of Christopher Clunis recommended 24-hour 'phone lines for people in crisis; faster assessments; and – somewhat bizarrely, given the existing card developed by Survivors Speak

Out – that the Royal College of Psychiatrists should develop a crisis card.

For users this does not mean the battle is won. There is not necessarily a consensus either on what is wrong with the *status quo* or on what change is required. For instance, Government and NHS management bodies are working to an agenda of reducing hospital care across different specialities, largely on financial grounds: the projected number of general acute beds for the year 2000 is 75,000 – half the number in 1980 (Newchurch and Company Ltd., 1992). The Government is also working to introduce increased controls over users, through supervision registers (from October 1994) and supervised discharge which would oblige users who are at some form of risk to take their medication, or fulfil other requirements, as a condition of discharge from hospital. Passing laws to oblige people to use services when the main problem is that services are often absent or inappropriate is victim blaming, and contrary to the stated Government policy of having a consumer-led, needs-driven health service. Users also want more access to early help, which is likely to be contradicted by a managerial emphasis on rationing which means only those with a diagnosis of 'severe and enduring mental illness' – or even only those showing sign of suicide risk, or risk of being violent, or of neglecting themselves – would get any service at all.

In order to define proposals for change which genuinely reflect users' concerns and ideas, MIND collaborated with MINDLINK and the 230 local MIND associations to undertake a consultation exercise on crisis and acute services. Comments were invited from MINDLINK members, 51 of whom chose to complete a brief questionnaire. The questionnaire was also sent to all 230 local MIND groups, 99 of whom responded (40%). The questions centred on what people thought about hospital acute units and non-hospital alternatives. The outcome of the consultation is combined with research evidence to define some avenues for development that accord with user and grassroots concerns.

Views on hospital acute units

When asked what services should be available to people in a mental health crisis (on top of GP services), no MINDLINK members and only 1% of local MIND groups thought the response should be hospital acute units only. Most (74% of MINDLINK and 87% of local MIND) wanted a combination of non-hospital services (e.g. crisis houses, crisis teams) and hospital services. However, a significant minority of MINDLINK respondents (22%) thought there should be non-hospital crisis services only: they saw no role for hospital acute units and, when asked what changes should be made to acute units, said things like:

> They should be converted to non-mental health usage.

> Move off hospital sites.

Far more people identified unhelpful than helpful things about acute units; one person said 'Sorry! nothing is helpful about acute units'. The criticisms centred on a number of specific themes.

The atmosphere and environment

Although a minority of people identified the positive quality of 'refuge', most comments highlighted problems of an institutional atmosphere, noise and lack of privacy. For instance:

> Oppressive, depressing and dehumanising environment.

> The row in the place is dreadful and a form of torture to some who require peace and a tranquil atmosphere.

> I nearly hanged myself on the ward it was so bad.

Users are not the only people to have noted that the atmosphere and environment in acute units are 'not conducive to healing', as one MINDLINK member put it:

> The hospital architecture of these units, often undifferentiated from clinical areas, can, as we experienced, be as harsh, undomestic and institutional as the corridors of the unlamented Victorian hospital.
>
> *(House of Commons Health Committee, 1985.)*

> The Edith Morgan Unit has a surprisingly institutional atmosphere. Some patients and community staff have spoken of the pervading atmosphere of boredom and aimlessness ... There is no warm atmosphere, with little or no evidence of personal belongings in either the ward or the dormitories.
>
> *(Health Advisory Service, 1991.)*

> You feel ill just walking into the place.
>
> *(RCN convenor commenting on the Central Middlesex Hospital in 1992.)*

Many acute units were built according to the requirements of Health Building Note 35 (1988) – only revised in 1993 – which reads like a description of the archetypal soulless institution:

> It is assumed that there will be central catering facilities and a central washing up service and that patients will receive food served from an insulated bulk trolley.

With a few exceptions – like the Grange in Newcastle which provides acute care in a large house – there have been almost no attempts made in the UK to design or adapt buildings to the needs of people in psychological crisis. They are expected to fit into a hospital, complete with swabbable floors and sluice facilities that are entirely unnecessary to people in distress. What people say they want is a homely, peaceful atmosphere – 'quiet places of repose' – and space to walk about.

> A hospital devoted to carying for people with physical conditions is not appropriate for people experiencing life crisis.
>
> *(MINDLINK member)*

A safe space?

Although a few respondents mentioned safety as a plus point about acute units, many others commented that they did not feel safe. Sometimes this was because of disturbed behaviour on the ward:

> Troublesome patients often not dealt with effectively.
>
> Not well enough to cope with this.

Sometimes it was because of harassment or abuse of women:

> Invasion of women's space by men.
>
> Sexual exploitation.

A series of inquiries into suicides and other untoward incidents in acute units – for instance, 10 deaths in 15 months at the Shrodells Unit in Watford, Hertfordshire; three suicides in a year, and 40 incidents of violence or threatening behaviour in two months, at the Central Middlesex Hospital – have pointed to contributory factors including overcrowding, poor communication and absence of adequate complaints procedures. In-patient suicides appear to be on the increase (Lloyd, 1992).

Women have spoken out increasingly about sexual harassment and abuse on acute wards (Darton *et al.*, 1994). Following the intervention of Esther Rantzen, who covered the issue in two editions of *That's Life* in 1994, the Royal College of Psychiatrists was prompted to change its view to one that accepted the need for choice, for women, of being in women-only space. It is clear that many women, including for example Muslim and Jewish women, simply do not feel comfortable enough to relax or recover in a mixed facility:

> Now at last I feel I can relax. I feel like I am on holiday.
>
> *(Asian woman after transfer to a single-sex ward, following intervention by a MIND advocacy worker who eventually won the argument that the woman could not recover her mental health in a mixed ward.)*

For others whose main language is not English, hospitalisation can be disorientating in the extreme:

> I visited someone in hospital and an Asian woman patient clung to me. She told me that Hindi was her first language and none of the ward staff could understand her. She hadn't been offered an interpreter and she kept touching my feet almost begging me to talk to her. How can they know what someone's mental state is if they don't understand your language?
>
> *(Southampton MIND, 1993.)*

Finally for some people being in hospital is not safe because the treatments given are not safe. Mr Majothi, admitted to hospital for 15 hours in 1992, died after being given 10 times the recommended safety level of a major tranquilliser. Others suffer adverse effects of treatment even within the safety levels: for instance, estimates of how many people taking neuroleptic drugs suffer from tardive dyskinesia range from 25 to 72% (Bergen *et al.*, 1989).

It would be extremely hard to argue that Britain's acute units generally offer a place of refuge and safety. As one young woman contacting Esther Rantzen put it:

> I'd feel safer sleeping on a park bench.

The regime

Some people valued the company and the support that they got in the acute ward – both from staff from other patients:

> If you have 'let yourself go' they help you get back together.

But others complained that they wanted more to do, better food and, particularly, more autonomy:

> Too little information and choice.

> Impossible to feel you are anything but a small patient in a large machine.

> Unable to make a cup of tea when you want to.

Amongst the changes people wanted to see in acute units were choice of consultant and treatment:

> I was told I would be sectioned if I didn't take the anti-depressants.
>
> *(Rogers et al., 1993)*

Some people also disliked the fact that they were 'cut off from normal life'. Sometimes this means that pressing problems at home – for instance, what is happening to the children or who is paying the rent – can be overwhelmingly anxiety provoking. The separation from children that is usually involved in hospital admission can be highly distressing, especially if a woman (or more rarely a man) feels that her parenting abilities are in question because of her mental state and that she may lose her children in custody or care proceedings. This fear is especially acute for 'non-traditional' mothers, who feel under scrutiny anyway: for instance, black single parents or lesbian mothers (Sayce, 1995).

The treatment

The above indignities could perhaps be argued to be tolerable if we were sure that treatment in hospital was effective. Some respondents valued the help on offer:

> Expert professionals on hand.

Most, however, were critical. They said there was little opportunity to talk or to address the causes of distress:

> Rigid ideas of mental illness – ignore human and social reasons for distress.

> Staff ignore you during the bad times.

> You're lucky to see a psychiatrist for more than five minutes a week.

> There's not action to solve problems. The person is merely drugged and ignored and when calm (i.e. accepting being driven to distraction) is allowed to leave eventually.

> Too much emphasis on drugs and ECT.

When asked what they would like to see changed about acute units a common response was more choice of treatment (psychological or physical), and more opportunity to explore the causes of distress.

These comments echo those of users surveyed in *Experiencing Psychiatry* (Rogers *et al.*, *1993)*.

> Some of them wanted to be helpful but they didn't know how to help me – they just knew how to give pills and ECT which wasn't helpful.

> I hated hospital life – it made me crack up even more.

Their views are partly confirmed by other types of research. Controlled trials to compare hospital and home-based care found that:

> No study found inpatient care to be better on any variable.
> *(Muijen et al.*, 1992.)

Even where people's symptoms do improve in hospital, the improvement is not sustained if they are discharged back to the same situation in which they broke down in the first place. For example, where people, who feel suicidal, improve in hospital...

> this does not reduce the risk of suicide on discharge unless social circumstances have also changed.
> *(Morgan & Priest, 1991.)*

It appears that community-based services have the potential to be more effective and more popular than acute hospital care. The benefits of home treatment for patient and relative satisfaction has been shown:

> Home treatment is feasible for most patients with acute psychiatric illness.
> *(Dean & Gadd, 1990)*

Birchwood has shown that cognitive therapy for people with acute mental health problems can reduce the length of the episode by 50% (unpublished paper to 1994 British Psychological Society conference). Clearly there are alternatives both to acute wards and to the drug regimes that usually prevail within them. It is not even the case that hospital care is necessarily cheaper. Indeed, giving people treatments that they do not want risks being a major waste of resources. One study found that, of 2149 people using acute psychiatric services, a quarter were estimated by professionals to take their medication never or rarely (Clifford and Webb, pers. comm.). Trials of psychiatric crisis intervention services and home treatment show savings of up 50% on conventional care, although for some individuals costs can be higher than hospital provision, and investment in choice is likely to make the community service at least as costly (Dean & Gadd, 1990).

Critics of community care are fond of calling it an under-researched experiment and demanding evidence of its effectiveness before any investment is made. If this level of scrutiny were demanded of the more traditional services of the hospital acute unit some highly challenging questions would be posed – and the current huge investment in acute hospital care would perhaps be stemmed.

Views of non-hospital crisis services

When MINDLINK and local MIND were asked for their views on non-hospital crisis services many said that they had never experienced them. Many of the comments are, therefore, based on what people imagine a crisis service to be. Often the things people said would be helpful about non-hospital crisis services were the exact opposites of what they found unhelpful about acute units. People thought the crisis would be seen in context:

> You'd be a person not a case.
>
> Not cut off from normal life.
>
> Relations could get involved.

There would be a chance of more autonomy:

> We could decide if we needed help.
>
> People should be offered the opportunity to define their experience and what they hope to achieve.
>
> Care organised around individuals, not hospital routines.

There would be more chance of a holistic response, rather than a medically dominated one:

> Need human help, not just medical.
>
> Less rigid divisions between professionals.

People also thought help could be given earlier to avoid longer treatment later. It is all too common that people are turned away from acute services when they ask for help because they are not 'ill enough', and then get beyond the point of wanting help – ending up getting treatment compulsorily or not at all.

On the other hand some people were concerned that the new service might repeat old problems:

> Same service in a different place?
>
> Depot injections are dehumanising.

Some were concerned that medical power might be replaced by the power of a different set of professionals:

> Will we be forced to talk about our feelings?

Some thought home treatment could be intrusive:

> Does this mean intrusion into people's homes without the resident's permission? With the intruder saying 'we're here to help'?

There might be a loss of anonymity with neighbours, or problems with getting too attached to a person from a time-limited 'crisis' team. There might be a feeling of insecurity if there were not enough 'containment'. Finally, loss of beds might mean a loss of resource priority for mental health and no support at all – sadly a realistic anxiety given the fact that beds have often closed with the money saved spent on acute medicine, meeting NHS deficits or other purposes of no use to mental health service users:

> It's our money from the asylums.
>
> *(Rogers et al., 1993.)*

Existing alternatives to acute hospital care

Despite the general picture of a total imbalance between hospital and community expenditure, there are some excellent examples of non-hospital crisis services in place or under development, as well as individual practitioners working in more imaginative ways:

> When I escaped from the hospital I went to the other end of the country where I met a GP who ... refused to enforce the section [authority to admit someone to hospital against their will] and treated me herself. She supported me on withdrawing from the medication and came to see me every day – talking to me and reinforcing my sense of self. She gave me practical tasks by which I could measure my progress.
>
> *(MINDLINK, 1993.)*

There are a small but growing number of alternatives to acute units, both in the statutory and the voluntary sectors. Some psychiatrists are coming out of their hospitals and treating people at home, retaining just a small number of beds. The home treatment service in West Birmingham explains its success by its comprehensive approach to meeting needs (not overly medical), its non-coercive nature and round the clock availability. It is able to respond flexibly to people's needs rather than slot them into an existing system: for instance, if someone in crisis needs to be able to contact the team, they can be lent a mobile phone; if someone needs immediate help with getting the electricity put back on or the children cared for, the team will assist people to ensure it happens; if someone needs to talk to someone in a language other than English it can be arranged. These creative solutions were often absent in the old institutions – and absent also in acute units.

In Newcastle the acute unit is a large house, offering residential and day care and a range of treatment approaches. It is less stigmatising than a hospital and has close links with the community mental health team. In Barnet, London, there is a long established crisis intervention service in which a three person multidisciplinary team visits the person or family to assist in working through the crisis and in enabling them to learn coping strategies for the future. Redbridge, Essex, crisis team has cards in their local accident and emergency unit to encourage those who have attempted suicide to use their services. Southampton MIND's Crisis Point provides someone to talk to by telephone or in person between 10 p.m. Saturday and 8.30 a.m. Sunday – 'they have said that they left feeling more relaxed and able to sleep, and a few have said that it saved calling out the duty doctor'. 'Choices' in Cambridge, a project for women and children who are being or have been sexually abused provides a crisis refuge and counselling.

Where these newer services have been evaluated the results are promising. A 24-hour helpline in Mid-Downs (southern England) was found to have reduced admissions (Health Advisory Service, 1990). An unstaffed flat in Bassetlaw, Nottinghamshire resulted in improved symptoms and praise for the 'peace and quiet of the flat' (Turkington, 1991). Home treatment is preferred to the traditional acute hospital service by both users and carers and can reduce admission by over 50% (Dean & Gadd, 1990).

The main key to positive development is that users are involved from the outset in running or planning the projects. It is important that different groups of users have a say, as relevant – for example, black people as well as white. According to the 1991 Census there are over three million black people in Britain, 5.5% of the total population (Centre for Research in Ethnic Relations, 1992). Issues that have been identified as relevant to black people using mental health service are increases in: diagnosis of schizophrenia (Harrison *et al.*, 1988; Knowles, 1992); use of medication and ECT (Sashidiran & Francis, 1993); forced custodial treatment (Browne, 1990); involuntary admissions (Moodley & Perkins, 1990); and likelihood of transfer whilst on remand (Cope & Ndegwa, 1990). The response of service developers to these issues has been inadequate (Jones, 1991). Good practice guidelines have been developed (Wilson, 1993), yet culturally inappropriate concepts of normality are still applied, such as the nuclear family (Webb-Johnson, 1991).

The dissatisfaction expressed by black people results in not willingly engaging with services before a crisis, having negative experiences of interventions and dropping out of care rapidly afterwards. Problems with these three stages of care were addressed in the development of the Sanctuary Project. The idea for this project initially evolved at the King's Fund Centre in London, a service development centre which promotes improvements in health and social care. Local consultation exercises were then undertaken. The philosophy and consultation process undertaken in developing the Project are discussed.

The Sanctuary Project is envisaged as a community mental health development, which will be more appropriate to the needs of black people than existing services. It is intended to help black people with serious mental health problems. Black users, carers and other community members will be centrally involved in the planning, running and evaluating of the service, with the aim of encouraging participation and a sense of ownership by the black community as a whole. An accessible 24-hour, seven-days a week service is envisaged, that offers short-stay facilities. People will be seen in their home or in the Sanctuary. Child-care will be a central component, since the experience of black women with psychiatry has been particularly negative – one research study found that Afro-Caribbean women are twice as likely as Afro-Caribbean men to be diagnosed as schizophrenic, and 13 times as likely as white women (Knowles, 1992). The aim will be for early engagement between the persons in crisis and the service, hence avoiding the involuntary and negative contact with police and psychiatrist that arises from high use of Section 136 of the Mental Health Act on black people (Ferguson, 1992).

Assessment will be holistic, rather than based on the medical model. It will avoid early diagnosis and use of drugs, emphasising instead information, counselling and other therapies. Counselling will be appropriate, meaning more than just by another black person, but also considering class, race, religion and gender issues (Bhugra, 1993). Any staff employed will be sensitive to these concerns. Complementary therapies, such as dance, drama, music, acupuncture and herbalism will be available. A time-out room will allow safe emotional expression. The option of medication will be available, but not as the central therapeutic approach. In particular, there will be no medical or nursing staff based at the Sanctuary. The therapy process will therefore have a different orientation to most existing psychiatric services, and the intention is that the experience of therapy be positive for the black person in crisis.

After the initial crisis contact, seeing the person soon (e.g. next morning) will allow on-going relationships and support to be established. Flexible and assertive outreach practices will be used, to work with black people whose previous experience has left them feeling marginalised by psychiatry (Phaure, 1991).

Consultation took place at a local level in the two London districts selected as sites for Sanctuary projects, under the direction of a steering group for each district. The purpose of consultation was to encourage involvement in and ownership of the Sanctuary Project by the local community, and for the project to be seen as complementary to, rather than in competition with, existing services. The key issues addressed were similarity in values and culture of agencies, agreement on roles and responsibilities, network awareness, all parties gaining from working together, and the absence of alternative resources (Smith *et al.*, 1993).

The steering groups comprised users, carers, advocacy workers, voluntary sector staff, mental health and social services managers, and a King's Fund representative. Public consultation meetings were then held at neutral settings, which is important if people are not to be disadvantaged (Christie & Blunden, 1991). The exercise generated new ideas, such as the need for two venues, one for peace and tranquillity, the other for help and information. The issue of feeling safe at the Sanctuary was highlighted by users, as was the need to educate GPs about cultural needs and alternative therapeutic options. Practical suggestions for involving black women in the project were made. Local issues were also raised, such as a request for the involvement of a particular worker. The consultation therefore was of practical benefit in operationalising the Sanctuary idea. However, the problems that occurred during the process may inform future consultation exercises.

It was difficult to encourage service users to attend these meetings. A danger of this is that poorly-attended stake-holder meetings can be used (wrongly) to justify decision-making as being based on users' views. Even when people do attend, while having had bad experiences of a system they may not know what they would like to see change, with the possibility that whatever suggestions are being discussed are approved in the absence of anything better. Furthermore, few people will have the confidence to speak, typically without training, in a public forum to people who they do not know or (necessarily) trust. The steering group therefore held meetings in various day centres, and liaised with organisations that work with black people.

A second issue in the consultation process was the difficulty in involving local service providers, such as GPs, who would ensure high visibility for the Sanctuary Project. This was where the lack of clinical staff on the steering group was a drawback. However, there is a trade-off between the number of people on the steering group and how quickly progress is made. The King's Fund representative had links with staff in one of the two districts, and it was noticeably easier to develop a vision for the Sanctuary in that district. This suggests that, even where there is a wish to avoid operating under the control of health or social services, it is still helpful to have informal links with practitioners during the consultation process. The ideal configuration is a small steering group, which has links with both community-level and formal services, and whose members have a vested interest in the development of new models of care for black people.

Several principles emerge from the consultation process. Discussions should flexibly encourage service user participation, and should go out to them, instead of expecting users to attend organised meetings. Training for service users in public speaking can increase participation. A steering group should be small but representative, and can facilitate both mental health staff and user group involvement. Individual workers can be used to gain access to the local networks of black people. If services are to address the needs of black people, or indeed any marginalised group within society, then meaningful local consultation and community involvement must take place.

The way forward for British crisis services

From experience with existing projects and consultation with service users, we can make recommendations for new services:

- As a first principle that it does not do harm.
- That it is as effective as possible.
- That it offers autonomy, including a choice of treatments, a choice of worker and a right not to be intruded upon.
- That it gives opportunities to talk through underlying causes of distress, and adopts a holistic, rather than mainly medical, approach.
- That it helps people with their problems where they arise, and does not unnecessarily cut people off from normal life.
- That it offers safety, including safety from abuse for women, black people and others; and including some genuinely safe containment in crisis houses – or in hospital-type care for the minority who want or need that.
- That it takes place in people's own environments or in environments geared towards mental health needs.
- That it manages people's dependence on others when in a crisis with sensitivity – for instance, by ensuring people can withdraw from the service gradually and be linked into other help, such as self-help or longer term professional support.
- That it can offer anonymity.
- That it safeguards resources from the hospitals for support for mental health service users.
- That it respects the support that users offer each other.

The potential pitfalls of non-hospital crisis services identified by users could be tackled by following the above principles – and by ensuring that the new services are developed by or with users.

Many respondents to MIND's consultation on crisis and acute services were attracted to the idea of a safe house (sanctuary, crisis house). Safety can mean safety to be out of control without coming to harm – for example, harming yourself or being oblivious to danger (such as traffic), or being emotionally destructive to those nearest to you. Safety can mean separate space for women, or black women, or black men and women. It can mean 'safety from psychiatry' to those who have had bad experiences of hospital, or safety from drugs. Someone commented that 'you don't want to be "quizzed to death" before being accepted – or rejected'.

Crisis services could be preventive – a place that people can turn to when they anticipate a crisis. For some people it is important that support should come from other users of mental health services – people who can offer peer support, 'fellow travellers'. Diverse users have diverse needs – for example as women, or Afro-Caribbean or Asian people. People using crisis houses may need to have their child(ren) with them or benefit from having their partner stay over. They may need the service to value their spiritual beliefs. Or to respect a lesbian or gay relationship. Or understand money worries.

There is demand both for residential services and support services which come to individuals at home. This is not preference alone – some people have to get away from their home when in a crisis, others are unable to. For other people it is having a complete rest that matters. Befriending, or telephone contact may be what is needed. One suggestion for people in rural areas was for the kind of phone-based alarm system developed for elderly and disabled people living alone to be adapted for those vulnerable to a 'mental health emergency'. A 'sitting service' was mentioned in the survey, where someone stays with the person in distress. In Prato, Italy, a co-operative organisation provides a rota of people to stay with the person in crisis round the clock until they are able gradually to withdraw support.

There is no doubt that a partial revolution has been brought about by user involvement. For the first time users in some areas have begun to have some real say in what is – and is not – developed.

> 250 people turned up to the public meeting and told the District General Manager where to put his DGH unit and his concrete jungle.
>
> *(Personal communication, on how Nottingham's plans to create another acute unit were foiled.)*

However, in some quarters a backlash is occurring, fuelled by concern about the management of risk in the community, especially since the Clunis inquiry. The Royal College of Psychiatrists in 1992 argued that the way to improve the nation's mental health under the Government's Health of the Nation programme was through more psychiatrists and more beds (Royal College of Psychiatrists, 1992). Old arguments re-surfaced about the need for psychiatric wards to be physically near to general medicine – arguments that were forcefully demolished, including by some psychiatrists, many years ago:

> Psychiatry has experienced a *rapprochement* with the rest of medicine. To ask psychiatry to move out of hospitals would be regarded as a disruption. Hence, data about the effectiveness of alternatives are not greeted with great enthusiasm by the profession.
>
> *(Mosher, 1983.)*

> Association with the general hospital in itself seems particularly lame as a solution. Such hospitals have continually to struggle to balance technical efficiency and humane care.
>
> *(Brown, 1973.)*

There is another concern: that progressive ideas will be co-opted by professionals, such that we end up with community crisis services that are coercive, intrusive and drugs-based. If the Royal College of Psychiatrists takes up the Ritchie Report's suggestion that it develops a crisis card, the result could be a less empowering version of the card already developed by Survivors Speak Out. Or co-option could be by the managers, who might introduce community crisis services as a cost-cutting measure, providing minimal service only to those at 'risk' and consigning users' hopes for early intervention and holistic care to the scrap-heap.

The next few years demand that professionals, managers and the voluntary sector support users in setting up the services which users state that they need. There could be broad public and professional support for this. A survey of the general public found that 76% believe that people with mental health problems should have a legal right to 24-hour crisis services (MIND/RSGB 1994), as do 89% of Directors of Social Services (MIND/Community Care, 1994). As one person in the consultation put it:

> Services must be run on the lines of a co-operative effort between users, professionals and voluntary agencies.

Exactly which agencies will fulfil which roles in the purchase and provision of these services remains to be established. But what is clear is that change of substance will only occur if users call the tune.

References

Barbour, K., Clegg, J., Conlan, E. & Smith, L. (1991) *Enquiry into the Need for a Mental Health Easy Access / Crisis Centre in Milton Keynes*. Milton Keynes, Sub-Group of Joint Advisory Group for Mental Health.

Beeforth, M., Conlan, E. Field, V., Hoser, B. & Sayce, L. (1990). *Whose Service Is It Anyway?* London, Research and Development of Psychiatry.

Bergen, J., England, E. A., Campbell, J. A., *et al.* (1989). The course of tardive dyskinesia on long-term neuroleptics. *British Journal of Psychiatry*, **154**, 523–8.

Bhugra, D. (1993). Setting up services for ethnic minorities. In *Dimensions of Community Mental Health Care*, ed. M. Weller, & M. Muijen. London, W. B. Saunders.

British Medical Association (1994). *Call for Community Care Charter One Year On*. Press Release, March 24.

Brown, G. (1973). The mental hospital as an institution. *Social Science and Medicine*, **7**, 407–24.

Browne, D. (1990). *Black People, Mental Health and the Courts: An Exploratory Study into the Psychiatric Remand Process as it Affects Black Dependants at Magistrates Courts*. London, NACRO.

Camden Consortium/GPMH (1988). Good practices in mental health and Camden Consortium. *Treated Well? A Code of Practice for Psychiatric Hospitals*. London, GPMH.

Centre for Research in Ethnic Relations (University of Warwick) (1992). *1991 Census Statistical Paper No. 1*. Centre for Research in Ethnic Relations.

Chamberlin, J. (1988). *On Our Own*. London, MIND.

Christie, Y. & Blunden, R. (1991). *Is Race on your Agenda?* London, King's Fund Centre.

Cobb, A. (1993). *Safe and Effective?* London, MIND.

Cope, R. & Ndegwa, D. (1990). Ethnic differences in admission to a regional secure unit. *Journal of Forensic Psychiatry*, **1**(3), 365–76.

Darton, K., Gorman, J. & Sayce, L. (1994). *Eve Fights Back*. London, MIND.

Davidge, M., Elias, S., Jayes, B., *et al.* (1993). *Survey of English Mental Illness Hospitals.* (Prepared for the Mental Health Task Force.)

Dean, C. & Gadd, E. M. (1990). Home Treatment for Acute Psychiatric Illness. *British Medical Journal*, **301**, 1021–3.

Ferguson, G. (1992). Race and mental health. *Community Psychiatric Nursing Journal*, **12**(6), 11.

Harrison, G., Owens, D., Holton, A., Neilson, D. & Boot, D. (1988). A prospective study of severe mental disorder in Afro-Caribbean patients. *Psychological Medicine*, **18**, 643–57.

Health Advisory Service (1990). *Report on Services for Mentally Ill People and Elderly People in the Mid-Downs Health District.* NHS Health Advisory Service, Department of Health Social Services Inspectorate.

Health Advisory Service (1991). *Report on Services for Mentally Ill People and Elderly People in the Torbay Health District.* NHS Health Advisory Service, Department of Health Social Services Inspectorate.

Health Building Note 35 (1988). *Accommodation for People with Acute Mental Illness.* London, HMSO.

House of Commons Health Committee (1985). *Second Report From the Social Services Committee 1985 Community Care with Special Reference to Adult Mentally Ill and Mentally Handicapped People.* London, HMSO.

House of Commons Health Committee (1993). *Community Supervision Orders.* London, HMSO.

Huxley, P. (1993). Social Services Response to Psychiatric Emergencies. *Psychiatric Bulletin*, **17**, 282–5.

Johnson, S. & Thornicroft, G. (1991). *Emergency Psychiatric Services in England and Wales.* Report to the Department of Health.

Johnstone, L., Metcalfe, M. & Owen, J. (1991). The First International Conference on Crisis Intervention Approaches in Mental Health. *Psychiatric Bulletin*, **15**(1), 36.

Jones, A. (1991). *Black Communities Care: Report of the Black Communities Care Project.* Leeds, NISW.

Knowles, C. (1992). Afro-Caribbeans and schizophrenia: how does psychiatry deal with issues of race, culture and ethnicity? *Journal of Social Policy*, **20**(2), 173–90.

Lloyd, G. (1992). *Confidential Report into Recent Suicides and Related Events at Lister Hospital, Stevenage.* (Made public October 1992.)

Mental Health Foundation (1993). *Mental Illness. The Fundamental Facts.*

MIND/Community Care (1994). Survey reported in *Community Care Magazine*, 30 April 1994.

MINDLINK (1993). Treatments consultations. (Written communications in consultation with MINDLINK members on treatment. Unpublished.)

MIND/RSGB (1994). *The Public's View of Mental Health Services.* MIND/RSGB Survey quoted in *Community Care Magazine*, 10 March 1994.

Moodley, P. & Perkins, R. (1990). Routes to psychiatric inpatient care in an inner London borough. *Social Psychiatry and Psychiatric Epidemiology*, **26**, 47–51.

Morgan, H. & Priest, P. (1991). Suicide and other unexpected deaths among psychiatric in-patients – the Bristol confidential inquiry. *British Journal of Psychiatry*, **158**, 368–74.

Mosher, L. R. (1983). Alternatives to psychiatric hospitalisations: why has research failed to be translated into practice. *New England Journal of Medicine*, **303**, 1579–80.

Muijen, M., Marks, I., Connolly, J. & Audini, B. (1992). Home-based care and standard hospital care for patients with severe mental illness: A randomised controlled trial. *British Medical Journal*, **304**, 749–54.

Murphy, E., Jenkins, J., Scott, J. & Rooney, P. (1991). *Proceedings of Community Mental Health Services – Models for the Future*. Conference Series No. 11, University of Newcastle Upon Tyne.

Newchurch and Company Ltd. (1992). *Acute Hospitals – A Case for Treatment*.

Phaure, S. (1991). *Who Really Cares?: Models of Voluntary Sector Community Care and Black Communities*. London, London Voluntary Service Council.

Ritchie, J. H., Dick, D. & Lingham, R. (1994). *Report of Inquiry into the Care and Treatment of Christopher Clunis*. London, HMSO.

Royal College of Psychiatrists (1992). *Mental Health of the Nation: The Contribution of Psychiatry*. Council Report CR16.

Rogers, A., Pilgrim, D. & Lacey, R. (1993). *Experiencing Psychiatry*. MIND/MacMillan.

Sashidharan, S. & Francis, E. (1993). Epidemiology, ethnicity and schizophrenia. In *Race and Health in Contemporary Britain*, ed. W. Ahmed. Milton Keynes, Open University Press.

Sayce, L. (1995). Good practices in mental health for women with children. In ed. C. Andrews, J. Copperman & Z. Nadirshaw. (In press.)

Sargeant, J. (1988). Bitter pills? *Openmind*, **34**, 4–5.

Smith, R., Gaster, L., Harrison, L., Martin, L., Means, R. & Thistlethwaite, P. (1993). *Working Together for Better Community Care*. Bristol, SAUS Publications.

Southampton MIND (1993). *Stress on Women Survey*. (Unpublished).

Turkington, D. (1991). The use of an unstaffed flat for crisis intervention and rehabilitation. *Psychiatric Bulletin*, **15**, 13–14.

Webb-Johnson, A. (1991). *A Cry for Change: An Asian Perspective on Developing Quality Mental Health Care*. London, Confederation of Indian Organisations.

Wilson, M. (1993). *Mental Health and Britain's Black Communities*. London, King's Fund Centre.

4

Legal aspects of mental health emergencies

IAN BYNOE, ADINA HALPERN AND CAROLINE BATES

Mental health law: an introduction

This chapter describes the legal powers which professionals may use in the mental health 'emergency'. The law is that in force in England and Wales and after outlining how this has developed, the various common law principles and statutory measures which may apply are presented. These may be used to restrain a person's behaviour, help secure an assessment of a person's condition or provide forced treatment in hospital. The chapter concludes with a brief examination of international trends in mental health law and some thoughts on future legal changes.

The development of mental health law can be seen as a convergence of two strands of legalism. The first sought to formulate principles and procedures to protect the public from the 'insane'. The second attempted to protect both the 'sane' from unjustified detention and persons with a mental disorder from detention that is unnecessary. The law has also been concerned to define and protect the rights of citizens who have to have their liberty restricted due to their mental condition.

By the mid-nineteenth century, a system had emerged for dealing with mental illness which strongly mirrored the social class of the person affected. Upper classes were confined in licensed private institutions, middle classes in registered hospitals, whilst those whose families could not finance such confinement were found in the workhouse or in public asylums. The aims of the respective institutions were containment and isolation rather than cure or rehabilitation and the law reflected this.

By the time the Mental Treatment Act was passed in 1930, social attitudes to mental illness and its treatment had changed sufficiently for a significant advance to take place, in part reflecting a more treatment oriented approach. For the first time, this legislation permitted voluntary admission to psychiatric hospital for treatment.

In 1957, the *Report of the Royal Commission on the Law relating to Mental Illness and Mental Deficiency* (Royal Commission, 1957) proposed changes of even greater significance. The resulting 1959 Mental Health Act sought to render an admission to hospital for psychiatric treatment no different from one for treatment for a physical condition, save where compulsion was needed due to the severity of the person's disorder or the risk which they posed to themselves or to others.

No special formalities were to be completed before a person could be admitted and compulsory admission would be mainly an administrative process operated by mental health professionals. Judicial committal would be largely restricted to those occasions when a criminal court wished to order treatment for a person convicted of an imprisonable offence.

The 1959 Act created a new mechanism for judicial oversight of the 'civil' detention of patients which has continued to the present. The Mental Health Review Tribunal, a three person body with legal, medical and lay membership, would in future hear patients' applications for discharge with powers of release for most categories of those detained for treatment.

In time, concerns grew that the 1959 Act inadequately protected patients' rights and that changes were required to render professionals more accountable. The campaign for reform led to the Mental Health Act 1983 – the present statute. This was reformist rather than radical both in spirit and effect. The main criteria for compulsory admission to hospital were retained thus enabling interventions to be justified on grounds of the patient's health alone or their safety or so as to protect others. Instead of narrowing the criteria, the Act shortened periods of detention thus increasing the frequency of independent review.

Where the 1983 Act clearly broke with the past was in the ways it increased formal professional accountability for decisions taken using its powers. It did not do this by creating a mass of detailed, complex and mandatory regulations but by creating a new agency, the Mental Health Act Commission, to oversee the care and treatment of detained patients; by requiring a code of professional practice to offer guidance to doctors, social workers, nurses and others on how they should use the Act and provide medical treatment to those who suffer from a mental disorder (Department of Health and Welsh Office, 1990, 1993); and lastly by obliging the approval of social workers before their use of legal powers.

The law that applies in Scotland derives from a separate statute, the Mental Health (Scotland) Act 1984, and remains distinctly different. It defines the concept of 'mental disorder' more narrowly, retains judicial commitment by the Sheriff before a patient detained under 'civil' powers can be compulsorily treated, and provides the Scottish Mental Welfare Commission with powers and a constitutional independence far greater than is given its southern equivalent.

Community settings now predominate as the places where people are being, and prefer to be, treated and cared for, and the old asylums are closing or are scheduled for closure. The hospital retains a role as the place for the assessment and stabilisation of acute phases of mental illness. Institutional treatment must also be retained for those requiring security or whose capacity for independent living is severely restricted.

However, patients who do not need a hospital place for either of these reasons will find in future that those who finance and manage mental health care services will expect them to live in 'ordinary' neighbourhoods, receiving assistance in their own homes. Such changes in policy and practice may call into question the relevance and adequacy of present laws and new and additional measures are about to be introduced, in particular a new legal status of 'aftercare under supervision', provided for in the government's Mental Health (Patients in the Community) Bill, presently before Parliament (Department of Health, 1993; Department of Health, 1994b). These will increase not reduce those powers which currently exist. It is to these that we will next turn.

Law and the mental health emergency: provisions

Common law provides very limited authority to detain or restrain a person who may be a risk to themselves or others or who may be or about to be committing a breach of the peace. It is worth considering such rules since they may have to be used urgently in the absence of specific authority under mental health legislation. Unless the law provides some common law or statutory defence allowing the use of physical force to restrain or confine a person then those responsible may be liable for the crimes or torts of assault, battery and false imprisonment.

Common law allows a person to take all reasonable steps to ensure that he or she does not come to any physical harm. This is the principle of self-defence and enables someone to use force to restrain a person whose behaviour causes them a risk of such harm. The force employed must be limited to what is necessary and appropriate in the circumstances.

A breach of the peace occurs whenever harm is actually done or likely to be done to a person or to property or where a person is in fear of being so harmed through an assault or other disturbance. Some harm, actual, likely or feared, must be present and where a person's words or behaviour lead to a reasonable expectation of violence then reasonable force can be used to restrain that person to prevent them from acting in this way. A person whose mental disorder causes conduct such as this can therefore be restrained for as long as the threat lasts.

Although there are no modern cases on the subject, there is considered to be a separate common law power to justify the apprehension and restraint of a person who is 'mentally disordered' and whose behaviour is dangerous (Department of Health and Welsh Office, 1993). Whilst the danger exists, this power only allows restraint that is reasonable and appropriate and which ends as soon as the danger has gone. This power is particularly relevant in health settings, as a justification for short-term physical restraint or sedation in an emergency.

s. 3(1) Criminal Law Act 1967 permits the use of force in the making of an arrest or in the prevention of crime. The force used must be 'reasonable in the circumstances'. It would, for example, allow a mentally disturbed person to be restrained if they were about to assault another person with a weapon. If force is used it must be necessary, in proportion to the harm to be avoided and can only last as long as the threat of harm exists.

The powers mentioned above are temporary and linked to concepts of self-defence and necessity. Mental health legislation provides powers which can last longer and which can be applied to significantly more circumstances. The Mental Health Act 1983, which applies only to England and Wales, provides a number of such powers which can be employed in the mental health emergency. These powers are not restricted to one class or category of professional or office holder and specific powers can be used respectively by police constables, nurses, junior hospital doctors, GPs, psychiatrists and social workers in addition to the patient's nearest relative, a status which is defined by law.

Most of these powers will only be exercisable where 'mental disorder' or 'mental illness' is believed to be present. Although the latter term is not further defined in the Act and therefore depends upon a clinical judgement as to its presence or absence, 'mental disorder' is defined.

Definition of mental disorder

'Mental disorder' means mental illness, arrested or incomplete development of mind, psychopathic disorder and any other disorder or disability of mind.

s. 1(2) Mental Health Act 1983

The emergency in a public place

There are specific powers granted to the police constable to take a person into custody and remove him or her to 'a place of safety', there to be examined by a doctor and interviewed by an approved social worker (s. 136(1) & (2) Mental Health Act 1983). The detention which follows use of this power can last for up to 72 hours. A 'place of safety' can be chosen from a range of premises such as a police station, hospital ward or accident and emergency (A & E) department. The assessment which takes place can lead to an admission to hospital under other powers which we shall outline later.

This power is the only one which is exercisable by a lay person alone. For it to be used, it only needs to appear to the constable that the person suffers from a 'mental disorder' and is in immediate need of care or control. The police power can extend to any place to which the public has access. It therefore extends to many enclosed spaces such as shops, recreational facilities and premises for public transportation.

There have been concerns about the manner in which the power has been exercised. In particular, it has been claimed that the police employ the power when this is not strictly justifed, that medical assessments are not undertaken with sufficient expertise, speed and thoroughness and that social work involvement is sometimes ignored or given too little priority. Some of these claims have without doubt been justified (Rogers & Faulkner, 1987; Bean *et al.*, 1991). In consequence, recent guidance on the use of this power now requires better standards of practice and accountability (Department of Health and Welsh Office, 1993). The principal requirements are as follows.

Good practice in use of police power of arrest

- A clear, written policy agreed between local police, health and social services authorities.
- Identification of the preferred local 'place of safety'.
- Attendance of a psychiatrist to examine detainee.
- Requirement for clear record keeping and regular monitoring, including for ethnicity.
- Clear guidance on the role and responsibilities of doctors and social workers to ensure a competent and speedy assessment.

Mental Health Act Code of Practice (1993) Chapter 10

The emergency in private premises

What power exists to deal with the situation where a person is in private premises? The police are granted the power to enter these premises but application for the magistrate's warrant conferring such an authority must be made by an approved social worker (s. 135(1) Mental Health Act 1983). The magistrate considers brief evidence from the social worker, in private and without any other party present. The evidence has to show, not that the situation constitutes an emergency, but that it is reasonable to believe that someone in the premises who is 'mentally disordered' is being ill-treated or neglected or is unable to care for themselves.

If a warrant is issued then it empowers a police constable to enter the named premises, if necessary by force, but only when accompanied by a medical practitioner and an approved social worker. After entering, the constable has the power to remove the person to a 'place of safety' to be detained there for further assessment.

In practice, this power is often used to enable a multidisciplinary assessment to take place in the premises entered under the warrant. If the person assessed needs admission to hospital this is likely to be effected under powers which specifically provide for this rather than through removal to a 'place of safety'. We shall describe those powers later.

Crime arrests and the mental health emergency

The police possess many powers in addition to those granted them under mental health legislation, many of which can be exercised without first obtaining a warrant. Some of these will be highly relevant to a mental health emergency where a person's behaviour during this also constitutes a suspected criminal offence, or 'breach of the peace'. The police will then arrest the person and detain them in custody for that offence, only later discovering that the person has some mental disorder which may need the attention of health or social services.

For example, the police have numerous statutory powers to arrest a person suspected of committing a criminal offence (e.g. Police and Criminal Evidence Act, 1984) and retain the power at common law to arrest a person to deal with or prevent a breach of the peace. As well, a constable has a power to enter and search any premises without a warrant to save 'life or limb' or prevent serious damage to property (s. 17(1)(e) Police and Criminal Evidence Act, 1984).

It is now the stated aim of government policy that a person suspected of a criminal offence but at the same time in need of treatment or care for a mental disorder should receive such treatment and care from health and social services rather than within the criminal justice system (Home Office, 1990). General guidance has been issued to all agencies in that system requiring action to reflect this policy. Specific directions have also been given to the police on cautioning and the treatment of mentally vulnerable suspects (Home Office, 1994), to prosecutors on prosecution policy (Attorney General's Office, 1994) and to the probation service on its co-operation with social services authorities (Home Office, 1993).

Health and social services authorities are expected to co-operate with the police and court system, providing psychiatric and social assessments when these are necessary. Recent government guidance has required mental health professionals in England to maintain registers of patients considered to be 'at risk' in the community and to enhance the care given to them under the Care Programme Approach (Department of Health, 1994a,b). The Mental Health (Patients in the Community) Bill, presently before Parliament, will lead some patients in addition having their aftercare 'supervised' in the community within a defined legal framework. It is likely that police action in future will be influenced by such statuses when they discover one or both affect someone they have arrested. Early intervention leading to an assessment and the provision of a hospital place on a compulsory or voluntary basis can greatly influence a police decision to charge a suspect, and, if so, whether or not to grant bail.

The police have two principal duties towards a person they have arrested and detained who may show signs of mental disorder (Code C, Police and Criminal Evidence Act 1984 Codes of Practice). Firstly, they must arrange the attendance of a responsible adult, such as a close relative or mental health professional, at the police station to ensure that the person is dealt with fairly and to aid in communication. Secondly, the police must arrange the attendance of a police surgeon to examine the person and assess his or her need for treatment. Clearly, the latter rule can potentially lead to an early intervention by health and social work professionals resulting in admission to hospital or arrangements for out-patient assessment or treatment.

The protections are of limited effectiveness in guaranteeing early diversion for the suspect needing health care. This is due to varying and inconsistent practice by police surgeons (Royal Commission, 1993) and divergent responses to requests for assessment by health and social work staff. However, if good practice and the effective targeting of resources can ensure that the police obtain an expert psychiatric assessment as soon as possible after a person has been arrested then later problems, in the court or prison system, will be avoided.

Before those problems and the measures which can be taken to avoid them are considered, it is important that a description of the powers of psychiatrists and social workers to intervene in order to deal with the mental health emergency is presented.

The emergency requiring admission to hospital for assessment

Where civil powers are employed, in contrast to the powers of the criminal court, a formal admission to hospital usually follows an assessment by two registered medical practitioners, one of whom is a psychiatrist, and an approved social worker. There are situations when only one medical assessment is needed and occasions when a person's nearest relative will wish to apply for their admission but these are not common. Where the purpose of hospitalisation is to assess a person's condition before deciding on diagnosis or specific treatment then the provisions are as shown below and are principally found in s. 2 Mental Health Act 1983.

Admission to hospital for assessment

Criteria

- Mental disorder of a nature or degree which warrants detention in a hospital for assessment (or for assessment followed by medical treatment) AND person ought to be detained in the interests of their own health or safety or with a view to the protection of others.

Procedure

- Two written medical recommendations (one from approved doctor).
- Application, subject to strict time limits, by approved social worker or patient's nearest relative.

Effect

- Patient detainable for up to 28 days, subject to compulsory treatment rules and entitled to apply to Tribunal for discharge.

Parts II, IV, and V Mental Health Act 1983

Sometimes, where there is an emergency, it would be undesirable to delay admission to hospital in order to comply with the requirements shown above. The Mental Health Act thus allows an emergency application to be made where, additionally, there is 'urgent necessity' demonstrated. The effect is to relax the procedural rules for admission and reduce the time the person can be detained from 28 days to 3 days. As well, there is no power to compel treatment for a patient during that period.

To permit a person's admission to hospital on the basis only of one medical opinion, which may not be from a psychiatrist, is controversial. There is concern, however, that the power has been used when psychiatrists have not co-operated with requests for assessments and not for occasions of true emergency. Use of the power has dropped dramatically, from 5640 in 1983 to 1868 in 1989–90, and the current guidance is strict, strongly discouraging its use save in exceptional situations (Department of Health and Welsh Office, 1993). The Code advice is summarised below. The emergency admission can be converted to a conventional admission for assessment after a second medical recommendation has been obtained.

Emergency admission: good practice guidance

- Power is for genuine emergency and should never be used for administrative convenience.
- Emergency arises where those involved cannot cope with mental state or behaviour of patient.
- Use where evidence of significant risk of mental or physical harm to patient or others and/or danger of serious harm to property and/or need for physical restraint of patient.
- Approved social worker must be satisfied that application is necessary and proper.
- Approved social worker to report unacceptable reasons for non-availability of second doctor.

Mental Health Act Code of Practice (1993) Chapter 6

Admission to hospital for treatment

Sometimes an urgent intervention will be necessary particularly in circumstances where the person's diagnosis and likely treatment are already well known to mental health professionals. Government guidance in England requiring the Care Programme Approach (Department of Health, 1990) and the placing of 'at risk' patients on a register may encourage more applications in the case of such patients. The power which is available differs in important respects from those already mentioned and is found in s. 3 Mental Health Act, 1983. There is no general principle of law or guidance in operation in England and Wales which requires a short-term assessment admission to precede one for treatment. Details are given below.

Admission to hospital for treatment

Criteria

- Mental illness, severe mental impairment, mental impairment or psychopathic disorder of nature or degree to make medical treatment in hospital appropriate.
- Necessary for health or safety of patient or protection of other persons that person be treated.
- Treatment cannot be provided without detention.

Procedure

- Two written medical recommendations (one from approved doctor).
- Application, subject to strict time limits, by approved social worker (ASW) or nearest relative.
- If ASW application, nearest relative must be consulted and not object.

Effect

- Patient detainable for up to six months, renewable for six months, then yearly.
- Patient subject to compulsory treatment rules and entitled to apply to Tribunal for discharge.

Parts II, IV and V Mental Health Act 1983

Current guidance on the use to be made of this power, suggests that it should be reserved for those occasions where there is little, if anything, remaining to be learned about the patient's condition or the nature of the treatment(s) which may alleviate it (Chapter 5, Mental Health Act Code of Practice). It would not therefore be appropriate to employ the power if emergency circumstances limit the ability of health or social work professionals to investigate the patient's past medical history or their present mental state to reach firm conclusions about either of these factors.

The emergency in prison

Current guidance, and to a limited extent the criminal law, aim to prevent the arrival in the prison system of any person who needs assessment or treatment as a psychiatric hospital inpatient (Home Office, 1990 and s. 4 Criminal Justice Act, 1991). The mental health care services provided to prisoners do not even approach standards found within National Health Service hospitals (Department of Health and Home Office, 1992) and it is now widely recognised that the NHS should be the place where such assessment or treatment is offered.

However, not only do the prisons receive men and women who should be in hospital but also a prisoner can, whilst awaiting trial or serving a sentence, develop a condition requiring a psychiatric intervention (Gunn *et al.*, 1990; Dell *et al.*, 1991). Courts and prison authorities have a number of options available to them in these circumstances. These are shown below.

Diversion from the criminal justice system

- Remand to hospital by court for assessment (s. 35).
- Remand to hospital by court for treatment (s. 36).
- Interim hospital order by court for treatment (s. 38).
- Hospital order by court for treatment (s. 37).
- Transfer of remand prisoner for urgent treatment (s. 48).
- Transfer of sentenced prisoner for treatment (s. 47).

Part III Mental Health Act 1983

Where it is appropriate for civil powers to be used to detain a person for assessment or treatment, nothing should prevent this happening even though the person may at the same time be subject to a charge before a criminal court. In that event, either representations may lead the court or the prosecution to discontinue the proceedings or the two systems will run in parallel, with bail being granted to the person detained in hospital until the case has ended.

The emergency on the hospital ward

Stopping a patient from leaving

An emergency may occur on the hospital ward. Commonly, this will be a patient attempting to leave the ward when it is felt that this should be prevented. As well there may be a patient's violent or disruptive behaviour calling for physical restraint, seclusion or emergency sedation. Such problems will not be limited to the psychiatric hospital and may occur in medical or surgical wards or in A & E departments which admit patients to beds. Each of these situations will be dealt with in turn.

Whilst an informal in-patient is free to refuse treatment and leave a hospital, there are circumstances in which such a person may be prevented from doing so and this may be prompted by their planning to leave. Under s. 5(2) of the 1983 Mental Health Act, the doctor in charge of a patient's treatment (or that person's nominee) may complete and sign a short report under which authority the patient can be detained for up to 72 hours. All the doctor must believe is that an application ought to be made in due course for the patient's formal admission to psychiatric hospital. A patient detained under this power can be transferred to another ward in the same hospital but not to another hospital altogether.

A senior nurse working in a psychiatric hospital has the power to prevent a patient leaving the ward (s. 5(4) Mental Health Act 1983). The circumstances in which this can be employed are shown below.

Senior nurse's holding power

- Patient is suffering from mental disorder to degree necessary for health or safety or for protection of others for him or her to be immediately restrained from leaving hospital.
- Not practicable to secure immediate attendance of doctor to sign report preventing leaving.
- Psychiatric nurse (registered, first level, trained) must record this.
- Patient then detainable for up to six hours to await doctor.

s. 5(4) Mental Health Act 1983

Emergency treatment

Whether or not a person can be treated against his or her will depends firstly on whether or not they are detained under the Mental Health Act 1983, and, if so, under which section of that Act. Secondly, it depends on the type of treatment(s) to be given.

For those patients to whom the statutory rules apply, treatments can be given in legally defined circumstances in the absence of a consent and despite a refusal to provide this from a patient with the capacity to do so. Where the statutory rules do not apply, then apart from the limited power to detain the person, the only authority is derived from the common law principle outlined above. This is now summarised in the current Mental Health Act Code of Practice (Department of Health and Welsh Office, 1993) and details are shown below.

Emergency power to treat under common law

On rare occasions involving emergencies, where it is not possible immediately to apply the provisions of the Mental Health Act, a patient suffering from a mental disorder which is leading to behaviour that is an immediate serious danger to himself or to other people may be given such treatment as represents the minimum necessary response to avert that danger.

Mental Health Act Code of Practice (1993) Paragraph 15.24

It will be noticed that this common law power of treatment is extremely restricted. This power, and only this one, will be available to treat a person who will not consent to treatment and who is subject to the police powers mentioned above, or is a patient admitted in an emergency for assessment or detailed under the medical or nursing holding powers. If treatment is therefore required for longer than allowed by emergency circumstances, it will be necessary to admit the patient under the Mental Health Act 1983, in order to apply the more extensive treatment powers available under that Act.

Where the absence of a patient's consent to proposed treatment is due, not to their refusing, but to their incapacity to give or withhold consent then a further common law principle applies which can sanction treatment. The person must truly lack capacity. In a recent case, the court adopted an approach which judged that the following abilities were needed: (1) comprehending and retaining treatment information; (2) believing it to be true; and (3) weighing it in the balance to arrive at choice (Re C. (Adult: Refusal of Treatment) [1994] 1 WLR 290). In addition, the intended treatment must be in the patient's 'best interests', that is:

- necessary to save life or prevent a deterioration or ensure an improvement in the patient's physical or mental health; and
- in accordance with a practice accepted at the time by a responsible body of medical opinion skilled in the particular form of treatment in question.

Mental Health Act Code of Practice (1993) Paragraph 15.19

These principles have been formulated particularly in relation to the provision of medical treatment for physical not mental disorders. The authors (IB, AH, CB) are aware of occasions when medical practitioners have justified the use, even of ECT, on a patient under this rule. Given the availability of extensive statutory authority and the importance of the protections to the patient which come with it, it is surely poor practice to have resort to this general power when the Act specifically offers a code for the giving of psychiatric treatment in such situations? Before going further, we therefore need to examine just what those rules are and to whom they can be applied.

The patients who are subject to the treatment rules under the 1983 Mental Health Act are shown below.

Patients subject to Mental Health Act treatment powers

- A patient detained under an admission for assessment (s. 2).
- A patient detained under an admission for treatment (s. 3).

- A patient remanded to hospital for treatment (s. 36).
- A patient detained under a hospital order (s. 37).
- A patient transferred from prison for treatment (ss. 47 & 48).

Parts II, III and IV Mental Health Act, 1983

These rules permit medical treatment for mental disorder to be given, in particular sanctioning medication for a period of three months from its first administration without special formalities, and ECT and medication beyond three months if special formalities are undertaken. The principal requirement is, that for treatment to take place, a second psychiatric opinion must be obtained from an independent psychiatrist appointed by the Mental Health Act Commission for this purpose. These formalities can be avoided if it is necessary to give 'urgent' treatment, such as in an emergency. The statutory definition of such treatment mirrors the common law principle but is significantly wider in its potential application. The provisions are summarised below.

Urgent treatment under the Mental Health Act 1983

- Treatment immediately necessary to save life.
- Treatment (not being irreversible) immediately necessary to prevent serious deterioration of condition.
- Treatment (not being irreversible or hazardous) immediately necessary to alleviate serious suffering.
- Treatment (not being irreversible or hazardous) immediately necessary and minimum interference necessary to prevent violent behaviour or danger to self or others.

s. 62(1) Mental Health Act 1983

As has been outlined above, only certain types of treatment attract special protections under the 1983 Mental Health Act for those who are detained under its authority, though only 'medical treatment for mental disorder' as defined in the Act can be given using its powers. As long as these other treatments are given for the mental disorder from which the person is suffering and are given by or under the direction of the person's Responsible Medical Officer (i.e. consultant in charge of treatment) then they will be lawful and there are no special legal rules relevant to emergency situations.

Guidance on the use of physical restraint, seclusion and 'timeout' is, however, given in the current Code of Practice (Department of Health and Welsh Office, 1993) and this will be highly important for health professionals, particularly nursing staff, responding to threatening, violent or self-harming behaviour. The advice is lengthy and detailed and cannot be summarised here. Its thrust is to restrict such interventions to the exceptional occasions where they are absolutely necessary; to limit seclusion only to those situations where a person is a risk to others; and to require local policies and procedures to ensure consistent practice and regular, sometimes independent, review of the justification for the use of such powers in a particular situation.

International trends and future changes

Although there has been a wide variety of legal frameworks governing mental health adopted by countries throughout the world some trends can be noticed. Two studies into international mental health practice undertaken by the World Health Organization (WHO) in 1955 and in 1977 demonstrated that during this period significant changes had occurred. There had been a marked trend towards voluntary rather than compulsory detention, and administrative methods for admission rather than judicial ones. The study noted an alteration in terminology with regard to mental disorder, and a conspicuous shift from surgical and electro convulsive treatment to the use of tranquillising medication. The increased use of treatment in the community and the reduction in use of large institutions was also detected by the WHO.

Another trend has been the emergence of new powers to require treatment in the community for patients who may have been treated in hospital and been discharged still needing supervision and medication, or, being an alternative to hospitalisation, imposed on the patient as the 'least restrictive' option. In the United States many states have legislated for such 'involuntary out-patient commitment'. It has been estimated that such out-patient treatment orders constitute up to 20% of all cases of compulsory psychiatric treatment in that country (Miller, 1985). This high proportion is due in part to factors specific to the United States and not necessarily the clinical benefits of their use. The criteria employed to justify such powers differ from state to state. Some systems require proof that the person will be dangerous unless admitted to involuntary treatment, others adopt lower thresholds for applying the powers. Most include a rule that the person in question lacks capacity to make their own treatment decisions. In keeping with the 'due process' approach common in the United States, such orders are created following a judicial procedure and judges keep under review the need for the orders to continue.

In Australia, Victoria was the first state to provide for compulsory powers for treatment in the community. Under the Mental Health Act 1986, a person can be placed under such powers after first being admitted to hospital so there are no special grounds formulated, although the admission may only be a token gesture and for as little as 30 minutes. A qualified psychiatrist signs the order, which must specify details of the treatment of the person. Non-compliance with the order can lead to its revocation and the forced return of the person to hospital as a detained patient. A Mental Health Review Tribunal must review the order shortly after its instigation. Use of this order has been fairly limited (Dedman, 1990).

New South Wales, in its Mental Health Act 1990, provided for both a Community Counselling Order and a Community Treatment Order. The process for creating both of these orders is a judicial one. The latter order is specifically created for those who it is perceived will fail to comply with counselling if this is ordered for them. Those using such powers must have regard to the principle of the least restrictive alternative, which must be satisfied if the order is to be made.

In its recent Mental Health (Compulsory Assessment and Treatment) Act 1992, New Zealand has been the latest country to create new powers for treatment in the community. This is in the context of a statute which assumes that the community will be the location for treatment unless 'the patient cannot be treated adequately as an out-patient'. There is a recognition that in applying restrictions on a person's liberty by requiring co-operation with treatment, the state has reciprocal obligations to provide services appropriate to the needs of the person affected. The mechanism for creating such orders is a judicial one and the court, before doing so, has to be satisfied that the 'Board provides through the institution or service named in the order care and treatment on an out-patient basis that is appropriate to the needs of the patient; . . .' (s. 28(4) (a) Mental Health (Compulsory Assessment and Treatment) Act 1992).

The legal changes being introduced by the Mental Health (Patients in the Community) Bill for patients in Great Britain follow this trend to create new powers for supervision and treatment in the community (Department of Health, 1993). Firstly, the arrangements for permitting detained patients to have leave of absence from hospital will be amended to allow for the continuation of this leave up to the end of a person's period of detention, not just for the maximum of six months currently allowed for in the present Mental Health Act. This proposal is modest and will have little impact since most of the 4500 admissions to hospital for treatment last for less than 12 months and this change will not affect them.

Secondly, the Bill will extend to six months or the end of their detention, whichever is the later, the period of time during which they can be returned to hospital if they leave it without permission whilst receiving compulsory treatment there. The present time limit is 28 days.

The creation of an entirely new legal status – in England, 'aftercare subject to supervision' and in Scotland, a 'community care order' – is the main change being introduced and is far more significant. The status is similar to the present arrangements for guardianship under the 1983 Act and may be applied for by the consultant psychiatrist in charge of the patient's treatment in hospital. That patient must have been admitted to hospital for compulsory treatment and in the view of those applying for or recommending it require supervision in the community following their discharge. That supervision has to be provided by a named individual according to a specific written care plan. The patient may be required to comply with conditions concerning, for example, where they will live. A patient failing or refusing to comply with supervision may be physically taken to hospital or other premises. In such circumstances, those responsible for supervision will be legally obliged to review their aftercare and whether those circumstances should prompt an admission to hospital, if necessary, a compulsory one.

In England, the new measure is associated with the creation of 'at risk' registers (Department of Health, 1994a) and the issue of fresh guidance on discharged patients (Department of Health, 1994b). These changes reflect a determined attempt by Government to apply a new procedural regime to the multidisciplinary assessment and supervision of patients. In part, it is responding to those who have severely criticised the current system for its lack of co-ordination, effectiveness and humanity (Ritchie *et al.*, 1994). In practice, a decision to place a person on a register or to require their discharge to be supervised will remain the prerogative of the consultant psychiatrist in charge of treatment. There is no sign that any of these changes will increase the formal accountability of health or social services authorities for the level or standard of services provided to someone, despite many claims that new powers will prove inequitable and ineffective unless more resources are made to match them.

Conclusion

This chapter has provided an outline of the powers available to health professionals and others in England and Wales to intervene in the mental health 'emergency'. Such powers are extensive, often generally and vaguely stated and can be employed with limited administrative burdens. The legal system sanctioning such compulsion is far from the 'due process' model found in the United States or other countries both in its philosophy and in the practical accountability needed for professional actions.

In such a system, there is all the more reason for practice to be consistently applied according to contemporary standards of human and civil rights. In the UK context, the importance of the Mental Health Act Code of Practice and training around its requirements in guaranteeing this cannot be underestimated. It may well be necessary for some Code guidance to become law when the Act is next amended in England and Wales.

Most mental health legislation narrowly concerns itself with providing the means of compelling compulsory treatment. There are as yet few signs of an interest in making the law an effective passport for a patient to receive adequate services. As the century moves to a close and community care though sometimes discredited is not abandoned, we must hope that imaginative and effective means are found for those who will depend upon it to have guaranteed the services which they need. The community seems so much less prepared to finance welfare provision now, particularly for those who carry the stigma of mental illness, and it must surely be right for politician's hands to be stayed by legally enshrined obligations.

References

Attorney General's Office (1994). *Code for Crown Prosecutors.* London, Attorney General's Office.

Bean, P., Bingley, W., Bynoe, I. *et al.* (1991). *Out of Harm's Way.* London, MIND.

Dedman, P. (1990). Community treatment orders in Victoria, Australia. *Psychiatric Bulletin*, **14**, 462–4.

Dell, S., Grounds, A., Robertson, G. *et al.* (1991). *Mentally Disordered Remand Prisoners*. Report to Home Office. (Unpublished.)

Department of Health (1990). *Caring for People*. The Care Programme Approach for People with a Mental Illness referred to the Specialist Psychiatric Services. HC(90)23/LASSL(90)11.

Department of Health (1993). *Legal Powers on the Care of Mentally Ill People in the Community. Report of the Internal Review*. London, Department of Health.

Department of Health (1994a). *Introduction of supervision registers for mentally ill people from 1 April 1994*. Health Service Guidelines (94)5. London, NHS Executive.

Department of Health (1994b). *Guidance on the discharge of mentally disordered people and their continuing care in the community*. Health Service Guidelines (94)27. London, NHS Executive.

Department of Health and Home Office (1992). *Final Summary Report of the Joint Review of Services for Mentally Disordered Offenders and Others Requiring Similar Services*. London, HMSO.

Department of Health and Welsh Office (1990). *Code of Practice laid before Parliament in December 1989 pursuant to s. 118(4) Mental Health Act 1983*. London, HMSO.

Department of Health and Welsh Office (1993). *Code of Practice published August 1993 pursuant to s. 118 Mental Health Act 1983*. London, HMSO.

Gunn, J., Maden, A. & Swinton, M. (1990). *Mentally Disordered Prisoners*. London, Institute of Psychiatry.

Home Office (1990). *Provision for Mentally Disordered Offenders*. Home Office Circular No 66/90. London, Home Office.

Home Office (1991). *Police and Criminal Evidence Act 1984 Codes of Practice*. London, HMSO.

Home Office (1993). *Community Care Reforms and the Criminal Justice System*. Home Office Circular No 29/93. London, Home Office.

Home Office (1994). *The Containing of Offenders*. Home Office Circular No. 18/94. London, Home Office.

Miller, R. D. (1985). Commitment to outpatient treatment: a national survey. *Hospital and Community Psychiatry*, **36**, 265–7.

Ritchie, J. A., Dick, D. & Lingham, R. (1994). *The Report of the Inquiry into the Care and Treatment of Christopher Clunis*. London, HMSO.

Rogers, A. & Faulkner, A. (1987). *A Place of Safety*. London, MIND.

Royal Commission (1957). *Report of the Royal Commission on the Law relating to Mental Illness and Mental Deficiency 1954–57*. Cmnd 169. London, HMSO.

Royal Commission (1993). *Royal Commission on Criminal Justice*. Cmnd 2263. London, HMSO.

5

The economics of mental health emergency services

PAUL McCRONE

Introduction

This chapter will explore the economic aspects of providing emergency mental health services in hospital and community settings. The methodology which lies behind the economic evaluation of emergency mental health care services will be discussed as will the areas of cost which are of relevance. It will identify both formal emergency services, and those programmes which incorporate emergency or crisis care within them. The key studies which have included an economic element will be reviewed.

Economic burden of mental health problems

Mental health care is resource hungry. In the UK mental health problems account for 10% of all health care expenditure, 23% of in-patient costs and 25% of pharmaceutical charges, and in addition are the cause of 14% of all days lost to the workplace (Davies & Drummond, 1990). As a consequence of the high expenditure on health care in general, governments in the UK and elsewhere have wanted to encourage cost containment within the health sector.

There are also economic consequences associated with the tragedy of suicide. Suicide is not easy to predict (Henry, 1993) and it cannot be said that the absence of emergency and crisis services will necessarily increase the suicide rate. However, one of the hopes of such services is that they will help to prevent suicide. This is matched at a national level with the UK government making a reduction in the suicide rate one of its targets in *The Health of the Nation* (Department of Health, 1991). In the United States it has been estimated that some 60% of suicides are the result of depression (Stoudemire *et al.*, 1986). From this, the authors calculated the cost of lost productivity caused by suicide amongst depressed people to be $4.2 billion. Suicides in the UK likewise have a major economic impact, as well as the effect that they have on families, friends and service providers.

Move to the community

Alongside the vast cost of mental health problems has been the move from institutional care towards care in the community (Griffiths, 1988; Thornicroft & Bebbington, 1989). This has major financial implications. No one body bears all the cost burden, but a multiplicity of agencies now have the responsibility of financing effective community care. This is very relevant with regard to the establishment of effective emergency services and crisis care which should play a major role in comprehensive community programmes.

If a comprehensive system of community mental health care is developed then there may be a containment of cost associated with acute disorders (Herz, 1985). However, the co-ordination and financing of community mental health services appears to lack co-ordination and effective resourcing (Torrey, 1990; Blom-Copper & Murphy, 1991; McCrone & Strathdee, 1994).

Need for emergency services

A number of model plans have been laid down for the development of comprehensive community mental health care services. Integral in these plans is the need to provide emergency and crisis services. The National Institute of Mental Health (1987) in the United States identify five types of crisis service that may be incorporated into a wider service: a 24-hour hotline, walk-in crisis centre, mobile outreach teams for in-home crises, crisis beds in community settings and in-patient beds to be used when community facilities are deemed to be unsuitable for clients. In the UK a survey of community mental health centres revealed that only 19% offered a crisis intervention service (Sayce *et al.*, 1991).

Why economics is important

Scarcity of resources

Economics has been dubbed 'the science of scarcity' and even 'the dismal science'. This may not be surprising. Most economic textbooks and commentaries on economic methodology begin by reminding the reader that there are not enough resources to go round to meet the requirements that we put on them. Economics is simply a way of examining how resources can be allocated in the face of such scarcity. Every health care decision made has an opportunity cost, in that the resources used could have been used elsewhere. Therefore, there will always be an opportunity foregone. It could be argued that if more resources were made available then there would not be a problem of scarcity. This would be true if demand remained constant. However, it is likely that a welcome increase in resources and improvement in technology, and treatment, would lead to increases in demand.

Resource allocation

The need to allocate resources efficiently is crucial. Given that resources are scarce it is important that maximum benefits to the users of services are achieved in the area of mental health care services. Decisions as to how resources should be allocated need to be informed with combined cost and outcome data (O'Donnell *et al.*, 1992).

Although economics is crucial in the process of programme planning and evaluation, it is often neglected or used in the wrong way. Reviews of the literature reveal that many studies do not include an economic component, and when they do costs are often inappropriately calculated and not correctly combined with outcomes (O'Donnell *et al.*, 1992; McCrone & Weich, 1995). This may lead to invalid conclusions guiding policy decisions.

Economic methodology

Many economic evaluations of mental health care programmes have been undertaken. However, the quality of them has not been high. It is crucial to adopt a robust methodology when calculating costs – as one would when measuring the level of functioning or establishing a diagnosis. Four rules of costing should be adhered to (Knapp & Beecham, 1990).

First, comprehensive cost measurements should be used. It is not enough to measure only the cost of the treatment programme itself. Other health services are received by the user and contact with these services may be affected by the intervention under examination. Also affected may be services provided by local government, voluntary agencies, and informal carers. The effects of a particular intervention may also extend to the employment status of the user and the amount of leisure time that he or she has. These aspects also have cost implications. Therefore, all relevant costs must be measured. Secondly, cost variations should be fully explored. Assessing a mental health scheme by observing average costs omits much information. The spread of costs around the mean will often be large, and it is unlikely that the distribution will be normal. This creates a requirement to explain why some users have higher service inputs (and hence costs) than others. Thirdly, it is important to compare like with like. To observe differences in outcomes that are a result of the service inputs requires that the users should be equally able to use either of the alternative programmes. Finally, costs must be combined with outcomes. Even though policy makers may be swayed by lower cost schemes, it may be that the more efficient intervention is also the most expensive. (Indeed the cheapest option may be to do nothing.) This can only be determined by examining costs in relation to outcomes. Likewise it would be inappropriate to omit costs from any evaluation. This error, however, is frequently made.

Type of economic evaluation

Cost minimisation analysis (CMA) is often used, but it is generally the most inappropriate form of evaluation. This should only be used if the outcomes of comparable treatments are known to be identical as only the costs are measured. Cost benefit analysis (CBA) has been incorporated into a wide range of evaluations in health economics as well as environmental and transport economics. Costs are measured in monetary terms, and benefits are also monetised. This latter aspect of CBA provides both advantages and disadvantages. If benefits are monetised then it is straightforward to compare them to costs, and it is readily observable whether costs are outweighed by benefits. This also allows for a comparison between widely differing programmes.

However, mental health care does not easily allow this to take place. Benefits tend to be more inclined towards aspects such as clinical state, social functioning and quality of life. To assign a monetary value to such outputs may not be possible or indeed appropriate. In contrast to CBA, cost-effectiveness analysis (CEA) makes no attempt to assign a monetised value to the outcome. Instead the aim is to achieve a maximum level of output (e.g. a change on a disability rating scale) for a given cost, or to achieve a given output for as low a cost as possible. In the majority of CEAs the measure of outcome will be programme specific and, therefore, comparisons between programmes of differing natures is not possible. Cost utility analysis (CUA) has similarities with CBA and CEA. Outcomes are not monetised, but they are measured in terms of a generic unit which allows for comparisons between say a mental health care programme and a new treatment for heart disease. The outcome measure is based upon the 'utility' that a user gains. Quality of life is generally used as a proxy for utility. The commonest form of CUA uses quality adjusted life years (QALYs) where the length of life and its quality are combined in a single measure. The cost per QALY can then be calculated to provide a relative measure of efficiency. Such a method has not been successfully applied in the evaluation of mental health care evaluations, and it may be very problematic to do so (Wilkinson *et al.*, 1990; Oyebode, 1994).

Identification of cost

The process of costing involves the identification of significant costs and to be clear as to where they fall. This is particularly important for policy making. Clearly we would wish to be as accurate as possible in calculating cost. However, research resources are themselves limited. Pragmatism is often required in deciding how extensively costs are measured (Challis *et al.*, 1993). Individual costs can be grouped under three headings. An intervention will create **direct costs**. These include psychiatric in-patient episodes, out-patient appointments, CPN contacts, etc., and of course emergency services. Other services, normally provided to a wide range of individuals and groups, will also be used by clients of mental health services. These create **indirect costs**. Included here are general practitioners (GPs), dentists, law and order agencies, etc. The cost of accommodation also forms an indirect cost. **Hidden costs** are seldom measured in economic evaluations. The three main types of hidden cost are: informal care, lost employment, and time spent travelling and waiting by the client. Many of the relevant costs are listed in Table 5.1. Some of the services will only be used by a handful of clients, and each client will probably only have contact with a few services. However, the list presented is not exhaustive.

The cost of a service input is determined by the number of times that a client has contact with the service during a defined time period, the duration of contacts and the unit cost of the service. Allen and Beecham (1993) provide a detailed account of this methodology.

Identification of cost burdens

As well as identifying the particular type of cost it is important to determine where the burden of cost falls. This is particularly relevant with regard to policy making decisions concerning the provision or otherwise of emergency or crisis services. Although the true economic cost is that which is borne by society as a whole, managers may only be concerned with the cost that accrues to their agency.

The provision or absence of emergency services is likely to have a cost effect to the individual. It may be that the client is in employment and thus the ability to receive emergency treatment may influence greatly his or her ability to maintain that position and resultant income. If there are no innovative emergency services available then the user in times of crisis may have no other option than hospital admission. One aspect of this that appears to be overlooked in the literature is the time sacrifice that the client makes as a result of a stay in hospital. Emergency treatment within a community setting would allow clients to determine how they should use their time which may have a significant economic value. The health of the client will be affected by the availability of appropriate services in a time of crisis. The lack of emergency services when the client requires them most could have long-term effects on their health.

Likewise, if there are no emergency services available to an individual who is facing a crisis then the result may be an increased dependence on the family network, if one exists. Family members have in some systems acted as case managers (Intagliata *et al.*, 1986). Informal care has a cost both in terms of time and emotions and should, therefore, be included in economic assessments (Netten, 1993).

The lack of an emergency service for people facing a crisis may

Table 5.1. *The range of service costs*

Direct costs	
Psychiatric hospital:	Community:
in-patient	community psychiatric nurse
out-patient	psychiatrist home visit
day-patient	community mental health centre
depot clinic	crisis house
emergency clinic	respite house
psychologist	drop-in
occupational therapy	day centre
Indirect costs	
Accommodation:	Law and order:
supported residential care	police
private accommodation	probation service
Family health services:	court
GP	solicitor
GP home visit	legal aid
optician	prison
chiropodist	Social services:
gynaecologist	field social worker
family planning clinic	field social worker home visit
nurse	home help
domiciliary nurse	meals on wheels
dentist	
	Employment:
General hospital:	job centre
in-patient	job club
out-patient	disablement rehabilitation officer
day-patient	careers advice
accident and emergency	Others:
physiotherapy	counsellor
dental services	social security officer
	education course
Hidden costs	
Informal care:	
lost employment of friends and relatives	
lost leisure time of friends and relatives	
User time:	
travelling	
waiting	
Lost employment:	
time off work due to mental health problem	
foregone potential employment	
lost production to economy	
Benefits:	
opportunity cost of welfare payments	

cause an increase in the cost burden that falls to different agencies. If someone has to be admitted in the absence of such a service then this will place increased demands on the resources of the hospital. Also GP contacts may be higher. The same scenario may be true for local authorities and voluntary agencies (e.g. the Samaritans).

Finally there exists the cost to society as a whole. Lack of effective crisis services may lead to prolonged health problems. This can cause a burden on society's resources and may also cause a reduction in potential production. The cost of lost employment is sometimes felt to be zero as it is assumed that the person with a mental health problem would inevitably be absent from the workforce. However, as Warner (1985) points out, in time of economic prosperity many people considered unfit for work are drawn into employment.

Costs of emergency services

An emergency service for people facing a crisis may take a number of forms. The service may be exclusively geared towards crisis care or this may just be one element of a wider package of support. The setting of the service may be in a psychiatric hospital, a general hospital, a residential home or elsewhere in the community.

Emergency clinic

Walk-in emergency clinics have reduced hospitalisation as one of their aims. Many such clinics operate during office hours only. The clinic at the Maudsley Hospital in South London differs in that it offers a 24-hour service. Studies that have examined the service (Lim, 1983; Haw *et al.*, 1987) have discovered that schizophrenia is the most common diagnosis of attenders, 33% of people with schizophrenia visited during the night, and although patients were offered follow-ups the uptake was low. A crucial point to establish is whether the emergency clinic results in fewer admissions, which could produce considerable cost savings. From a sample of 102 mental health service users, with a psychotic disorder, in the Maudsley catchment area, 16 had contact with the emergency clinic during a six-month period. Of these, 14 also had in-patient episodes. By contrast, of the 86 people who had no contact with the emergency clinic, only 16 were admitted during the six months. It can be seen that there is no evidence to suggest that attending the emergency clinic has led to a reduced likelihood of admission. It has been suggested that assessment at home, however, could lead to fewer admissions (Burns *et al.*, 1993).

Crisis housing and residential treatment for acute illness

Bond *et al.* (1989) compare two types of crisis service. One initiative purchased accommodation from hotels and boarding houses. The alternative was a crisis house with eight beds. In both settings the majority of users (two-thirds) avoided being admitted during a four-month follow-up. The direct treatment costs of the first option were 69% of the direct costs of the crisis house. However, with hospital services and government assistance included, the total costs were virtually the same.

One particular evaluation of a crisis housing intervention is unique in its comprehensive approach to costing. The 'Quarterway House' proved to be similar in outcome to standard hospital treatment but resulted in 20% lower costs (Dickey *et al.*, 1986). Cost data were collected for direct services and a wide range of secondary services. Excluded were hidden costs.

In California, in 1978, Psychiatric Health Facilities were created. These were a residential alternative to in-patient care for people with acute mental health problems. A legal requirement was that the new facilities must maintain a minimum amount of services and operate at a cost of 40% below comparable general hospital services. The average daily costs of all the facilities in California were 43% less than the hospital costs. Rappaport *et al.* (1987) noted that although the costs were higher prior to this initiative, the actual number of days spent in the facilities was on average higher than the number of days spent in hospital.

An intensive community-based residential programme for clients with acute disorders was found to have higher unit costs than standard care, but overall costs were lower (Bedall & Ward, 1989). However, this study lacked sophisticated cost and outcome measures.

Case management and assertive outreach

Case management is a method for the distribution and co-ordination of services, both clinical and social, for and in liaison with the client. This calls for great skill and expertise. Care needs to be provided to the individual within an environment of limited resources and competing alternatives (hence the need for economic evaluation). One of the areas which case management focuses upon is crisis care for those people facing emergencies.

The most well known case management service has been the 'Training in Community Living' programme in Madison, Wisconsin, USA (Stein & Test, 1980; Test & Stein, 1980). This was an assertive form of case management which offered support to clients in their own home. An economic evaluation of the project (Weisbrod *et al.*, 1980) revealed that the intervention was associated with higher costs and more benefits than traditional care. This study employed a relatively comprehensive approach to costing and also took the form of a CBA where the benefits were monetised.

A similar programme was set up in Australia where clients were either in receipt of traditional hospital and after care, or else they received comprehensive community care and 24-hour crisis cover (Hoult *et al.*, 1983). Mainly direct treatment costs were measured, which showed that the traditional care cost 26% more than community care. This was mainly due to the reduced utilisation of in-patient services by the community care group. However, there was a (non-significant) higher number of people in this group who had attempted suicide during the study period.

The Maudsley Daily Living Programme (DLP) was set up in South London in the late 1980s. This was an innovation to provide services to clients who were facing emergency admission. The DLP consisted of a multidisciplinary team offering intensive home-based support involving case management. One of the main aims of the service was to provide crisis intervention. The project was, and is being, evaluated (Marks *et al.*, 1988; Marks, 1992; Muijen *et al.*, 1992). The users of the DLP and their families preferred the care offered in this community setting compared to a group of clients who had been randomly assigned to standard care. Clinical and social outcomes did not differ. After a start-up period the DLP made a 25% cost saving over traditional care.

Clearly with any intervention it would be advantageous to observe the long term effects on outcome and cost. A study in the United States has examined the effects of intensive case management after five years of continuous use (Borland *et al.*, 1989). The clients had chronic conditions and were treatment resistant. The number of days which clients spent in hospital was reduced. This was offset though by the increased number of residential care days in the community. Fewer contacts were made with the emergency services after the five-year period.

Partial hospitalisation

Partial hospitalisation provides care to clients who have acute mental health problems and would normally be admitted for some time. It is an intermediate setting between in-patient and community care.

Studies have shown that the direct costs of brief hospitalisation followed by aftercare are lower than traditional in-patient care (Washburn *et al.*, 1976; Endicott *et al.*, 1978; Hertz *et al.*, 1979). There have been few reported differences in clinical or social outcome, although satisfaction with services has been found to be higher in the experimental setting (Washburn *et al.*, 1976).

Day treatment has been evaluated as a treatment option for people with acute mental health problems. Results have been mixed. Dick *et al.* (1985) found that direct costs were lower for day-treatment users with non-psychotic disorders when compared to a group of clients receiving standard in-patient care. However, with a group of people in the Netherlands who had schizophrenia the costs were higher (Wiersma *et al.*, 1991). Neither of these studies discovered significant differences in outcome.

One proposed form of emergency care in the United States is the short procedure unit (Dubin & Fink, 1986). This often avoids the requirement for hospital admission. Rather the service allows for intensive out-patient contacts, family crisis therapy and tranquillisation. Although cost savings are suggested there has been no full evaluation of the concept.

Use of emergency service by particular client groups

The different levels of emergency service utilisation by current substance abusers, past substance abusers and those who have never abused substances have been compared (Bartels *et al.*, 1993). Current substance abusers were twice as likely to use emergency services as were past and non-abusers. Overall the use of emergency services was considered to be low. This was felt to be due to the existence of intensive case management programmes and residential support.

In-home crisis services for children and their families have been initiated, particularly in the United States, and have undergone evaluation. One crisis intervention providing an intensive programme lasting for four to six weeks showed that huge savings in hospital time and costs were possible (Grant Bishop & McNally, 1993). However, there was no extensive costing described and to claim that the scheme is cost-effective just on the grounds of bed days saved is premature.

People suffering from dementia often require constant support and supervision. This places enormous pressure on the client's family. One alternative to standard day care and family support is group living, where houses are permanently staffed. Within the house the client would have his or her own flat and possessions. One such scheme has been evaluated in Sweden (Wimo *et al.*, 1991). It was discovered that people in a group-living home required fewer hospital services, including emergency care.

Conclusion

Emergency services have been developing in the UK, the United States and elsewhere for many years. The existence of them is required for those people who need care and support over and above that provided by conventional mental health services (Hillard, 1994). The range of services has risen sharply, and in the United States there has been some focus upon particular client groups such as the elderly and victims of domestic violence (Ellison *et al.*, 1989). The great importance of emergency and crisis services in a community mental health service means that cost-effectiveness information is required. This is especially relevant if successful programmes are to be replicated.

In Britain, there has been an enhanced demand for cost information since the creation of the internal market. Programme evaluations will need to incorporate an economic component in the future. It can be seen from the above review that a number of such evaluations have taken place. However, more often than not the evaluations have lacked a structured methodology and cost figures may be misleading. It is essential that more rigour be employed in such exercises if economic data is to be exploited effectively.

References

Allen, C. & Beecham, J. (1993). Costing services: ideals and reality. In *Costing Community Care: Theory and Practice*, ed. A. Netten, & J. Beecham. Aldershot, Ashgate.

Bartels, S.J., Teague, G.B., Drake, R.E., *et al.* (1993). Substance abuse in schizophrenia: service utilization and costs. *The Journal of Nervous and Mental Disease*, **181**, 227–32.

Bedell, J. & Ward, J.C. (1989). An intensive community-based treatment alternative to state hospitalization. *Hospital and Community Psychiatry*, **40**, 533–5.

Blom-Cooper, L. & Murphy, E. (1991). Mental health services and resources. *Psychiatric Bulletin*, **15**, 65–8.

Bond, G.R., Witheridge, T.F., Wasmer, D. *et al.* (1989). A comparison of two crisis housing alternatives to psychiatric hospitalization. *Hospital and Community Psychiatry*, **40**, 177–83.

Borland, A., McRae, J. & Lycan, C. (1989). Outcomes of five years of continuous intensive case management. *Hospital and Community Psychiatry*, **40**, 369–76.

Burns, T., Beadsmoore, A., Bhat, A.V., *et al.* (1993). A controlled trial of home-based acute psychiatric services. I: Clinical and social outcome. *British Journal of Psychiatry*, **163**, 49–54.

Challis, D., Chesterman, J. & Traske, K. (1993). Management: costing the experiments. In *Costing Community Care: Theory and Practice*, ed. A. Netten & J. Beecham. Aldershot, Ashgate.

Davies, L.M. & Drummond, M.F. (1990). The economic burden of schizophrenia. *Psychiatric Bulletin*, **14**, 522–5.

Department of Health (1991). *The Health of the Nation*. London, HMSO.

Dick, P., Cameron, L., Cohen, D., *et al.* (1985). Day and full-time psychiatric treatment: a controlled comparison. *British Journal of Psychiatry*, **147**, 246–50.

Dickey, B., Cannon, N.L., McGuire, T.G., *et al.* (1986). The Quarterway House: a two-year cost study of an experimental residential program. *Hospital and Community Psychiatry*, **37**, 1136–43.

Dubin, W.R. & Fink, P.J. (1986). The psychiatric short procedure unit: a cost-saving innovation. *Hospital and Community Psychiatry*, **37**, 227–9.

Ellison, J.M., Hughes, D.H. & White, K.A. (1989). An emergency psychiatry update. *Hospital and Community Psychiatry*, **40**, 250–60.

Endicott, J., Herz, M.I. & Gibbon, M. (1978). Brief versus standard hospitalization: the differential costs. *American Journal of Psychiatry*, **135**, 707–12.

Grant Bishop, E.E. & McNally, G. (1993). An in-home crisis intervention program for children and their families. *Hospital and Community Psychiatry*, **44**, 182–5.

Griffiths, R. (1988). *Community Care: An Agenda for Action*. London, HMSO.

Haw, C., Lanceley, C. & Vickers, S. (1987). Patients at a psychiatric walk-in clinic – who, how, why and when. *Bulletin of the Royal College of Psychiatrists*, **11**, 329–32.

Henry, J. A. (1993). Debits and credits in the management of depression. *British Journal of Psychiatry*, **163** (suppl. 20), 33–9.

Herz, M. I., Endicott, J. & Gibbon, M. (1979). Brief hospitalization: two-year follow-up. *Archives of General Psychiatry*, **36**, 701–5.

Herz, M. I. (1985). Treatment strategies for reducing costs of acute psychiatric hospitalization. *International Journal of Partial Hospitalization*, **3**, 81–90.

Hillard, J. R. (1994). The past and future of psychiatric emergency services in the US. *Hospital and Community Psychiatry*, **45**, 541–3.

Hoult, J., Reynolds, I., Charbonneau-Powis, M., *et al.* (1983). Psychiatric hospital versus community treatment: the results of a randomised trial. *Australian and New Zealand Journal of Psychiatry*, **17**, 160–7.

Intagliata, J., Willer, B. & Egri, G. (1986). Role of the family in case management of the mentally ill. *Schizophrenia Bulletin*, **12**, 699–708.

Knapp, M. & Beecham, J. (1990). Costing mental health services. *Psychological Medicine*, **20**, 893–908.

Lim, M. (1983). A psychiatric emergency clinic: a study of attendances over six months. *British Journal of Psychiatry*, **143**, 460–6.

Marks, I. (1992). Innovations in mental health care delivery. *British Journal of Psychiatry*, **160**, 589–97.

Marks, I., Connolly, J. & Muijen, M. (1988). The Maudsley Daily Living Programme. *Psychiatric Bulletin*, **12**, 22–4.

McCrone, P. & Strathdee, G. (1994). Needs not diagnosis: towards a more rational approach to community mental health resourcing in Britain. *The International Journal of Social Psychiatry*, **40**, 79–86.

McCrone, P. & Weich, S. (1995). Mental health care costs: paucity of measurement. *Social Psychiatry and Psychiatric Epidemiology*, (In press.)

Muijen, M., Marks, I. M., Connolly, J., *et al.* (1992). The Daily Living Programme: preliminary comparison of community versus hospital-based treatment for the seriously mentally ill facing emergency admission. *British Journal of Psychiatry*, **160**, 379–84.

National Institute of Mental Health (1987). *Toward a Model Plan for a Comprehensive Community Based Mental Health System.*

Netten, A. (1993). Costing unpaid care. In *Costing Community Care: Theory and Practice*, ed. A. Netten & J. Beecham. Aldershot, Ashgate.

O'Donnell, O., Maynard, A. & Wright, K. (1992). Evaluating mental health care: the role of economics. *Journal of Mental Health*, **1**, 39–51.

Oyebode, F. (1994). Ethics and resource allocation: can health care outcomes be QALYfied. *Psychiatric Bulletin*, **18**, 395–8.

Rappaport, M., Goldman, H., Thornton, P., *et al.* (1987). A method for comparing two systems of acute 24-hour psychiatric care. *Hospital and Community Psychiatry*, **38**, 1091–5.

Sayce, L., Craig, T. K. J. & Boardman, A. P. (1991). The development of community mental health centres in the UK. *Social Psychiatry and Psychiatric Epidemiology*, **26**, 14–20.

Stein, L. I. & Test, M. A. (1980). Alternative to mental hospital treatment: I. Conceptual model, treatment program, and clinical evaluation. *Archives of General Psychiatry*, **37**, 392–7.

Stoudemire, A., Frank, R., Hedemark, N., *et al.* (1986). The economic burden of depression. *General Hospital Psychiatry*, **8**, 387–94.

Test, M. A. & Stein, L. I. (1980). Alternative to mental hospital treatment: III. Social cost. *Archives of General Psychiatry*, **37**, 409–12.

Thornicroft, G. & Bebbington, P. (1989). Deinstitutionalisation – from hospital closure to service development. *British Journal of Psychiatry*, **155**, 739–53.

Torrey, E. F. (1990). Economic barriers to widespread implementation of model programs for the seriously mentally ill. *Hospital and Community Psychiatry*, **41**, 526–31.

Warner, R. (1985). *Recovery from Schizophrenia: Psychiatry and Political Economy.* London, Routledge & Keegan Paul.

Washburn, S., Vannicelli, M., Longabaugh, R., *et al.* (1976). A controlled comparison of psychiatric day treatment and inpatient hospitalization. *Journal of Consulting and Clinical Psychology*, **44**, 665–75.

Weisbrod, B. A., Test, M. A. & Stein, L. I. (1980). Alternative to mental hospital treatment: II. Economic benefit-cost analysis. *Archives of General Psychiatry*, **37**, 400–5.

Wiersma, D., Kluiter, H., Nienhuis, F. J., *et al.* (1991). Costs and benefits of day treatment with community care for schizophrenic patients. *Schizophrenia Bulletin*, **17**, 411–19.

Wilkinson, G., Croft-Jeffreys, C., Krekorian, H., *et al.* (1990). QALYs in psychiatric care? *Psychiatric Bulletin*, **14**, 582–5.

Wimo, A., Wallin, J. O., Lundgren, K., *et al.* (1991). Group living, an alternative for dementia patients. A cost analysis. *International Journal of Geriatric Psychiatry*, **6**, 21–9.

6

Suicide prevention

David Kingdon and Rachel Jenkins

Introduction

A brief summary of the epidemiological evidence of suicide, the risk factors and the strategies for preventing it is presented. This chapter begins by considering the widespread beliefs that prevention of suicide is an activity with relatively little prospect of success (Morgan, 1993) and even one which is ethically misguided: why should anyone who wishes to do so be prevented from ending his or her own life? As social circumstances, such as unemployment, are important determinants of suicide risk, is there very little that can realistically be done by individuals – even in specialist mental health services – to reduce incidence?

Reduction in avoidable mortality is an aim of most health services and the many other government departments which deal with safety issues. For instance, death from road traffic accidents – transport and environmental departments determine safety standards on roads and in vehicles, adding considerably to the cost and inconvenience of the passenger, e.g., structural modification to vehicles, safety barriers on motorways and seat-belts in front and rear of cars. Health services have also improved techniques for managing accidents, e.g., improvements to ambulances and developments in surgical and intensive care technique. In England, this has been successful such that road traffic deaths have now been reduced to around 4000 per year. More deaths occur from suicide which, until recently, has received relatively little direct preventative attention. Suicide rates have remained at much the same level throughout the twentieth century.

But is suicide comparable? An important element in considering this is whether suicide is usually a choice which individuals have the right to make or whether it is the result of circumstances, including suffering from a mental illness, which distort judgement and are potentially remediable. The evidence from psychological morbidity studies is that mental disorder, including alcohol (and other drug dependence) and personality disorder, is very common. Barraclough *et al.* (1974) and Robins *et al.* (1959) have estimated rates of 90% with mental disorder; 'rational' suicide, therefore, appears to be very unusual. Circumstances are nevertheless frequently cited in which suicide seems a logical step to take and prevention attempts to be inappropriate. These include where someone is suffering from a terminal physical illness, experiencing persistent severe pain, be under unremitting stress, or have committed a very serious criminal or otherwise dishonourable act. However, in most instances, appropriate management of terminal illness or chronic pain – including treatment of associated depressive symptoms – can markedly alleviate suffering such that the remaining period of life can be experienced without the severe distress inducing suicidal intent. Although exceptionally such alleviation is not possible, the hospice movement has demonstrated that this is much less inevitable than most people, including medical and nursing staff, have previously considered. The way in which life circumstances are perceived is also of considerable importance. Maintenance of hope (Beck & Steer, 1989) may be of particular significance, along with straightforward environmental manipulation, and can be a focus of therapeutic effort. There may remain some circumstances in which suicide is an appropriate choice for the individual concerned – once other alternatives have been exhausted – but for the overwhelming majority, this cannot be the case and it is as reasonable to attempt to prevent suicide as it is to attempt to prevent other causes of death.

National Prevention Programmes

Can we reasonably expect to influence suicide rates? International opinion over the past decade has increasingly come round to the opinion that we should at least attempt to do so. The WHO (World Health Organization) 'Target 12' aims to stop the rise in suicide as part of 'Health for the year 2000'. The main components of suicide prevention strategies have been described by Diekstra (1989) as:

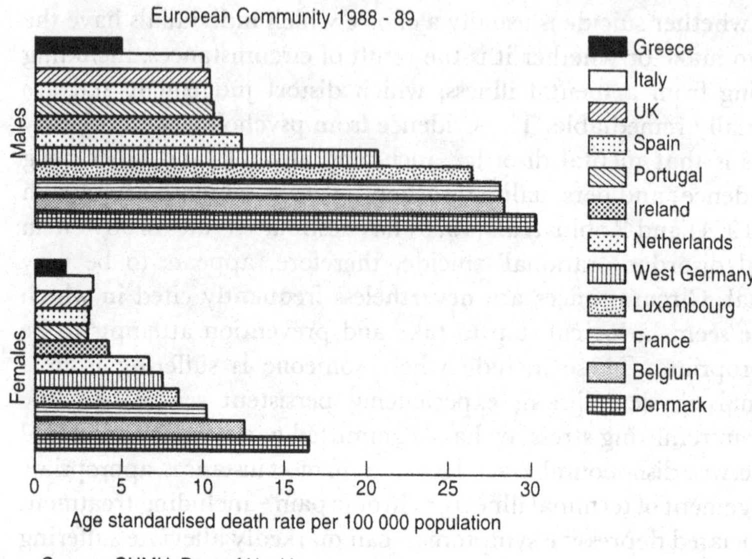

Fig. 6.1. Deaths from suicide and self-inflicted injury

- design and implementation of national research programmes;
- the improvement of services;
- the provision of information and training on suicide prevention to relevant professional groups, organizations and the general public;
- formulation of strategies and techniques to deal with special risk groups.

Such strategies have been developed in a number of European countries (see Fig. 6.1 for comparative suicide rates in the European Union), notably in Scandinavia and the Netherlands. In England, mental illness has been selected as one of five key areas for priority action under *The Health of the Nation* initiative (Department of Health, 1993a). Two of the three targets established involve reduction of suicide:

- To improve the health and social functioning of mentally ill people.
- To reduce the overall suicide rate by at least 15% by the year 2000 (from 11.0 per 100,000 population in 1990 to no more than 9.4).
- To reduce the suicide rate of severely mentally ill people by at least 33% by the year 2000 (from the estimate of 15% in 1990 to no more than 10%).

Crucial to any attempt at prevention must be an understanding of the epidemiology and risk factors involved on which to build a broad multi-faceted strategic approach (Department of Health, 1993b).

Epidemiology

In England and Wales, suicide accounts for approximately 1% of all deaths and 5% of all days lost through death before the age of 65. There were 5541 deaths in 1992 from suicide (and 'open verdicts', which are included as this reduces the variation between coroners). Figure 6.2 shows the number of recorded suicides from 1901 to 1989 for males and females based on a three-yearly moving average (Charlton *et al.*, 1992). Falls during the world wars and the rise in the inter-war depression, peaking in 1932, are striking. The highest annual total level of suicides (male and female combined) was reached in 1963 with the preceding increase for women more pronounced than for men. Both rates then fell until the early 1970s when the male rate began to rise again; this divergence of trends has not previously occurred and remains unexplained. The rapid and continuing rise in suicide amongst young men (75.8% in those aged 15–24 from 1982–91) is particularly notable and worrying. There is also concern about suicide rates amongst particular ethnic groups, especially young women from the Asian subcontinent (Standardised Mortality Rate = 273 in age range 15–24 and 160 in age range 25–34) who contrast with male and females from other age groups originating from the subcontinent and with those from the Caribbean, generally, in whom rates are markedly lower (Soni Raleigh & Balajaran, 1992).

Methods used for suicide have varied: between 1948 and 1950, poisoning by domestic gas accounted for recorded suicides in 41% of men and 60% women, but by 1968–70, poisoning by solid or liquid substances had become the most common method (Charlton *et al.*, 1992). This was still the case for women in 1988–90 but poisoning by other gases (principally car exhaust fumes) had become the commonest method for men. The disappearance of domestic gas has had a marked effect on overall rates (see Fig. 6.3) with some partial apparent replacement in males but not in females.

International comparisons are also useful. Much research has been done in Scandinavia and comparisons between countries with a high rate of suicide, such as Denmark and Greenland, and those with a low rate, such as Norway and Faroe Islands, have highlighted cultural

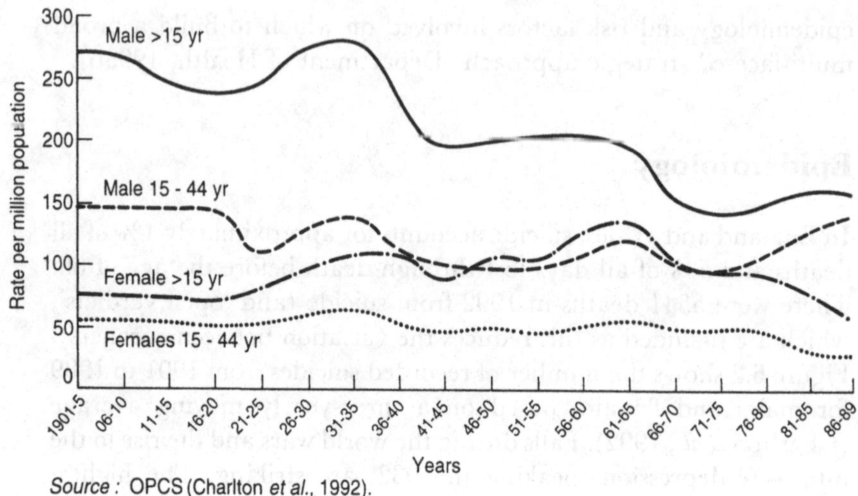

Source : OPCS (Charlton *et al.*, 1992).

Fig. 6.2. Suicide rates, England and Wales, 1901–89

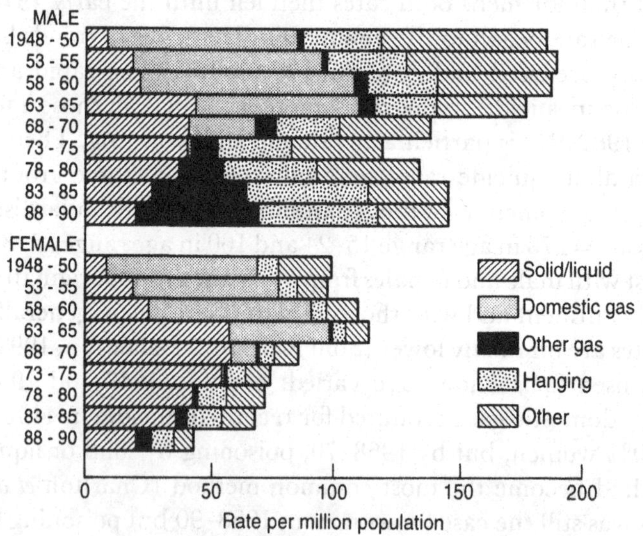

Source: OPCS (Charlton *et al.*, 1992)

Fig. 6.3. Distribution of recorded suicides by sex, year of death and method (England and Wales)

differences (Retterstøl, 1992) particularly in relation to social integration – rapidly changing roles and alienation may be of significance amplified by increases in alcoholism, violence and a general feeling of hopelessness.

Risk factors

Most programmes have established risk factors in the population and then developed programmes tailored for individual groups. In England, risk rises with age (except that it is particularly high in young males): it is four times higher amongst men than women (Charlton *et al.*, 1992); it is associated with unemployment (Moser *et al.*, 1984) and it is higher in social class V (unskilled workers) than any other social class; it is highest amongst the divorced, followed by widows, widowers and people who have never married, and it is lowest amongst married people; it is associated with mental and physical illness, social isolation and family history; and it varies with the seasons, being highest in April, May and June.

As unemployment and other social circumstances outside the control of health services affect rates, social policies towards improving job prospects and reducing family breakdown may be relevant, but this does not preclude other strategies being developed and it is these strategies upon which the remainder of this chapter will concentrate.

Targeting at-risk groups

In England and Wales certain occupational groups have high rates of suicide (see Table 6.1). Ready access to means of suicide seems particularly important – doctors and vets have access to lethal drugs and farmers to guns. Strategies which target these occupational groups have been developed – for farmers by involving groups such as the National Farmers Union, Country Landowners Association and the Samaritans; for doctors by the development of a National Sick Doctors Scheme. Support services have also been developed for students. Work has also been proceeding within the prison service in developing suicide prevention policies following concern at the rapid increase in suicide rate during the 1980s. This has included improving reception procedures and standards for psychiatric assessment and care; the use of 'buddies' – i.e., fellow prisoners who are given training and supervision – and the Samaritans; and training of prison doctors and officers. (Suicide rates in prison peaked in 1990, at $107/10^5$ average daily population, but dropped to below $90/10^5$ average daily population in 1991 and 1992.) Adapting services to the needs of

Table 6.1. *Suicides by occupation (male deaths ages 16–64) during 1979–90. The 10 highest and lowest proportional mortality rates (PMRs)*

Occupation	*Suicides and undetermined deaths* PMR	*No. deaths*
Vet	364	35
Pharmacist	217	51
Dental practitioner	204	38
Farmer	187	526
Medical practitioner	184	152
Therapist n.e.c.	181	10
Librarian, information officer	180	30
Typist, Secretary	171	16
Social and behavioural scientist	170	11
Chemical scientist	169	70
Civil Service, Executive officers	44	17
Drivers, motormen, etc., railways	43	24
Bus inspectors	42	5
Managers in building and contracting	38	34
Civil Service administrators HEO-Grade 6	37	14
Transport managers	36	31
Glass and ceramics furnacemen	34	4
Machine tool setter operators	29	5
NCOs and other ranks – armed forces	27	12
Education officers, school inspectors	15	1

individual groups would seem the most likely strategy to succeed.

Strategies aimed at reducing risk for different age groups also may be successful. Deaths amongst young men are causing particular concern and the accelerating rise suggests new factors are involved, but as yet these can only be a matter of conjecture. General social change such as unemployment and divorce may be related, although the effect is certainly not direct. For unemployment, a lag effect may be present but evidence that regional rates of suicide and unemployment are poorly correlated suggests that the relationship is a complex one (Charlton *et al.*, 1987; Crombie, 1989). European figures suggest a linkage with male rates (Pritchard, 1988) although Denmark and West Germany have been exceptions to this. Clearly, targeting unemployed young men, as a whole, specifically with suicide prevention measures would be a massive task and unlikely to be cost-effective. It is not yet known whether recent or long-term unemployment differentially influences rate, which might in part explain the regional variations, and influence risk assessment and management.

The circumstances under which suicide occurs in young men needs further investigation but a typical scenario is one where the young man has a row, perhaps with family or a girlfriend, goes out and may consume alcohol with its depressant effects. He then returns and puts the garden hose on the exhaust of his or the family car, leads it into the car, sits down and drifts off into oblivion. Alternatively he may simply go up to his room and be found having hanged himself. It is particularly tragic because it frequently appears to be due to an impulsive act (Hoberman & Garfinkel, 1988), a transient mood state, and is, and seems, to families left behind, so meaningless. There may have been some persistence of low mood or irritability because of problems, for example with school or work, or lack of work, but communication of distress has either not occurred or not been understood.

Significant co-factors in teenage suicide include hopelessness, running away, reckless behaviour, self-damage, panic symptoms, recent loss and social isolation. In 50%, symptoms have been present for three years or more and, for unknown reasons, one-third to one-quarter die within two weeks of their birthday. Specific programmes have been directed at teenagers, and such initiatives have been reviewed by Lester (1992). He examined state government initiatives in the United States which he found to be associated with a beneficial effect on teenage suicide rates, but it is of note that he found the reverse for school-based suicide prevention programmes.

Older people are also at increased risk, particularly after a bereavement. Isolation and physical illness are also added factors. Some districts with large populations of older people, e.g., Scarborough (item in *Health Services Journal*, 1992), have been developing strategies with voluntary agencies to target this group.

Mental disorders are also known to raise the risk of suicide – 15% of those with affective disorders, 10% with schizophrenia and up to 10% with anorexia nervosa are estimated to ultimately commit suicide. Alcohol and drug dependence and personality disorders lead to similar rates. Even in younger age groups, identifiable psychiatric symptomatology (most commonly minor affective symptoms) has been identified in over 90% of suicides (Graham & Burvill, 1992).

Suicide attempts raise the risk of completed suicide by 100 times in the succeeding year and provide an opportunity for intervention.

This may be particularly important in the UK, as monitoring of hospital-treated deliberate self-harm in Oxford and Edinburgh has shown their rates to be well above the European median (Platt, 1992). Apart from specific strategies targeting individual risk factors, a combination of such risk factors might be expected to be more effective. Retrospective analysis of suicidal behaviour in depressed in-patients followed up over 18 years (Duggan *et al.*, 1993) and of suicide following attempted suicide (Hawton & Fagg, 1988), has suggested that severe dysphoria, past alcoholism, long-term hypnotic medication and chronic physical illness are the most predictive. Personality features such as hostility (Farmer & Creed, 1989), dependency (Berglund *et al.*, 1987) and obsessionality (Murthy, 1969) and experience of early loss (Adam *et al.*, 1982) are associated with suicidal behaviour. Moreover, these have been assembled into methods for producing reliable and specific risk assessment measures (e.g., Pallis *et al.*, 1982; Beck & Steer, 1989). Using the measure developed by Pallis and colleagues, 91% of a group of suicides and 83% of attempted suicides were assigned to the correct groups. However, prospective success of such measures has been less successful (Pokorney, 1983). Nevertheless in practice, suicide assessments by clinicians will tend to include such relevant factors and differentially weight them. On the conclusion of such assessment rests whether a person is referred to hospital, admitted and later discharged, and psychiatric management determined which can involve compulsory admission under the Mental Health Act 1983.

Attitude change

There are many popular misconceptions about suicide, which are potentially remediable and might improve the general population's understanding of suicidality, leading to earlier and more appropriate presentation of psychological concerns. Whilst this is difficult to demonstrate in practice, making information readily available to counter such misconceptions through well targeted mental health promotion has begun (Department of Health, 1993a) but will need to be built-on at the local level.

Such misconceptions include the belief that 'those who talk about it never do it' and, conversely, that asking about suicide might make it more likely. Psychological autopsy studies found that over two-thirds had expressed suicidal ideas and a third had expressed clear suicidal intent (Robins *et al.*, 1959; Barraclough *et al.*, 1974). Two-thirds had recently consulted their GP; 40% in the previous week (although this may not be the case with those under 35; Vassilas & Morgan, 1993); half had a psychiatric history (Seagar & Flood, 1965; Vassilas & Morgan, 1993), a quarter being current psychiatric out-patients (Morgan & Priest, 1991) with a half of these having seen a psychiatrist in the previous week. Four-fifths were on psychiatric medication and one in six left a note. There is therefore the potential for intervention to occur if risk assessment and management is considered. This could include other professionals who have contact with individuals at risk, e.g., probation service, social workers, counselling services, personnel managers, teachers and police, all of whom may be able to be of assistance or who could act as a link to those who can.

There is also little recognition that suicide is only rarely a choice made unclouded by depression – it is often seen as a 'rational choice'. Psychological autopsies (Barraclough *et al.*, 1974; Hawton, 1987; Hawton & Fagg, 1988) have suggested that as many as nine out of ten are likely to have some form of mental disorder especially depression and also alcoholism and schizophrenia. Treatments are available for each and need to be utilised but sometimes lack of knowledge of the skills of other professionals can mean patients are not referred. As Goldberg (in Birley, 1987) has cautioned, 'those who work only in the environment of their own profession [or in isolation] tend to develop the idea that if someone cannot be helped by their own brand of intervention then they cannot be helped at all and can therefore be discharged to suffer on their own'. A further important message, which is not clearly understood, even by GPs, is that mood can be significantly improved and suicidal risk reduced even in the face of seemingly overwhelming life events and circumstances such as severe physical illnesses.

The final major and particularly important misconception is that: 'If they want to do it, they will do it anyway'. Unavailability of 'acceptable' means, treatment of depression, life events and social supports can all intervene and remove, or significantly reduce, risk. Patients who have been fortuitously intercepted during a determined suicidal attempt and who have recovered and gone on to live meaningful existences are relatively common in clinical practice.

The influence of the media may be of some significance, both positively in its potential for education and negatively in terms of perpetuation of stigmatisation and 'copycat' attempted and completed suicide (Platt, 1994). Certainly caution is necessary in its use as part of a suicide prevention strategy. Bulusu and Anderson (1984) reviewing suicides prior to 1982 have suggested that the increase in use of car exhaust fumes as a suicide method may lie in the 'snowball' effect of people discovering this as a method. There is concern that education about the dangerousness of paracetamol overdosage may have similar effect (see later).

Treatment of depression

Improved management of depression generally, but particularly in general practice, is very important to any suicide prevention strategy. Suicide remains a rare event for the individual GP who may have a patient commit suicide only once in three or four years and this has led some commentators to conclude that they cannot play an important role in prevention (Diekstra & van Egmond, 1989). However, the position of the GP has been described as 'analogous to ... the car manufacturer, who contributes to reducing traffic accidents not by identifying potentially dangerous customers but by building safety into the product' (Lindesay, 1993). Effective treatment of depression is clearly important in its own right, as well as probably contributing to preventing suicide. There is good evidence that GPs recognise only about 50% of those who are depressed and that, when recognition is improved, improvement in management and symptomatology occurs. Consensus guidelines on recognition and management of depression have been developed and endorsed by the Royal Colleges of Psychiatrists and General Practitioners (Paykel & Priest, 1992) and detailed guidance on assessment and management of suicide risk has recently been produced by the Health Advisory Service (Morgan, 1994). Components of training (for GPs and health and social care workers in general; Diekstra & van Egmond, 1989) include provision of:

- Information on the epidemiology of suicide and attempted suicide and acute and chronic risk factors of suicidal behaviour.
- Information on and training in the skills necessary to identify people with a high risk of suicidal behaviour.

- Training in interview techniques, treatment and after-care of suicidal people, relatives of people who have committed suicide and the families of people who have made an attempt.
- Training in appropriate referral of suicidal people to other health workers.

Logically following such guidelines could be expected to have an effect on suicide rates and there is evidence from Sweden that such effects are possible. Rutz and colleagues (1992) described a small study of a comprehensive GP education programme about depression which occurred in the early 1980s in Gotland, which seemed to lead to a decrease in hospital admissions, sickness certification for depression and, somewhat unexpectedly, the suicide rate which was more than halved against previous local and national trends. There is also work from Hungary (Rihmer *et al.*, 1992) which has the highest levels of suicide internationally which suggests that treatment of depression can affect suicide rates. They provided further evidence supporting the importance of adequate antidepressant therapy in the treatment of depression (Peet, 1992), particularly the use of lithium carbonate.

It is of course possible to read too much into studies in countries with varying suicide rates and results from Sweden suggest that the education programme has to be sustained; but nevertheless it is supportive of such programmes. The 'Defeat Depression' campaign run by the Royal Colleges of Psychiatrists and General Practitioners has drawn on this evidence. It has developed training packages for GPs. Management guidelines based on the Colleges' consensus statement have also been distributed and a senior GP Fellow has been funded to work with regional trainers.

Reducing access to means

Another major area which may assist in bringing down suicide rates deals with changes to reduce the availability of certain methods used in suicide. There is evidence from the United States in relation to availability of guns and other means to suicide (Marzuk *et al.*, 1992), and the UK in relation to the replacement of coal gas by non-toxic North Sea gas (Kreitman, 1976) that this is of importance. In 1993, MOT tests for motor vehicles introduced emission standards in relation to toxicity of exhaust fumes and although, as yet, these are probably insufficient to lower the levels of carbon monoxide (CO) in exhaust fumes significantly towards non-toxic levels, they will still prolong the time required for asphyxiation and therefore the time available for intervention. Such changes in emission standards in the United States in the late 1960s are reported as leading to a reduction in deaths from CO poisoning (Clarke & Lester, 1987). Statutory introduction of catalytic convertors in all new cars at the beginning of 1994, seems likely to have an even greater effect as was recently reported (Tarbuck & O'Brien, 1992). This is of importance because of their significance as a suicide method. In young women, whilst rates are dropping overall, 'other gas' (predominantly CO poisoning) is beginning to rise. In young men, a rise in hangings and, particularly, 'other gas', accounts for the rapid, and very worrying, increase occurring.

Other public health and safety measures, for example, in relation to the availability of paracetamol, require consideration. Deaths have risen during the 1980s to around 200 annually. The routine addition of methionine or an emetic has been proposed and such tablets are available but at increased prices. Limiting dosages in individual packs (to 8 g) is reported to have been successful in France (Garnier & Bismuth, 1993). Alternatively, education about its dangerous effects might be considered but this could be hazardous as it might, in effect, be an advertisement for an accessible suicide method. For example, a television programme which demonstrated the adverse effects of paracetamol in a fictional context may have actually led to an increase in such overdoses presenting to one A & E department although early presentation to services was characteristic.

The use of antidepressants also raises difficult questions: in 1990, nine million prescriptions were written for antidepressant drugs making them the most costly (£55 million) in the central nervous system therapeutic class of drugs and the introduction of new serotonergic selective re-uptake inhibitors (SSRI) since that time will have significantly increased this. However, the tricyclic antidepressants are the commonest drugs used to commit suicide. Therefore it has been argued that, given equivalence of effect, the SSRIs – or safer tricyclics such as lofepramine – should be used instead because of their markedly reduced toxicity (Montgomery *et al.*, 1992), This would thus limit access to a convenient means of committing suicide for actively depressed patients who are at greatest overall risk. Whether it would reduce suicide rates overall for those prescribed antidepressants has, however, yet to be demonstrated.

Prevention techniques at specific suicide points have been considered although demonstration of overall effectiveness is problematic. Examples include, fencing off railway lines and bridges near psychiatric hospitals, installation of telephones to The Samaritans on Beachy Head and consideration of safety-netting on Clifton Suspension bridge in Bristol. The new Jubilee Underground line in London will have perspex covers and doors along the platforms, similar to those in Japan, which open at the same time as the train doors do so to prevent accidents and, presumably, also suicides.

Services responses

The development of mental health services (contributing to achievement of the first general Health of the Nation target) can be expected to assist by producing local accessible services with effective supervision systems. Measures to provide early intervention (Merson *et al.*, 1992) and improve the support and supervision of patients with severe mental illness in the community, by implementation of the care programme approach (Department of Health, 1993a), care management and the development of effective information systems can assist in ensuring that when suicidal risk emergences, the person is in contact with a key worker who they know, can talk to and who can ensure that appropriate reassessment and management occurs. The availability of a key worker to carers can mean that they can pass on concerns – as often they will be the first to become aware of changing mood and emerging danger – and they can then see action taken.

Psychiatric morbidity in general medical and surgical units, especially in A & E departments (Johnson & Thornicroft, 1994), is high amongst people presenting with physical symptoms (Hawton, 1987), especially epilepsy, or after attempted suicide or self-harm. However, whilst management of the physical symptoms and prevention of death is a focus of concern, treatment of psychological distress and prevention of suicide frequently is not. Assessment of suicidal risk (Hawton, 1987; Hawton & Fagg, 1988) can readily be developed, as recognised in the 1984 DHSS notice revising guidance to districts on such procedures (DHSS, 1984). Studies (cited in Johnson &

Thornicroft, 1994) comparing psychiatrists, physicians, social workers and general and psychiatric nurses suggest that, provided they receive appropriate training, they are equally effective. However, attitudes to patients who have survived self-harm are usually negative (Ramon *et al.*, 1975) and specific in-service training is only available in a minority of districts (Johnson & Thornicroft, 1994). In consequence, suicide assessment may be cursory or neglected, although this can be improved by use of structured assessment forms (Blacker *et al.*, 1992). Changing such attitudes may be a major component in improving risk detection.

Early results also suggest that providing availability of a contact point may also be an important and effective means of reducing suicidal behaviour. The Samaritans, with 22,400 volunteers and 198 branches in the UK and Eire, have seen a 49% rise in calls over the past decade (1981–91; Armson, 1994) although any effects that they may have in preventing suicide have proved methodologically difficult to demonstrate. This may be in part because their widespread recognition and availability have made it virtually impossible to establish adequate control areas to measure effect and the need to maintain caller confidentiality precluded follow-up comparison.

The ready availability of admission and community support facilities when risk is sufficient to require them is also very important (Morgan, 1992) and with this, clear agreed policies for managing suicidal people in the community and hospital. Clearly defined observation policies are particularly important (Morgan & Owen, 1990) as risk on acute units has been estimated to be 50 times that of the general population (Fernando & Storm, 1984). Ensuring staff are aware of findings that unresolved life events and 'alienation' can also be of significance (Morgan & Priest, 1991). The importance of appropriate, co-ordinated discharge planning needs to be stressed in this context. The principle of referral by mental health teams back to GPs when an episode of care, in hospital or as an out-patient is over, needs to be developed.

Suicide after discharge from psychiatric in-patient care is raised, particularly in the first month (Goldacre *et al.*, 1993). Reasons suggested include perceived lack of support, reduced supervision, relapse because of renewed exposure to problems in the home environment, withdrawal of drug therapy, or the fact that the patient is still unwell. The general trend towards reduced lengths of stay is also noted.

Suicide is clearly distressing to families, friends and relatives and providing appropriate support at an early stage is of great importance. Timing of the offering of assistance by professionals, whether primary or secondary care staff, is important but will vary with individual circumstances. In these circumstances, considered multidisciplinary discussion would seem essential and many services already have procedures for seeing this happens. It can allow a coherent constructive care plan to be drawn up. Specific tasks can be agreed. Support can be given to staff, from the most junior to the most senior involved. The circumstances leading up to the suicide should be discussed as part of this and some lessons may be drawn. At a later stage, more detailed examination of events may be possible but the immediate response needs to be supportive and constructive.

Audit

Such local multidisciplinary audits are being set up in many services (Morgan & Priest, 1991) and may produce more information generally and for the individual services concerned about suicides of those in contact with them. Participation in such audits by members of the primary health care team can add to their value. Primary health care teams may also gain from grouping together to review suicides occurring in a number of practices.

At a national level, the Confidential Enquiry into Homicides and Suicides by Mentally Ill People has been established, led by the Royal College of Psychiatrists in conjunction with other professional groups. This will allow for a more dispassionate analysis of events than can occur at a local level. As with other confidential enquiries, such as those into maternal and peri-operative deaths, information will be collected from professional staff on a voluntary and confidential basis to allow a complete examination of relevant events. The intention will be to elicit avoidable causes of death and determine best practice by detailed examination of the circumstances surrounding such events. It has now been collecting data about suicides of people in contact or recently discharged from psychiatric contact since June 1993. Its first report providing statistical data and detailing conclusions and initial recommendations will be published in 1995.

Conclusion

Suicide prevention requires a broad variety of approaches and as *The Health of the Nation* says: 'it is essential to stress that everyone has a part to play if the strategy is to be successful'. So this is not just for the NHS to deliver, although, as discussed, the NHS, particularly mental health services and primary care, have a major role to play. There are important roles for government departments, the media, the NHS, purchasers and providers of health services, the Health Education Authority, local authorities, employers and voluntary organisations.

Research has already provided the basis for coherent strategies but more detail is needed. For example, Italian research (Crepet, 1992) has shown that between 1978 and 1989 suicide rates amongst those seeking a job for the first time rose by 25%, among the employed by 37% and amongst those seeking a new job by 594%. If this type of work were replicated in the UK, it might assist in targeting those individuals particularly at risk.

The potential for reducing suicide rates by development and dissemination of effective strategies, particularly in primary and secondary care, is therefore considerable. There is now much greater attention to this area than has previously been the case; the debate is finally moving from a nihilistic questioning of **whether** we should be trying to prevent suicide to **how** we can use the methods available, continue to evaluate them, and develop new ways of reducing the occurrence of these tragic events.

Acknowledgements

These are due to Donald Brooksbank, Central Health Monitoring Unit (for Fig. 6.1) and other colleagues in the Department for their assistance with this chapter.

References

Adam, K. S., Bouckoms, A. & Streiner, D. (1982). Parental loss and family stability in attempted suicide. *Archives of General Psychiatry*, **39**, 1081–5.

Armson, S. (1994). The Samaritans: befriending the suicidal. In *The Prevention of Suicide*. ed. R. Jenkins *et al.* London, HMSO.

Barraclough, B., Bunch, J., Nelson, B. & Sainsbury, P. (1974). A hundred cases of suicide: clinical aspects. *British Journal of Psychiatry*, **125**, 355–73.

Beck, A. T. & Steer, R. A. (1989). Clinical predictors of eventual suicide: a 5 to 10 year prospective study of suicide attempters. *Journal of Affective Disorders*, **17**, 203–9.

Berglund, M., Krantz, P., Lundqvist, G. & Therup, L. (1987). Suicide in psychiatric patients. *Acta Psychiatrica Scandinavica*, **76**, 431–7.

Birley, J. L. T. (1987). Psychiatrists and Psychologists: Working together for planning services in the post-Griffiths era. *Psychiatric Bulletin of the Royal College of Psychiatrists*, **11**, 210–11.

Blacker, C. V. R., Jenkins, R. & Silverstone, T. (1992). Assessment of deliberate self-harm on medical wards. *Psychiatric Bulletin*, **16**, 262–3.

Bulusu, L. & Anderson, M. (1984). Suicides 1950–1982. *Population Trends*, **35**, 11–17.

Charlton, J. R. H., Bauer, R., Thankore, A. *et al.* (1987). Unemployment and mortality: a small area analysis. *Journal of Epidemiology and Community Health*, **41**, 107–13.

Charlton, J., Kelly, S., Dunnell, K., *et al.* (1992). Trends in suicide deaths in England and Wales. *Population Trends* 69. London, HMSO.

Clarke, R. V. & Lester, D. (1987). Toxicity of car exhaust and opportunity for suicide: comparison between Britain and the United States. *Journal of Epidemiology and Community Health*, **41**, 114–20.

Crepet, P. (1992). Suicide trends in Italy. New epidemiological findings. *European Psychiatry*, **7**(1), 1–7.

Crombie, I. K. (1989). Trends in suicide and unemployment in Scotland 1976–86. *British Medical Journal*, **298**, 782–4.

Department of Health (1993a). *'Sometimes I Think I Can't Go On Any More'*. Heywood, DH publications.

Department of Health and Social Security (1984). *The Management of Deliberate Self-Harm*. (Health notice HN(84)25). London, DHSS.

Department of Health/Social Services Inspectorate. (1993b). *The Health of the Nation. Key Area Handbook: Mental Illness*. Heywood, Department of Health.

Diekstra, R. F. W. (1989). Suicide and attempted suicide: An international perspective. *Acta Psychiatrica Scandinavica*, **80** (suppl. 354), 1–24.

Diekstra, R. F. W. & van Egmond, M. (1989). Suicide and attempted suicide in general practice 1979–1986. *Acta Psychiatrica Scandinavica*, **79**, 268–75.

Duggan, C. F., Sham, P., Lee, A. S. & Murray, R. M. (1993). Can future suicidal behaviour in depressed in-patients be predicted? *Journal of Affective Disorder*, **22**(3), 111–18.

Farmer, R. & Creed, F. (1989). Life events and hostility in self-poisoning. *British Journal of Psychiatry*, **154**, 390–5.

Fernando, S. & Storm, V. (1984). Suicide among psychiatric patients of a district general hospital *Psychological Medicine*, **14**, 661–72.

Garnier, R. & Bismuth, C. (1993). Liver failure induced by paracetamol. *British Medical Journal*, **306**, 718.

Goldacre, M., Seagroatt, V. & Hawton, K. (1993). Suicide after discharge from psychiatric inpatient care. *Lancet*, **342**, 283–6.
Graham, C. & Burvill, P. W. (1992). A study of coroner's records of suicide in young people, 1986–88 in Western Australia. *Australian and New Zealand Journal of Psychiatry*, **26**(1), 30–9.
Hawton, K. (1987). Assessment of suicide risk. *British Journal of Psychiatry*, **150**, 145–53.
Hawton, K. & Fagg, J. (1988). Suicide, and other causes of death, following attempted suicide. *British Journal of Psychiatry*, **152**, 359–66.
Health Services Journal (1992). News. In brief. 27 August, p. 8.
Hoberman, H. M. & Garfinkel, B. D. (1988). Completed suicide in youth. *Canadian Journal of Psychiatry*, **33**, 494–502.
Johnson, S. & Thornicroft, G. (1994). General medical services. In *The Prevention of Suicide*. ed. R. Jenkins *et al.* London, HMSO.
Kreitman, N. (1976). The coal gas story: UK suicide rates 1960–71. *British Journal of Preventative and Social Medicine*, **30**, 86–93.
Lester, D. (1992). State initiatives in addressing youth suicide: Evidence for their effectiveness. *Social Psychiatry and Psychiatric Epidemiology*, **27**(2), 75–7.
Lindesay, J. (1993). Suicide in the elderly. *Geriatric Medicine*, [June], 48–52.
Marzuk, P. M., Leon, A. C., Tardiff, K. *et al.* (1992). The effect of access to lethal methods of injury on suicidal rates. *Archives of General Psychiatry*, **49**, 451–8.
Merson, S., Tyrer, P., Onyett, S. *et al.* (1992). Early intervention in psychiatric emergencies: a controlled clinical trial. *Lancet*, **339**, 1311–14.
Montgomery, S. A., Montgomery, D. B., Green, M. *et al.* (1992). Pharmacotherapy in the prevention of suicidal behaviour. *Journal of Clinical Pharmacology*, **12** (2, suppl.), 275–315.
Morgan, H. G. (1992). Suicide prevention. Hazards on the fast lane to community care. *British Journal of Psychiatry*, **160**, 149–53.
Morgan, H. G. (1993). Suicide prevention and 'The Health of the Nation'. *Psychiatric Bulletin*, **17**, 135–6.
Morgan, H. G. (1994). *Suicide Prevention. The Assessment and Management of Suicidal Risk*. An NHS Health Advisory Service Thematic Initiative. London, HMSO.
Morgan, H. G., Owen, J. H. (1990). *Persons at Risk of Suicide. Guidelines on Good Clinical Practice*. Nottingham, Boots.
Morgan, H. G. & Priest, P. (1991). Suicide and other unexpected deaths among psychiatric in-patients. The Bristol confidential inquiry. *British Journal of Psychiatry*, **158**, 368–74.
Moser, K. A., Goldblatt, P. O., Fox, A. J. & Jones, D. R. (1984). Unemployment and mortality: comparison of the 1971 and 1981 longitudinal study census samples. *British Medical Journal*, **294**, 86–90.
Murthy, V. N. (1969). Personality and nature of suicide attempts. *British Journal of Psychiatry*, **115**, 791–5.
Pallis, D. J., Barraclough, B. M., Levey, A. B. *et al.* (1982). Estimating suicide risk among attempted suicides: 1. the development of new clinical scales. *British Journal of Psychiatry*, **141**, 37–44.

Paykel, E. S., Priest, R. G. (1992). Recognition and management of depression in general practice: consensus statement. *British Medical Journal*, **305**, 1198–202.
Peet, M. (1992). The prevention of suicide in patients with recurrent mood disorder. *Journal of Psychopharmacology*, **6**(2), 334–9.
Platt, S. (1992). Epidemiology of suicide and parasuicide. *Journal of Psychopharmacology*, **6**(2), 291–9.
Platt, S. (1994). The media response. In *The Prevention of Suicide*. ed. R. Jenkins *et al.* London, HMSO.
Pokorney, A. D. (1983). Prediction of suicide in psychiatric patients. *Archives of General Psychiatry*, **40**, 249–57.
Pritchard, C. (1988). Suicide, unemployment and gender in the British Isles and European Economic Community (1974–1985). Social Psychiatry and Psychiatric Epidemiology, **23**, 85–9.
Ramon, S., Bancroft, J. H. J. & Skrimstone, A. M. (1975). Attitudes to self-poinsoning among physicians and nurses in a general hospital. *British Journal Psychiatry*, **127**, 257–64.
Retterstøl, N. (1992). Suicide in Nordic countries. *Psychopathology*, **25**, 254–65.
Rihmer, Z., Szanto, K. & Barsi, J. (1992). Suicide prevention; fact or fiction. *British Journal of Psychiatry*, **161**, 130–1.
Robins, E., Gassner, S., Kayes, J. *et al.* (1959). The communication of suicidal intent: a study of 134 consecutive cases of successful (completed) suicide. *American Journal of Psychiatry*, **115**, 724–33.
Rutz, W., von Knorrling & Walinder, J. (1992). Long-term effects of an educational program for general practitioners given by the Swedish Committee for the prevention and treatment of depression. *Acta Psychiatrica Scandinavica*, **85**, 83–8.
Seagar, C. P. & Flood, R. A. (1965). Suicide in Bristol. *British Journal of Psychiatry*, **3**, 919–32.
Soni Raleigh, V. & Balajaran, R. (1992). Suicide and self-burning among Indians and West Indians in England and Wales. *British Journal of Psychiatry*, **161**, 365–8.
Tarbuck, A. F. & O'Brien, J. T. (1992). Suicide and vehicle exhaust emissions. *British Medical Journal*, **304**, 1376.
Vassilas, C. A. & Morgan, H. G. (1993). General practitioners' contact with victims of suicide. *British Medical Journal*, **307**, 300–1.

7

Using the crisis

MAX BIRCHWOOD AND VAL DRURY

The prevention of relapse and the ensuing crisis is one among many needs of people with a psychosis; it is nevertheless important as each relapse brings with it an increased probability of future relapse and residual symptoms (McGlashan, 1988) as well as accelerating social disablement (Hogarty *et al.*, 1991). Even an ideal combination of pharmacological and psychosocial intervention in the context of assertive outreach does not eliminate the potential for relapse (Stein, 1993).

These facts are not lost on those who themselves experience recurring psychotic symptoms. A survey by Mueser and colleagues (1992) found that patients expressed a strong interest in learning about 'early warning signs of the illness and relapse' and was ranked second in importance out of an agenda of over 40 topics. Their thirst for knowledge and understanding on this matter would seem to be driven by a perceived need for control rather than mere curiosity. In a study of 'secondary' depression in schizophrenia, Birchwood *et al.* (1993) found that 'perceived control over illness' was the variable most closely linked to depression, more so than illness variables, locus of control or self-evaluative beliefs derived from culture-bound stereotypes of mental illness. Fear of mental disintegration is understood to be among the best predictors of suicide and parasuicide in this population (Caldwell & Gottesman, 1990). The propensity of patients to seek control of psychotic disorder is now well understood (Brier & Strauss, 1983; Kumar *et al.*, 1989; Strauss, 1989) and the question is raised as to the possibility of empowering individuals with real control over an event they fear most: relapse. Considerable attention is paid in the literature to prevention of relapse or crisis whether using pharmacological (Hogarty, 1993), or psychosocial methods (Hogarty *et al.*, 1991). This is entirely appropriate in view of the damage relapse can cause, but it does emphasise the notion of relapse as a failure leaving little consideration to the potential opportunities it can provide for adjustment and change. For example, in initiating contact between vulnerable people and Mental Health Services (Stein, 1993), engaging families in psycho-education (Birchwood & Smith, 1990; Tarrier, 1991), promoting the value of maintenance medication (Hoge, 1990) and to initiate a process of 'integrating' the psychotic experience into the sense of self rather than denial or sealing over (McGorry, 1992).

In this chapter we will devote most of our attention to describing two ways in which the crisis can lead to tangible benefit. The first is in initiating contact and motivating client and family to engage in a psycho-educational process to promote recovery, and second as an opportunity to acquire specific information about the early symptoms of relapse, using them in order to rehearse and facilitate early intervention on the occasion of a future putative crisis.

Using the crisis: improving strategies for self-management

DSM III R (APA, 1987) recognises that relapse when defined as the re-emergence or exacerbation of positive symptoms is often preceded by subtle changes in mental functioning up to four weeks prior to the event. Not only is this perceived as a loss of well-being by the individual but it appears to trigger a set of restorative manoeuvres as McCandless-Glincher *et al.* (1986) show in their study.

McCandless-Glincher *et al.* (1986) studied 62 individuals attending for maintenance therapy, and inquired about their recognition of and response to reduced well-being. The patients were drawn from those routinely attending two medical centres; their age range (20–75 years), with a mean illness duration of 28 years, suggests that such a group would be well represented in ordinary clinical practice. Sixty-one said they could recognise reduced well-being; of these only 13 relied entirely upon others to identify symptoms for them. Nine were assisted by others and 36 identified the problem themselves. The majority (50 out of 61) of patients initiated some change in their behaviour when they recognised reduced well-being; including engaging in diversionary activities, seeking professional help and resuming or increasing their neuroleptic medication. Only three of this group had ever been encouraged to self-monitor by mental health professionals, and a further seven had received encouragement from relatives. Thus, these schizophrenic patients had initiated symptom-monitoring and a range of responses almost entirely on their own initiative. The study by Kumar *et al.* (1989), comes to rather similar conclusions.

In essence, there may be a relatively untapped pool of information which is not accessed adequately enough to initiate early intervention, except perhaps by individuals themselves. If individuals can recognise and act on symptoms suggestive of reduced well-being, then it is possible that patterns of early ('prodromal') symptoms heralding relapse may be apparent and identifiable, and may offer further avenues for relapse management in partnership with the individual with the psychosis.

Does a prodrome herald psychotic relapse?

Clinical, retrospective and prospective studies have and continue to address this question. In this section we shall concentrate on the last two and consider the implications of the clinical studies in trying to interpret the empirical investigations.

Psychiatric services are by and large organised to respond to crises such as relapse; this constrains our ability to develop clinical experience of prodromal changes. Thus the first systematic studies of the prodrome adopted the simple expedient of asking the patient and his relative or carer.

The interview study by Herz and Melville (1980) in the United States attempted systematically to collect data retrospectively from patients and relatives in this manner. It is widely regarded as definitive since they interviewed 145 schizophrenic sufferers (46 following a recent episode) as well as 80 of their family members. The main question, 'could you tell that there were any changes in your thoughts, feelings or behaviours that might have led you to believe you were becoming sick and might have to go into hospital?', was answered affirmatively by 70% of patients and 93% of families. These and the results of a similar British study (Birchwood *et al.*, 1989) are shown in Table 7.1.

Generally the symptoms most frequently mentioned by patients

Table 7.1. *Percentage of relatives reporting early signs*

Category	Birchwood *et al.* (1989) (n=42)		Herz and Melville (1980) (n=80)	
	%	Rank*	%	Rank*
Anxiety/agitation				
Irritable/quick tempered	62	2(eq)	—	—
Sleep problems	67	1	69	7
Tense, afraid, anxious	62	2(eq)	83	1
Depression/withdrawal				
Quiet, withdrawn	60	4	50	18
Depressed, low	57	5	76	3
Poor appetite	48	9	53	17
Disinhibition				
Aggression	50	7(eq)	79	2
Restless	55	6	40	20
Stubborn	36	10(eq)	—	—
Incipient psychosis				
Behaves as if hallucinated	50	7(eq)	60	10
Being laughed at or talked about	36	10(eq)	14	53.8
'Odd behaviour'	36	10(eq)	—	—

* There were many other symptoms assessed. Percentage reporting only shown for parallel data.

and family members were dysphoric in nature: eating less, concentration problems, troubled sleep, depressed mood and withdrawal. The most common 'early psychotic' symptoms were 'hearing voices', 'talking in a nonsensical way', 'increased religious thinking' and 'thinking someone else was controlling them'.

There is considerable agreement about the nature of these 'early signs' although somewhat less in their relative salience. Both studies (Herz & Melville, 1980; Birchwood *et al.*, 1989) concur in finding 'dysphoric' symptoms the most commonly prevalent. In the Herz and Melville (1980) study, although more families than patients reported the presence of early signs, there was considerable concordance between patients and families in the content and relative significance of early symptoms. There was substantial agreement between patients that non-psychotic symptoms such as anxiety, tension and insomnia were part of the prodrome but less agreement as to the characteristics of the earliest changes. Fifty per cent of the patients felt that the characteristic symptoms of the prodrome were repeated at each relapse. A number of these patients also reported that many of the non-psychotic symptoms persisted between episodes of illness, an important issue to which we shall return below.

Both studies carefully questioned respondents about the timing of the onset of the prodrome. Most of the patients (52%) and their families (68%) in the Herz and Melville study felt that more than a week elapsed between the onset of the prodrome and a full relapse. Similarly, Birchwood *et al.* found that 59% observed the onset of the prodrome one month or more prior to relapse, and 75% two weeks or more; 19% were unable to specify a time scale.

The true predictive significance of prodromal signs can only be clearly established with prospective investigations. Such studies need to examine three issues: (a) whether prodromes of psychotic relapse exist, (b) their timing in relation to full relapse and (c) how often the 'prodromes' fail as well as succeed to predict relapse (i.e. 'sensitivity' and 'specificity'). The clinical implications of this research will largely depend on the degree of specificity which early signs information affords. In particular a high false positive rate will tend to undermine the use of an early intervention strategy, in particular that which uses a raised dose of neuroleptic medication since in such cases, patients will have been needlessly exposed to additional medication.

In the course of a study comparing low and standard dose maintenance medication, Marder *et al.* (1984a,b) assessed 41 patients on a range of psychiatric symptoms at baseline, two weeks later, monthly for three months and then every three months. Relapse was defined as the failure of an increase in medication to manage symptoms following a minor exacerbation of psychosis or paranoia. Thus under this definition, it is not known how many genuine prodromes were **aborted** with medication and whether those that responded to medication were similar to those that did not. Patients were assessed using a standard psychiatric interview scale (brief psychiatric rating scale – BPRS: Overall & Graham, 1962) and a self-report measure of psychiatric symptoms (SCL-90: Derogatis *et al.*, 1973). Changes in scores 'just prior to relapse' were compared with the average ('spontaneous') change for a given scale during the course of the follow-up period. Marder *et al.* (1984a) found increases in BPRS depression, thought disturbance and paranoia and SCL-90 scores for interpersonal sensitivity, anxiety, depression and paranoid ideation prior to relapse. They note that the changes they observed were very small (equalling 2 points on a 21-point range) and probably not recognisable by most clinicians. A discriminant function analysis found the most discriminating ratings were paranoia and depression (BPRS) and psychoticism (SCL-90). They suggest: 'such a formula if used in a clinic could probably predict most relapses although there would be a considerable number of . . . false positives' (page 46). While this study strongly supports the presence of the relapse prodrome, it was unable to control for timing. The last assessment before relapse varied from between 1 and 12 weeks, weakening the observed effects. One would anticipate the prodrome to be at its maximum in the week or two prior to relapse; assessments carried out prior to this would measure an earlier and weaker stage of the prodrome, or miss it entirely.

A subsequent report (Marder *et al.*, 1991) studied 50 schizophrenic patients monitored weekly for non-psychotic prodromal episodes. This study compared different methods of monitoring for prodromes using experimenter-administered scales (BPRS: anxiety–depression cluster and their individualised prodromal scale), systematically varying the sensitivity of their instruments and observing the impact on their predictive efficacy. Thus Fig. 7.1 plots the hit rate against the rate of false positives under varying degrees of change in the prodrome scale from 10 to 50 points. This shows that using a change score of 3, 50% of relapses are accurately predicted with a 20% false positive rate; this was achieved only when patients with a relatively stable mental state were included.

Subotnik and Nuechterlein (1988) considerably improved upon the Marder *et al.* studies (1984a,b, 1991) by administering the BPRS fortnightly to 50 young, recent onset schizophrenic patients diagnosed by RDC (research diagnostic criteria). Twenty-three patients relapsed and their BPRS scores at two, four and six weeks prior to the relapse were compared with their scores in another six-week period not associated with relapse and with scores of a non-relapse group (N=27) over a similar period. This research found that BPRS anxiety–depression (which includes depression, guilt and somatic concern) and thought disturbance (hallucinations and delusions) were raised prior to relapse with the latter more prominent as relapse approached (two to four weeks prior to relapse). The contrast with the **non**-relapsed patients revealed a rise in low-level 'psychotic'

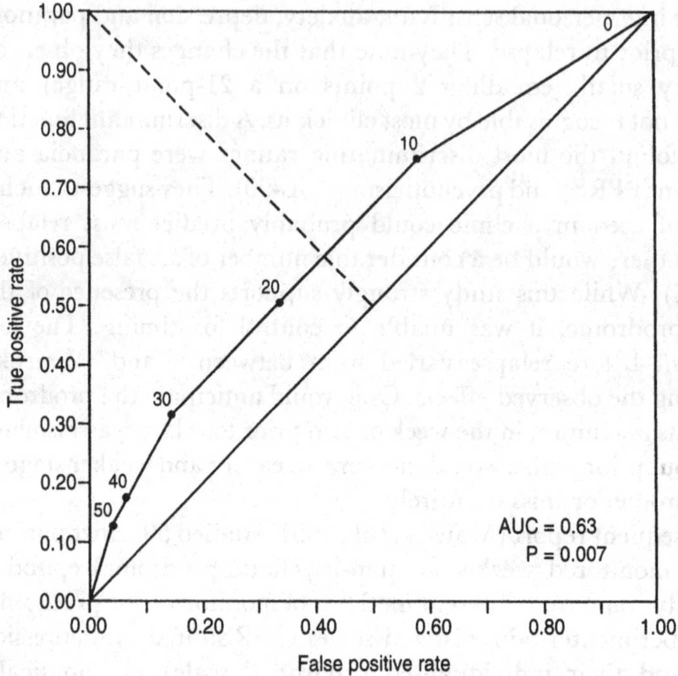

Fig. 7.1. The effect of changing thresholds for prodrome declaration on the true detection rate and false positives. (From Marder et al., *1991.)*

symptoms as part of the prodrome, but not of the non-psychotic items (depression, somatic concern, guilt, etc.). This suggests that the non-psychotic symptoms are sensitive to relapse but not specific to it. If, however, they were followed by low-level psychotic symptoms, this study suggests that relapse is more probable. Subotnik and Nuechterlein (1988, p. 411) note: 'mean elevations in prodromal symptoms were small ... 0.5–1.00 on a 7-point scale ... but in three patients no prodromal symptoms were present ... in several others they did not begin to show any symptomatic change until 2–4 weeks prior to relapse ... thus lowering the magnitude of the means'. These support clinical observations that the nature and timing of prodromal signs are like relapse itself – not universal, but include considerable between-subject variability. Nevertheless Subotnik and Nuechterlein reported that a discriminant function using two BPRS 'psychotic' scales correctly classified 59% of relapses and 74% of non-relapse periods, suggesting a false positive rate of 26%.

Hirsch and Jolley (1989) in the course of an early intervention study measured putative prodromes ('neurotic or dysphoric episodes') in a group of 54 patients with DSM-III schizophrenia using the SCL-90 and Herz's Early Signs Questionnaire (ESQ; Herz *et al.*, 1982; Herz, 1985, pers. comm.). Patients and their key workers received a one-hour teaching session about schizophrenia, particularly concerning the significance of the 'dysphoric' syndrome as a prodrome for relapse. It was hoped that this would enable them to recognise 'dysphoric episodes'. All subjects were symptom-free at the onset of the trial. At each dysphoric episode, the SCL-90 and the ESQ were administered and then weekly for two further weeks; otherwise each was rated monthly. Relapse was defined as the re-emergence of florid symptoms including delusions and hallucinations. Seventy-three per cent of the relapses were preceded by a prodromal period of dysphoric and neurotic symptoms within a month of relapse. These prodromes were defined clinically but confirmed by SCL-90 scores which were similar to those reported by the other two prospective studies and included depression, anxiety, interpersonal sensitivity and paranoid thinking. Interpretation of this study is complicated by the design, in which half the subjects received active and half placebo maintenance medication and all patients showing signs of dysphoric (prodromal) episodes were given additional active medication (Haloperidol, 10 mg per day). Dysphoric episodes were much more common in the placebo (76%) than in the active group (27%) but the prompt pharmacological intervention does not allow us to ascertain whether these dysphoric episodes were part of a reactivation of psychosis (i.e. true prodromes) aborted by medication and to what extent these included 'false positives' related, perhaps, to the use of placebo.

A further prospective study (Birchwood *et al.*, 1989) used a scale designed to tap the specific characteristic of the prodrome rather than that of general psychopathology. Construction of the scale was informed by the retrospective study reported in the same paper. Two versions of the scale were used for completion by both the patient **and** a chosen observer (e.g. relative, carer, hostel worker). It was reasoned that the behavioural observations by the observers might provide additional information if the individual under-reported or lost insight. **Changes** in baseline levels were readily apparent, which is particularly important if the individual experiences persisting symptoms.

The authors (Birchwood *et al.*, 1989) reported an investigation of 19 young schizophrenic patients diagnosed according to the broad CATEGO 'S' class (Wing *et al.*, 1974). All, except one, were on

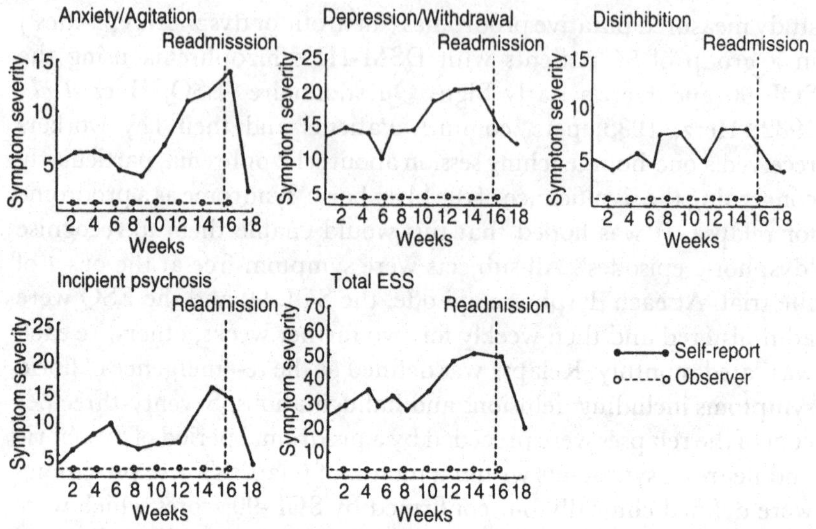

Fig. 7.2. A prodrome detecting using the ESS (early signs scale)

maintenance medication and monitored in the context of a routine clinical service and were not involved in a drug trial. Eight of the 19 relapsed in the course of nine months and of these, 50% showed elevations on the scales between two and four weeks prior to relapse. A *post hoc* defined threshold on their scale (> or <30) led to a sensitivity of 63%, specificity of 82% and an 11% rate of false positives.

Figure 7.2 shows a case example of a young male who relapsed 16 weeks following discharge. In this case the first change was that of dysphoria/withdrawal which was apparent five weeks prior to relapse. One to two weeks later he became steadily more agitated and within two weeks of relapse, low level ('incipient') psychotic symptoms appeared. Disinhibition was unaffected. Further examples may be found in Birchwood *et al.* (1992).

The concept of the relapse signature

The prospective studies have raised a number of questions. They have confirmed the existence of prodromes of psychotic relapse and find a true positive rate in the region of 50–60% with a false positive rate of up to 25%; however, their limitations have not enabled a clear picture to emerge of the true predictive significance of apparent early warning signs. Patients in the Hirsch and Jolley (1989) and Subotnik and Nuechterlein (1988) studies were generally symptom free; there was somewhat more variability in residual symptoms than in the Birchwood *et al.* (1989) and Marder *et al.* (1984a,b, 1991) studies. Residual symptoms will tend also to be associated with an unstable mental state: Marder *et al.* (1991) found better prediction when 'unstable' patients were excluded. In view of the large numbers of patients with even moderate residual symptoms, this issue deserves serious and careful examination. If the work of Birchwood *et al.* (1989) is borne out, then group studies in the mould of Subotnik and Nuechterlein (1988) would be inherently limited as they could not capture the apparent quantitative and qualitative differences between patients in their early signs or symptoms. This is supported by Subotnik and Nuechterlein's finding that greater prediction came when patients were compared against their own baseline rather than that of other patients. It may be more appropriate to think of each patient's prodrome as a personalised **relapse signature** which includes core or common symptoms together with features unique to each patient. If an individual's relapse signature can be identified, then it might be expected that the overall predictive power of 'prodromal' symptoms will be increased. Identifying the unique characteristics of a relapse signature can only be achieved once a relapse has taken place; with each successive relapse further information becomes available to build a more accurate image of the signature. This kind of learning process has been acknowledged by patients (Brier & Strauss, 1983) and could be adapted and developed by professionals and carers as well. In the next section we detail a method to build an image of the 'relapse signature'.

The relevance of individual and illness factors

An issue not directly examined in the prospective studies concerns the existence of a prodrome of relapse where the individual continues to experience significant residual symptoms. Where the patient experiences continued negative symptoms such as anergia and withdrawal, a prodrome presumably may involve an apparent **exacerbation** of these symptoms as shown in some of the cases in Fig. 7.1. Where individuals continue to suffer from symptoms such as delusions and hallucinations, a 'relapse' will involve an exacerbation of these symptoms; whether these relapses will also be preceded by prodromes of a similar character is unknown.

Patients participating in the prospective studies generally were young (18–35 years) with a relatively brief psychiatric history. Such individuals may be more prone to relapse and tend to be recruited at acute admission or because they were thought to be appropriate for low dose or intermittent drug strategies (cf. Hirsch & Jolley, 1989). The application of this methodology to older, more stable individuals is another important area for further investigation.

Collaborative early intervention

Engagement and education

Early intervention rests on a close co-operation between patient, carer/relative and professionals. In common with many interventions, an ethos of trust and 'informed partnership' between these groups must be developed (Smith & Birchwood, 1990). Education about prodromes and early intervention opportunities needs to be provided which might be given in the context of general educational intervention about psychosis (Birchwood *et al.* 1991; Smith *et al.*, 1992), and as the experience of Jolley *et al.* (1990) illustrates, this requires psycho-education to be a continuous feature of this relationship.

Discrimination of false positives from true positives may be facilitated through provision of clear cues. Firstly, the client's prodrome derived from the initial interview and any further clarification that comes from further early episodes (see below) should be documented in case notes and retained by the client and carer, preferably written using the clients own words. Secondly, this should contain information about timing as well as content, and include actions that the client might take to verify the prodrome and to engage in restorative manoeuvres, including contacting the relevant professional. Thirdly, the 'relentless and remorseless' feature of prodromes is a useful 'rule of thumb'; changes may be anticipated continuously over several days and not just one or two. Example of prodrome charts are provided later on in this chapter.

Suitable clients

Individuals with a history of repeated relapse or who are at high risk, for reasons of use of non-adherence or with a maintenance regime, recovery from a recent relapse, living alone or in a high expressed emotion family environment, may be appropriate to participate in early intervention as will those who fear relapse and are demoralised by their apparent inability to control it. For those with severe drug-refractory positive symptoms, discriminating a prodrome against such a background is likely to prove extremely difficult (indeed its very existence is questionable) and early intervention becomes less meaningful in this context. The absence of insight may preclude an individual's acceptance of an early intervention strategy; indeed the ultimate test will be the individual's acceptance of the approach, which in our experience has much to do with his or her dislike of the dislocation which relapse/readmission can cause, as well as fear of the experience itself. The availability of a close relative or carer to maximise information about prodromal signs and provide support can be helpful but must be selected in collaboration with the individual.

Identifying the time window and provisional relapse signature for early intervention

Four problems need to be overcome if our knowledge about prodromes is to have clinical application. Firstly, the identification of 'early signs' by a clinician would require intensive, regular monitoring of mental state at least fortnightly which is rarely possible in clinical practice. Secondly, some patients choose to conceal their symptoms as relapse approaches and insight declines (Heinrichs, 1985; Heinrichs & Carpenter, 1985). Thirdly, many patients experience persisting symptoms, cognitive deficits or drug side-effects which may obscure the visibility of the prodromes. Indeed the nature of a prodrome in patients with residual symptoms (in contrast to those who are symptom free) has not been studied and is important since in clinical practice the presence of residual symptoms is extremely common. Fourthly, the possibility is raised that the characteristics of prodromes might vary from individual to individual and this information may be lost in scales of general psychopathology and the group designs of research studies.

With regard to the latter, provisional information about the nature and duration of an individual's prodrome or 'relapse signature' may be obtained through careful interviewing of patient (and if possible relatives and other close associates) about the changes in thinking and behaviour leading up to a recent episode. Where this is fed back, it may enable a more accurate discrimination of a future prodrome.

Such an interview (used by the authors) is shown in Table 7.2. This involves five stages. The first establishes the date of onset of the episode and the time between this and any admission. The second establishes the date when a change in behaviour was **first** noticed; and in the third and fourth stages the sequence of subsequent changes is established using specific prompts if necessary. Finally, the prodrome is summarised. Figure 7.3 represents the outcome of one such interview which was drawn by the client herself.

Monitoring and intervention

In our work, individuals engage in a process of monitoring using the ESS (early signs scale) described earlier.

This has four objectives:

1. To develop a baseline measure against which changes can be discerned and compared.
2. To reinforce the discrimination of the changed perceptual, cognitive and affective processes through use of appropriate labels.
3. To educate individuals, their carers and professionals about the precise nature of the 'relapse signature' using information from a monitored prodrome.
4. To promote client's engagement in services, and to share responsibility for prodrome detection between individual and professionals.

Thus monitoring is not conceived as a lifetime activity but a relatively short-term manoeuvre to learn about prodromes, to engage patient and professional in meaningful activity to enhance control and to demonstrate that control can be achieved.

In the next stage, decision rules are discerned to operationally define the onset of a prodrome; these include a quantitative change on the ESS scales and/or the appearance of individualised prodromal signs. This then is an entirely client driven and controlled system as is the intervention.

Early intervention seeks to intervene as early as possible in the process of relapse on the basis of information that relapse is probable. Where a pharmacological intervention is indicated, a targeted and time-limited oral dose of neuroleptics may be chosen in advance in

Table 7.2. *Early signs interview: relatives' version*

Stage One: Establish date of onset/admission to hospital and behaviour at height of episode
'On what date was X admitted to hospital?'
Prompt: date, day, time; contemporary events to aid recall.

'When did you decide (s)he needed help?'
Prompt: date.

'What was X's behaviour like at that time?'
Prompt: What kind of things was (s)he saying?
What kind of things was (s)he doing?

Stage Two: Establish date when change in X was first noticed
'So X was admitted to hospital weeks after you decided (s)he needed help...'.
'Think back carefully to the days or weeks before then'

'When did you first notice a change in X's usual behaviour or anything out of the ordinary?'
Prompt: Nature, time of change.

'Were there any changes before then, even ones which might not seem important?'

Stage Three: Establish sequence of changes up to relapse
'I'd like to establish the changes that took place after that up to (date) when you decided X needed help'.

'What happened next (after last change)?'
Prompt: Was this a marked change?
When did this happen?
Can you give me some examples?
Repeat question until point of relapse is reached.

Stage Four: Prompting for items not already elicited
'During this build up to her/his relapse/admission to hospital...'.
'Was (s)he usually anxious or on edge?'
Prompt: When did you notice this?
Prompt items from relevant Early Signs checklist.
'Did (s)he seem low in his/her spirits?'
Prompt: As above.

'Did (s)he seem disinhibited (excitable, restless, aggressive, drinking, etc.)?'
Prompt: As above.

'Did (s)he seem suspicious or say/do strange things?'
Prompt: As above.

Stage Five: Summary
'Let me see if I'm clear on what happened before X's admission'
'X was admitted on (date), (number) weeks after you decided (s)he needed help; (s)he was (describe presentation)'.

'You first noticed something was wrong on (date) when (s)he (describe behaviour) ... then (s)he began to...'.
(Complete description of prodrome)

'Have I missed anything out?'

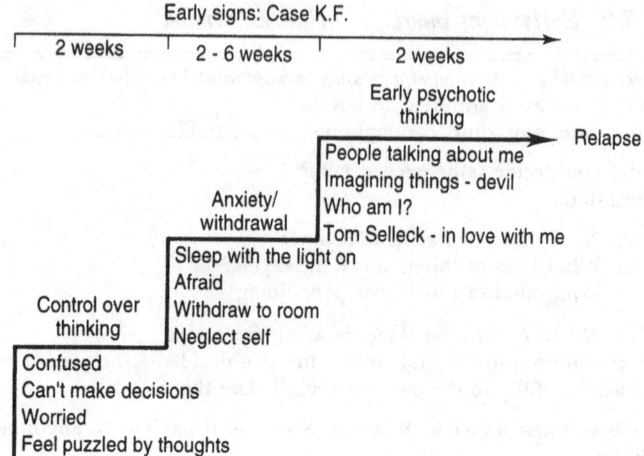

Fig. 7.3. One client's representation of her relapse signature (some details have been changed)

consultation with the client. Figure 7.4 gives a case example. In the first example (Fig. 7.4a) S.H. achieved a baseline score of 13 on the ESS scale: his decision rule was a 20-point increase on the ESS scale including the presence of idiosyncratic signs: racing thoughts, inefficient and confused thinking, poor concentration and a 'giggly' affect. He self-administered a targeted dose of 20 mg Stelazine which was to be increased by 50% if an improvement was not observed within one week. His record clearly shows a steady improvement over six weeks with no breakthrough of either hallucinations or delusions.

A sense of ownership over these data should be fostered between professionals, patients and their families so that responsibility for initiating early intervention is a shared one; for example in the authors' work, regular updated copies of the graphs are available to participants, some of whom are taught to interact with the computer-based system. Educating patients and relatives about early signs of relapse, collaboration in monitoring, feeding back to them information from the early signs interview, and any detected prodromes should significantly raise the likelihood of future early detection and therefore intevention.

Clarifying the relapse signature

Impending or actual crises present an important opportunity to 'sharpen the image' of the signature for client, carer and professional;

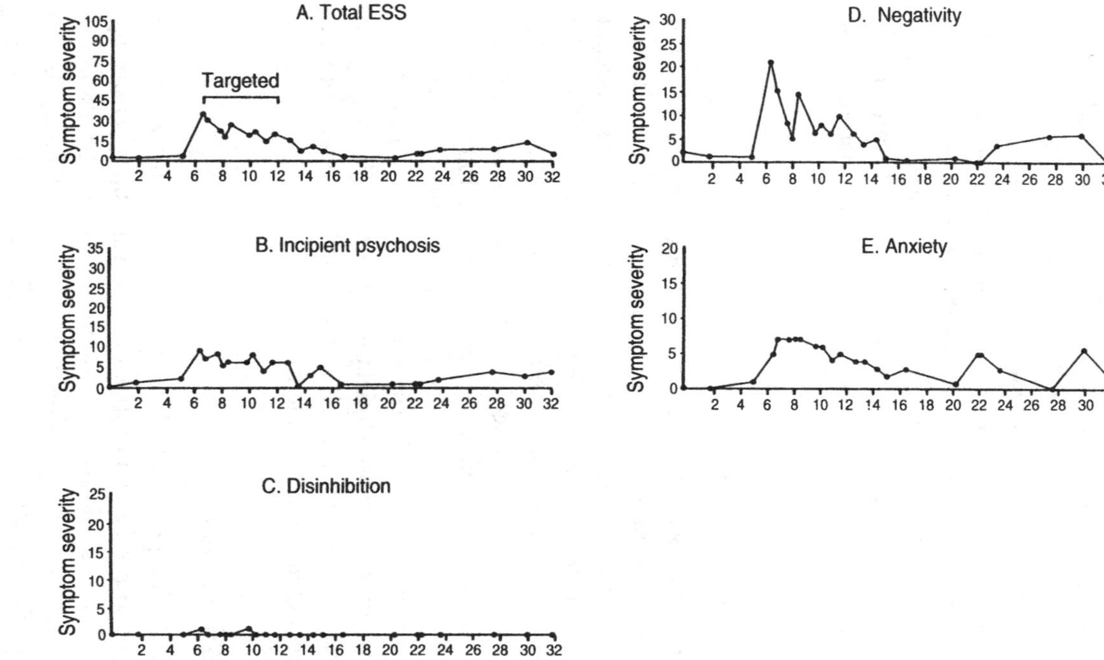

Fig. 7.4. Impact of early pharmacological intervention: a case example

in this respect the crisis can be reframed as an opportunity to acquire information that can facilitate control and prevention. Figure 7.5 illustrates a client (T.F.) who showed early relapse on more than one occasion. The prodromes of these episodes are juxtaposed in the Figure. Considerable consistency in the nature and timing of the early symptoms is apparent, consistent with the 'signature' concept. In the case of T.F. the record clarifies that the time window is at least two weeks; the onset of 'psychotic thinking' coincides with increases in agitation and withdrawal. Two weeks prior to this, T.F. showed clear evidence of an **improvement** in these indices (agitation/withdrawal) followed by an abrupt deterioration. This then was incorporated into his signature, 'raising the question' of early relapse. The presence of the following qualitative aspects serve to reduce likelihood of a false positive.

Support and counselling

Once a prodrome has been declared, the individual and family need intensive support. The psychological reaction to a loss of well-being, and the possibility that this may herald a relapse, places a significant strain on both parties, which, if unchecked, could accelerate the decompensation process. The availability of support, quick access to the team, the use of stress management and diversionary activities may help to mitigate these effects (Brier & Strauss, 1983).

Weekly, daily, or even in-patient contact can be offered, serving to alleviate anxiety, emphasising the shared burden of responsibility. In routine clinical practice most clinicians value the opportunity to utilise day care where admission is not deemed necessary but an element of decompensation is evident.

Potential difficulties

Notwithstanding its potential therapeutic value, the notion of self-monitoring does raise a number of concerns about sensitising patients and carers to disability, promoting the observations as critical responses, burdening individuals at frequent intervals, or increasing the risk of self-harm in an individual who becomes demoralised by an impending relapse. There is as yet no evidence that self-monitoring is likely to increase the risk of self-harm; indeed, florid and uncontrolled relapse may be more dangerous and more damaging.

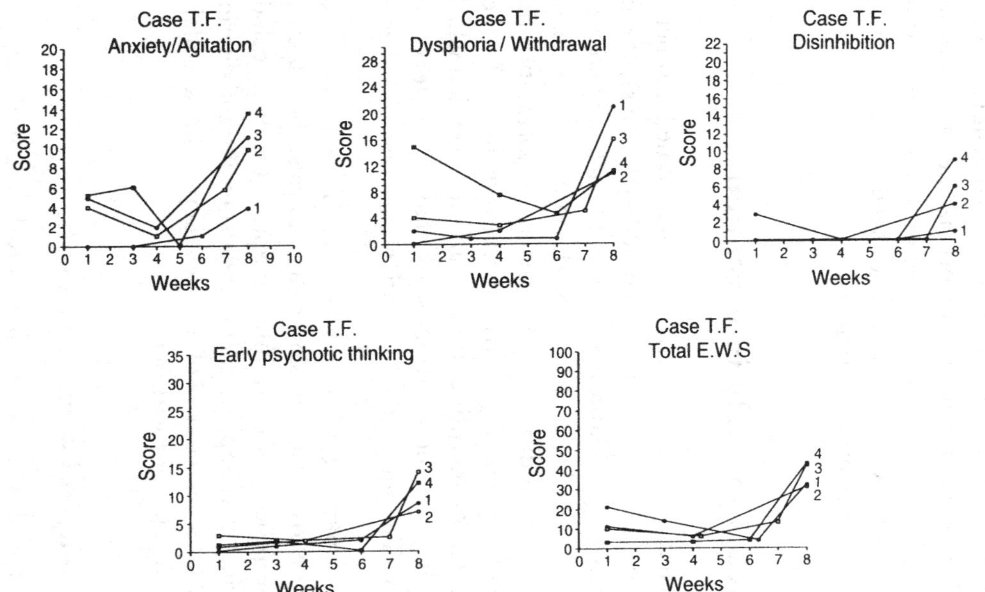

Fig. 7.5. Stability of the early relapse signature between episodes: a case example (1: relapse 1; 2: relapse 2; 3: relapse 3; 4: relapse 4)

Engaging patients and carers more actively in the management of the illness may also promote a sense of purposeful activity and have therapeutic benefits *per se*. However, it is probable that a substantial group of patients, who retain very little insight or lose insight very early in decompensation, may be unable or unwilling to entertain self-monitoring; and are also least likely to consent to observation by another. Family education and support may permit key people in the individual's life to monitor and recognise specific early warning signs, and to initiate preventative strategies such as seeking professional help promptly if relapse is predicted.

The efficacy of early intervention

In the opening section of this chapter it was argued that percived loss of control over 'illness' (relapse, residual symptoms), the life goals they affect as well as relapse itself can lead to deleterious outcomes for people with a psychosis (depression/demoralisation, suicide, raised relapse risk). In addition to any further opportunities that early pharmacological and/or cognitive intervention may offer the control of relapse, the collaborative ethos of early intervention which places the individual in the 'driving seat' may promote control and self-efficacy. The important evaluative questions then become:

- Can pharmacological interventions initiated at the onset of apparent early symptoms slow down or arrest the relapse process?
- Does the process of early intervention (education, collaborative monitoring, etc.) improve clients understanding and discrimination of prodromes and control of relapse and promote a 'collaborative' style of engagement with services?

Pharmacological early intervention

All the reviewed drug studies have involved withdrawing patients from maintenance regimes, monitoring clinical state and providing brief pharmacotherapy at the onset of a prodrome. This paradigm has been chosen with the goal of minimising drug exposure and therefore side effects without prejudicing prophylaxis, rather than as a means of further controlling relapse. This issue will be returned to at the conclusion of this section.

Three well controlled studies have been reported (Table 7.3) using this paradigm (Carpenter *et al.*, 1990; Jolley *et al.*, 1990; Gaebel *et al.*, 1994). Jolley *et al.* (1990) studied 54 stabilised, symptomatic and thus highly-selected patients who were randomly assigned to active or placebo maintenance therapy conditions, with both receiving early drug intervention at the onset of a prodrome which involved the administration of 5–10 mg daily of Haloperidol. Patients received a brief educational session on entry to the study about prodromes and early intervention as reliance was placed on patients to recognise their early signs of relapse and to contact the clinical team. Outcome at one year revealed that significantly more patients experienced prodromal symptoms in the intermittent group (76%) than in the control group (27%), which was accompanied by an increased rate of relapse in the intermittent group (30% versus 7%) although there was good evidence that 'severe' relapse was not affected and was indeed low in both groups. Nevertheless, the large difference between the number of prodromes and number of relapses, does suggest that prompt action can abort relapse in many instances. During the first year of the study, 73% of relapses were preceded by identified prodromal symptoms; during the second year this fell to 25%, as reliance was placed on patients and families to identify and seek assistance for prodromal symptoms, this suggests 'that the single teaching session at the start of the study does not provide patients and families with an adequate grasp of the intermittent paradigm ... ongoing psycho-educational intervention should be an essential component of further studies' (Jolly *et al.*, 1990, p. 841).

Carpenter *et al.* (1990) report the outcome of a study of similar design to Jolley *et al.* (1990) with largely similar outcomes. Gaebel *et al.* (1994) found the rate of two-year relapse under maintenance and targeted conditions as 23% compared to 48% under targeted conditions alone ($p < .001$). However, in their study not only was the intermittent regime less effective, it was also less popular: 50% refused to continue with the regime (vs. 20% in continuous treatment), presumably due to the higher rate of prodromes and hospitalisation, and perhaps patients also found the responsibility placed on them to recognise relapse an excessive one.

The methodology used to identify relapse prodromes has relied heavily upon patients' skill and their initiative to alert services. Jolley *et al.* (1990) have suggested that a brief educational session is insufficient for patients to sustain a grasp of the prodrome concept

Table 7.3. *Pharmacological early intervention studies*

	No Maintenance		Maintenance and Targeted			Targeted only	
	Gaebel (1994)	Jolley *et al.* (1990)	Carpenter *et al.* (1990)	Gaebel (1994)	Jolley *et al.* (1990)	Carpenter *et al.* (1990)	Gaebel (1994)
	%	%	%	%	%	%	%
Relapse – 1 yr		7			30	–	–
– 2 yr	63	12	36	23	50	53	49
Readmissions – 1 yr		7			13		
Prodromes	50*	27	1.6/year	30*	76	3.18/year	90*
Side effects		55	?		24	?	
Drug-free period		0	0			48	
Non-adherence	56**		19	56**		51	56**

* Percent of relapse accurately predicted.

** Drop out across three conditions combined (no data for each condition).

and early intervention; and the high dropout rate noted by Carpenter *et al.* (1990) underlies its unpopularity. This experience suggests that this responsibility is viewed best as one that is very clearly shared between patient, carer and services.

Experimental designs ask specific questions and hitherto the early intervention studies have asked only limited questions, namely whether a targeted regime alone yields comparable prophylaxis to one which combines maintenance and targeting with the benefit of minimising side-effects. The answer to this is clearly negative.

For present purposes, therefore, our question then becomes, can a 'standard' dose maintenance medication regime combined with a targeting paradigm control relapse to an adequate degree?

The study of Jolley *et al.* (1990) found an unusually low rate of relapse over two years in the group receiving continuous and targeted regimes (12%) suggesting a possible additive effect. Marder *et al.* (1984a,b, 1987) studied patients assigned to a low (5 mg) or standard (25 mg) dose maintenance regime of Fluphenazine Decanoate over two weeks and at the first sign of exacerbation the dose was doubled. If this failed, patients were considered to have relapsed, which occurred in 22% taking the lower dose and 20% on the higher dose, with fewer side-effects in the former. Marder *et al.* (1984a,b, 1987) found that lower doses carried a greater risk of relapse, but these were not 'serious' and were eliminated once the clinician was permitted to double the dose at the onset of a prodrome (the survival curves of the dosage groups were not different under targeted conditions). These data suggest two conclusions. Firstly, by using pharmacotherapy alone, in maintenance and targeted forms, relapse can be reduced to between 12 and 22% over two years; and secondly this can be achieved with a low dose regime.

However, opportunities for early intervention do not rest on this consideration alone. There is first of all the problem of medication non-adherence (Hoge, 1990). Studies of clients' attitudes to medication show that the prevailing view is ambivalent: a necessary evil (Pan & Tantam, 1989). This resistance is linked partly to the experience of dysphoria and other drug side-effects (Hogan *et al.*, 1985) and to a perception that treatment is coercive and disempowering.

Non-adherence has been associated with youth (Davis, 1975), compulsory detention (Buchanan, 1992) and to its excessive use among black groups (Sashidharan, 1993). Early intervention approaches that are essentially client-driven may find favour with

Table 7.4. *Analysis of admissions and days in admission two years pre- and post-trial entry. (Those entering the trial after a first admission are excluded.)*

N=35 patients	Pre-trial entry	Post-trial entry
No. (%) of patients admitted	26 (74)	9 (26)
Total no. of admissions for group	31	10
No. of compulsory admissions	13	1
Days in hospital	2781	729

those who are disaffected by prescriptive approaches. In the wider arena of psychosocial interventions, a titration of drug dose against family intervention has been reported (Falloon *et al.*, 1985; Hogarty *et al.*, 1988); a collaborative approach to early intervention if successful may similarly offer options that allows medication to be used more sparingly than at present, thus maximising its efficacy and attractiveness.

Collaborative early intervention

Collaborative early intervention described here is an attempt to confer in a practical sense empowerment in relation to relapse by placing the individual in the 'driving seat' determining if and how intervention should take place. We (Birchwood, Smith, McGovern & Macmillan, unpub. data) are presently in the midst of a trial of this approach but we are able to present indirect evidence that the impact of collaborative early intervention is a positive one.

Table 7.4 shows a comparison of 35 patients taking part in our early intervention project two years prior to and post trial entry (i.e. non-first episodes). This shows a sharp decline in rates of readmission including compulsory admission and time spent in hospital. We believe the style of service provision is facilitating the engagement with services of a difficult client group who were selected as young, high relapse risk and predominantly inner-city resident. We are also collecting data on a group of clients who have spent two years in the early intervention programme comparing them with a case matched control group on their ability to discriminate and clarify their prodrome; their understanding of the significance of these symptoms and upon their attribution of these symptoms (Davis & Birchwood, unpub. data).

Using the crisis: engaging client and family in a recovery process

Concept of recovery

In clinical practice, recovery from an acute episode is often seen to be accomplished when florid symptoms have ameliorated, a decision frequently relying heavily on subjective judgment.

More precise criteria for recovery have been sought by those researchers and clinicians carrying out empirical studies to compare the outcome of people suffering from psychotic disorders. Research findings suggest the recovery process is only partly negotiated at the remission of positive symptoms, with considerable further recovery realisable especially in the area of social functioning (Brier & Strauss, 1984). One of the phases of social recovery Brier and Strauss call 'convalescence' may last from a few weeks up to a full 12 months post discharge and appears to be contingent upon the availability of supportive, unconditional relationships. Other researchers have attempted to divide the recovery process into 'syndromic' and 'functional' recovery (Dion *et al.*, 1988; Tohen *et al.*, 1992) where the former refers to remission of positive symptoms for a minimum period of six weeks and the latter refers to reinstatement of the patient's occupational status and living circumstances six months prior to the episode. In a sample of 102 in-patients admitted for the first time for a psychotic disorder, Tohen *et al.* (1992) found that whilst 80% had recovered syndromically at six months, only 50% had recovered both functionally **and** syndromically.

Recovery from acute psychosis also involves enormous psychological adjustment and is likely to be hampered by the traumas associated with acute hospital in-patient care such as unfamiliar, stressful and overstimulating ward atmospheres (Kellam *et al.*, 1967), enforced hospitalisation and pathways to care which involve the police and judiciary (e.g. McGorry, 1992).

Consequently, only some patients are able to integrate or understand their psychotic experiences in relation to their other beliefs and experiences, with many patients choosing to 'seal over' or ignore the significance or even the very existence of their psychotic experiences (McGlashan *et al.*, 1975). Absence of the necessary information and support to facilitate the patient's understanding of their illness may contribute to alienation of patients from services, poor medication compliance and as McGorry (1992) suggests, to marked patient deterioration in the first few years after onset and to 'post psychotic collapse' – a state of extreme physical under-activity not necessarily associated with low mood that appears after florid symptoms have remitted (Mino & Ushijima, 1989).

Models of acute care

As recovery has multidimensional aspects and is a difficult path to negotiate effectively, one would expect to find an elaborate system of acute care in operation to facilitate the process, however, nothing could be further from the truth. Psychosocial models of acute care are sadly lacking, with patients being offered little more than medication and 'asylum' in many instances. Where occupational therapy, recreation activities and counselling are available there is rarely an empirical or theoretical base for such intervention. It is not uncommon in our experience for relatives and patients who received routine service provision to comment 'we left hospital as ignorant (about the illness) as we came in'. Homecare models of treatment provide acute care in a more pleasant and familiar environment – the patient's home – but although there has been a shift towards this approach (Burns *et al* 1993), clinical and social outcomes were not significantly different to standard hospital care in two recent studies (Muijen *et al.*, 1992; Burns *et al.*, 1993).

Engagement in psychosocial intervention

Despite the upheaval caused by an acute psychotic episode, it may be an unrivalled opportunity to engage individuals and their families in services. Families are often 'hungry' for information about the course of the illness and how best to cope with difficult and disruptive behaviour when they have just witnessed a relapse or first episode of psychosis.

Families were found to be more willing to enrol in family intervention programmes during times of symptom exacerbation in their relative during hospital admission (Tarrier, 1991) than at times of symptom remission when their relative was living in the community, for which non-compliance rates can be as high as 35% (Smith & Birchwood, 1990).

As well as being more amenable to intervention during an acute admission or period of 'home treatment', patients and their families are also more accessible for education and support, being to some extent a 'captive audience'. Moreover, it may be their initial formal contact with psychiatric services so presenting the first occasion for comprehensive assessment and mobilisation of appropriate help. It has been found that patients with good pre-morbid adjustment, whose carers had received family intervention, were more likely to have symptom reduction and a better level of functioning at discharge and at six-months follow-up than patients whose families had not received such input (Glick *et al.*, 1985). Provision of information about schizophrenia is known to significantly reduce family burden (Sidley *et al.*, 1991; Birchwood *et al.*, 1992) and to be related to significant improvements in the patient's social functioning as perceived by their relatives when measured six months after the intervention (Birchwood *et al.*, 1992).

Psychosocial recovery programme

Thus we believe that the challenge for acute care is to use the crisis as constructively as possible to promote recovery within an ethos of partnership with services. In a study by the authors (Birchwood *et al.*, 1991) an attempt has been made to do just this. Fifty-eight acutely ill patients with a clinical diagnosis of non-affective psychosis were randomly selected from those individuals having a first or subsequent contact with mental health service for an acute psychosis. In addition to routine service provision and monitoring, 20 of these patients were asked to engage in four psychosocial procedures that had two main themes: cognitive therapy for positive symptoms, and provision of a stress limiting and supportive milieu. Another group of 20 patients were asked to engage in recreational pursuits away from the ward for a matched number of hours, and the remaining 18 received minimal monitoring of their symptomology.

The four psychosocial procedures consisted of:

1. Individual cognitive therapy in the context of a supportive interview which involves eliciting evidence for delusional beliefs and beliefs about auditory hallucinations with subsequent challenging of that evidence in reverse order of importance to the belief. This was conducted in an atmosphere of 'collaborative empiricism' as described by Chadwick and Lowe (1990) and Chadwick and Birchwood (1994). This was followed up by empirically testing the belief where appropriate.
2. Group cognitive therapy methods in the context of education about the etiology, nature and treatment of psychotic illness. This

was a manoeuvre to promote 'universality' and to gain insight into their own beliefs by observing the inconsistencies and irrationality in the way others' beliefs hold together.

3. Family education and support conducted with the family. This was an attempt to respond to individual family needs and to reduce family intolerance of difficult behaviour, family anxiety and family impatience for a quick solution or 'cure'. Specific guidance was given with regard to helpful ways of interacting with the patient during the acute episode and how to help the patient manage his/her symptoms. The relapse signature was derived as described previously and fed back to clients and carers.
4. A meaningful activity programme in a relaxed atmosphere away from the ward, to encourage social networking and improve self-esteem.

Along with the principal aim of reducing 'exposure' to florid psychosis using cognitive methods, patients are encouraged to share and understand their experiences in an accepting and empowering manner; families are encouraged to learn more effective ways of problem-solving and to reduce maladaptive ways of coping, and the long-term benefits of contact with services through, for example early signs monitoring, are highlighted. Individuals are encouraged to re-establish their sense of self and to challenge defeatist cognitions such as 'I am a schizophrenic – I am the illness' (Birchwood *et al.*, 1993). The process of recovery can be most effectively negotiated when the individual is aware of their active role in managing the future course of the illness, when their strengths can be harnessed to bring about a process of change and personal growth which can protect them from the damaging effects of stigma (Davidson & Strauss, 1992) and when the individual's conflicts and needs so often manifested in florid symptomatology have been addressed (McGlashan *et al.*, 1975). The following case example, from the above study, demonstrates the last point.

A 25-year-old girl whose life had begun to revolve around a fantasy relationship with a radio DJ, was experiencing ideas of reference, telepathy and auditory hallucinations which supported her delusional belief. After she had received an intensive period of cognitive and supportive therapy she was able to express her new found strength and understanding thus:

'I feel I was pursuing something through the whole episode – perhaps it was the meaning of life. I thought the meaning of life was the

> fourth-dimension of the gods and spirits. I intellectualised about aloneness, separateness and oppression, but really all I want to say is that I'm lonely, I want a boyfriend – I couldn't say these things before. My whole life became the radio – I had no other friends – real life became suspended. I'm sure it won't happen like that again'.

She like many of the other patients receiving the intervention have achieved good recovery and they recognise the importance of service involvement. From the data available at the time of writing it would appear that patients receiving the intervention achieve qualitatively different recoveries to those receiving recreational activities and routine service provision with 65% of those in the intervention group achieving a full recovery or complete remission of positive symptoms compared with 35% in the recreational activity control group (see Table 7.5, overleaf). Furthermore, those in the intervention group were more likely to have ongoing involvement with services, have taken advantage of pre-vocational training or be working, be compliant with medication and avoided readmission and relapse.

Conclusions

Recovery from an acute psychotic episode is a much longer and more complex process than hitherto fully appreciated (McGorry, 1992; Davidson & Strauss, 1992) lasting for up to a full 12 months post discharge and beyond (Brier & Strauss, 1984). Social, psychological and illness factors appear to interact to affect the speed and quality of the recovery. The challenge for professionals involved in acute care is to rise to the potential of the crisis by involving patients and families long-term in services in a collaborative rather than passive way and to facilitate an enduring recovery which increase patients' self-knowledge, understanding and mastery of their illness (Davidson & Strauss, 1992). Changing the model of acute care is likely to need considerable change in approach and training.

Table 7.5. *Outcome of patients receiving cognitive intervention compared with recreational activity controls*

	Control (n = 20) %	Cognitive intervention (n = 19) %
Attending out-patient department	60	80
Other involvement with services	25	70
Medication complicance	55	95
Completed prevocational training or working	35	50
Early relapse or readmission	30	15
Full remission of positive symptoms	35	65

References

American Psychiatric Association (1987). *Diagnostic and Statistical Manual of Mental Disorders*. 3rd edn. Washington DC, American Psychiatric Association.

Birchwood, M., Mason, R. & Macmillan, J. (1993). Depression, demoralisation and control over psychotic illness. *Psychological Medicine*, **23**, 387–95.

Birchwood, M. & Smith, J. (1990). Relatives and patients as partners in the management of schizophrenia: a service model. *British Journal of Psychiatry*, **156**, 654–60.

Birchwood, M., Smith, J. & Cochrane, R. (1991). Specific and non-specific effects of educational intervention for families living with schizophrenia: a comparison of three methods. *British Journal of Psychiatry*, **160**, 806–14.

Birchwood, M., Smith, J. & Macmillan, F. (1992). Early intervention. In *Innovations in the Psychological Management of Schizophrenia*, ed. M.J. Birchwood, and N. Tarrier, Chichester, Wiley.

Birchwood, M., Smith, J., Macmillan, F., Hogg, B., Prasad, R., Harvey, C. & Bering, S. (1989). Predicting relapse in schizophrenia: the development and implementation of an early signs monitoring system using patients and families as observers. *Psychological Medicine*, **19**, 649–56.

Brier, A. & Strauss, J. S. (1983). Self control in psychiatric disorders. *Archives of General Psychiatry*, **40**, 1141–5.

Brewin, C. (1988). *Cognitive Foundations of Clinical Psychology*. Lawrence Erlbaum Associates.

Buchanan, A. (1992). A two year prospective study treatment compliance in patients with schizophrenia. *Psychological Medicine*, **22**, 787–97.

Burns, T., Beadsmoore, A., Bhat, A., Oliver, A. & Mathers, C. (1993). A controlled trial of home-based acute psychiatric services. I. Clinical and social outcome. *British Journal of Psychiatry*, **163**, 49–54.

Caldwell, C. B. & Gottesman, I. (1990). Schizophrenics kill themselves too. *Schizophrenia Bulletin*, **16**, 571–90.

Carpenter, W. I., Hanlon, T. E., Heinrichs, D. W., Summerfelt, A. T., Kirkpatrick, B., Levine, J. & Buchanan, R. W. (1990). Continuous versus targeted medication in schizophrenic outpatients: outcome results. *American Journal of Psychiatry*, **147**, 1138–48.

Chadwick, P. & Birchwood, M. (1994). Challenging the omnipotence of voices: a cognitive approach to auditory hallucinations. *British Journal of Psychiatry*, **164**, 190–201.

Chadwick, P. & Lowe, C. (1990). Measurement and modification of delusional beliefs. *Journal of Consulting and Clinical Psychology*, **58**, 225–32.

Davidson, L. & Strauss, J. (1992). Sense of self in recovery from severe mental illness. *British Journal of Medical Psychology*, **65**, 131–45.

Davis, J. M. (1975). Overview: maintenance therapy in psychiatry. I. Schizophrenia. *American Journal of Psychiatry*, **132**, 1237–45.

Derogatis, L., Lipman, R. & Covi, L. (1973). SCL – 90: An outpatient psychiatric rating scale – preliminary report. *Psychopharmacology Bulletin*, **9**, 13–17.

Dion, G., Tohen, M., Anthony, B. & Waternaux, C. (1988). Symptoms and functioning of patients with bipolar disorder six months after hospitalisation. *Hospital and Community Psychiatry*, **39**, 652–7.

Falloon, J. R. H., Boyd, J. L. & McGill, C. W. (1985). Family management in the prevention of morbidity of schizophrenia. *Archives of General Psychiatry*, **42**, 887–96.

Gaebel, V., Frick, W. & Kopeke, M. (1994). Early neuroleptic intervention in schizophrenia. *British Journal of Psychiatry*, **163**, 8–12.

Glick, I., Clarkin, J., Spencer, J., Haas, G., Lewis, A., Peyser, J., Demane, N., Good-Ellis, M., Harris, E. & Lestelle, B. (1985). A controlled evaluation of in-patient family intervention. *Archives of General Psychiatry*, **42**, 882–7.

Heinrichs, D., *et al.* (March 1985). Early insight and the management of schizophrenic decomposition. *The Journal of Nervous and Mental Disease*, **173**, p. 133.

Heinrichs, D. W. & Carpenter, W. T. (1985). Prospective study of prodromal symptoms in schizophrenic relapse. *American Journal Psychiatry*, **143**, 3.

Herz, M. I., Glazer, W., Mirza, M., Mostest, M. & Hafez, H. (1989). Treating prodromal episodes to prevent relapse in schizophrenia. *British Journal of Psychiatry* (Supp. 5), 123–7.

Herz, M. & Melville, C. (1980). Relapse in schizophrenic. *American Journal of Psychiatry*, **137**, 801–12.

Herz, M. I., Szymonski, H. V. & Simon, J. (1982). Intermittent medication for stable schizophrenic outpatients. *American Journal of Psychiatry*, **139**, 918–22.

Hirsch, S. & Jolley, A. (1989). The dysphoric syndrome in schizophrenia and its implications for relapse. *British Journal of Psychiatry* (Supp. 5), 46–50.

Hogan, T. P., Awed, A. G. & Eastwood, M. R. (1985). Earls subjective response and prediction of outcome to Neuroleptic drug treatment in schizophrenia. *Canadian Journal of Psychiatry*, **30**, 246–8.

Hogarty, G. E. (1993). Prevention of relapse in chronic schizophrenic patients. *Journal of Clinical Psychiatry*, **54**(3), 18–23.

Hogarty, G. E., Anderson, C. M., Reiss, D. J. *et al.* (1991). Family psycho-education, social skills training and maintenance chemotherapy in the after care treatment of schizophrenia. II Two-year effects of a controlled study on relapse and adjustment. *Archives of General Psychiatry*, **48**, 340–7.

Hogarty, G. E., McEvoy, J. P. & Munetz, M. (1988). Dose of Fluphenazine, familial expressed emotion and outcome in schizophrenia. *Archives General Psychiatry*, **45**, 797–805.

Hoge, S. K. (1990). A prospective multicentre study of patients refusal of anti-psychotic medication. *Archives General Psychiatry*, **47**, 949–56.

Jolley, A. G., Hirsch, S. R., Morrison, G., McRink, A. & Wilson, L. (1990). Trial of brief intermittent neuroleptic prophylaxis for selected schizophrenia outpatients: clinical and social outcome at two years. *British Medical Journal*, **301**, 847–42.

Kellam, S., Goldber, S., Schooler, N., Berman, A. & Schmelzer, J. (1967). Ward atmosphere and outcome of treatment of acute schizophrenia. *Journal of Psychiatric Research*, **5**, 145–63.

Kumar, S., Thara, R. & Rajkumar, S. (1989). Coping with symptoms of relapse in schizophrenia. *European Archives of Psychiatry and Neurological Sciences*, **239**, 213–15.

Marder, S. R., Mintz, J., Van Putten, T., Lebell, M., Wirsching, W. & Johnstone-Cronk, K. (1991). Prodromal symptoms of schizophrenia: an application of receiver–operator methodology. *Psychopharmacology Bulletin*, **27**, 79–82.

Marder, S., Van Putten, T., Mintz, J., Labell, M., Mckenzie, J. & Faltico, G. (1984a). Maintenance therapy in schizophrenia: new findings. In *Drug Maintenance strategies in schizophrenia*, ed. J. Kane, Washington D.C., American Psychiatric Press.

Marder, S., Van Putten, T., Mintz, J., McKenzie, J., Lebell, M., Fztico, G. & May, R. P. (1984b). Costs and benefits of two doses of fluphenazine. *Archives of General Psychiatry*, **41**, 1025–9.

Marder, S., Van Putten, T., Mintz, J., McKenzie, J., Lebell, M., Fztico, G. & May, R. P. (1987). Low and conventional dose maintenance therapy with Fluphenazine Decanoate. *Archives of General Psychiatry*, **44**, 518–21.

McCandless-Glincher, L., McKnight, S., Hamera, E., Smith, B. L., Peterson, K. & Plumlee, A. A. (1986). Use of symptoms by schizophrenics to monitor and regulate their illness. *Hospital and Community Psychiatry*, **37**, 929–33.

McGlashan, T. (1988). A selective review of recent North American follow-up studies of schizophrenia. *Schizophrenia Bulletin*, **14**, 515–42.
McGlashan, T., Levy, S. & Carpenter, W. (1975). Integration and sealing over clinically distinct recovery styles from schizophrenia. *Archives of General Psychiatry*, **32**, 1269–72.
McGorry, P. (1992). The concept of recovery and secondary prevention in psychotic disorders. *Australian and New Zealand Journal of Psychiatry*, **26**, 3–17.
Mueser, K. T., Bellack, A. S., Wade, J. H., Sayers, S. Z. & Rosenthal, L. K. (1992). An assessment of the educational needs of chronic psychiatric patients and their relatives. *British Journal of Psychiatry*, **160**, 668–73.
Mino, Y. & Ushijima, S. (1989). Post psychotic collapse in schizophrenia. *Acta Psychiatrica Scandinavica*, **80**, 368–74.
Muijen, M., Marks, I., Connolly, J., *et al.* (1992). Home-based care and standard hospital care for patients with severe mental illness: a randomised controlled trial. *British Medical Journal*, **304**, 749–54.
Overall, J. E. & Graham, D. R. (1962). The brief psychiatric rating scale. *Psychological Reports*, **10**, 99–812.
Pan, R. & Tantam, D. (1989). Clinical characteristics, health beliefs, and compliance with maintenance treatment: a comparison between regular and irregular attenders at a depot clinic. *Acta Psychiatrica Scandinavia*, **7**, 564–70.
Robert, G. (1991). Delusional belief systems and meaning in life: a preferred reality. *British Journal of Psychiatry*, **159** (supp 14), 19–28.
Sashidharan, S. (1993). Afro-Caribbeans and schizophrenia: the ethnic vulnerability hypothesis examined. *International Review of Psychiatry*, **5**, 129–44.
Shepherd, G., (1990). Case management. *Health Trends*, **22**, 59–61.
Sidley, G., Smith, J. & Howells, K. (1991). Is it ever too late to learn? Information provision to relatives of long-term schizophrenia sufferers. *Behavioural Psychotherapy*, **19**, 305–20.
Smith, J. & Birchwood, M. (1990). Relatives and patients as partners in the management of schizophrenia. *British Journal of Psychiatry*, **156**, 654–60.
Smith, J., Birchwood, M. & Haddrell, A. (1992). Challenging schizophrenic patients' construction and understanding of her illness: the effect of residual symptoms. *Journal of Mental Health*, **1**, 61–70.
Stein, L. I. (1993). A system approach to reducing relapse in schizophrenia. *Journal of Clinical Psychiatry*, **54** (Supp.), 7–12.
Strauss, J. S. (1989). Subjective experiences of schizophrenia: toward a new dynamic. *Schizophrenia Bulletin*, **15**, 179–88.
Strauss, J. S. (1991). The person with delusions. *British Journal of Psychiatry*, **159** (Suppl. 14, 57–61.
Subotnik, K. L. & Nuechterlein, K. H. (1988). Prodromal signs and symptoms of schizophrenic relapse. *Journal of Abnormal Psychology*, **97**, 405–12.
Tarrier, N. (1991). Some aspects of family interventions in schizophrenia.

1: Adherence to intervention programmes. *British Journal of Psychiatry*, **159**, 475–80.

Tohen, M., Stoll, A., Strakowowski, M., Faedda, G., Mayer, A., Goodwin, D., Kolbrener, M. & Madigan, A. (1992). The McClean first episode psychosis project: six-month recover and recurrence outcome. *Schizophrenia Bulletin*, **18**(2), 283–93.

Wing, J. K., Cooper, J. & Sartorious, N. (1974). *The Description and Classification of Psychiatric Symptomatology: An Instruction Manual for the PSE and CATEGO Systems*. Cambridge University Press: London.

8

Community assessment of crisis

KIM SUTHERBY AND GEORGE SZMUKLER

Introduction

In Britain, crisis assessments have traditionally either been provided by a consultant carrying out a domiciliary visit in the patient's home or by a psychiatric trainee in the hospital setting. With the growth of community mental health services other options are now available. In this chapter the effects of a change from a unidisciplinary medical assessment to multidisciplinary assessments, and the change of setting from hospital to community are briefly discussed. The remainder of this chapter considers those aspects of a crisis assessment that are particularly relevant or altered by the change to a community setting, and the often conflicting ethical principles encountered in the practice of community psychiatry.

Multidisciplinary assessments compared to a unidisciplinary medical assessment

In the traditional hospital based service the consultant domiciliary visit was generally the only form of community outreach available. Although originally intended as a joint visit between consultant and general practitioner (GP), such joint visits now rarely occur (Littlejohns, 1986; Donaldson & Hill, 1991). Consultant domiciliary visits (DVs) are most commonly requested in the specialities of psychiatry and geriatrics (Smith & Blythe, 1971), and requests for psychiatric DVs have increased by two-thirds over the past 20 years (Sutherby, K., Strathdee, G. & Macdonald, A. J. D. Domiciliary visits in the South East Thames Region: twenty years of change. Unpublished research report, 1994).

Specialist multidisciplinary crisis intervention and home treatment teams are still uncommon at present, existing in only 15% of districts, while only 3% of districts have such teams available 24 hours a day (Johnson & Thornicroft, 1991). Two members of a multidisciplinary team typically carry out visits, thus they are able to provide a range of skills in the assessment, and improve safety. The aim of a crisis intervention team is usually to provide home-based assessment and treatment, and they claim to be able to provide more detailed assessments of cases, more liaison with other services and have an increased number of sessions with clients and carers (Coles *et al.*, 1991; Burns *et al.*, 1993). Although the rapid response and comprehensive care provided by such teams is often very popular with GPs, some are unhappy to accept liaison and advice from non-medical professionals (Dening, 1992). In contrast, a home visit by a consultant fulfils the need for an experienced medical opinion and can provide more continuity of care for patients with a long-term mental illness. However, it is more likely to result in hospital or out-patient follow-up than home-based treatment (Sutherby *et al.*, 1992).

There has been little research so far comparing multidisciplinary crisis assessments with that of the traditional medical assessment either in the community or hospital. Colligham *et al.* (1993) looked at the reliability of diagnostic assessments made by two community psychogeriatric teams, who used standardised assessment schedules and presented all cases at the weekly team meeting where an initial diagnosis was made. When these diagnoses were compared with independent formal assessments made by research psychiatrists there was a level of agreement ranging from 90–99%. There was no significant difference between medical and non-medical team members in their diagnostic accuracy, and increased accuracy was associated with longer experience of team-working regardless of the team members' background.

The hospital setting compared to the community setting for an assessment

The change of environment for assessments from hospital to community can facilitate a change in the service philosophy and the professional–patient interaction. Traditional hospital-based services have been criticised for being inflexible – patients are either expected to accept the limited service available or receive no care, or, at worst management decisions are made to fit the routine of the institution (Rassaby & Rogers, 1987). When patients are assessed in the home or community they can more easily be seen in their social context and services developed to fit their needs. Jones *et al.* (1987) followed up 200 patients after they were seen for non-urgent home assessments by a multidisciplinary team. They found that the majority (80%) felt that the assessors had gained a better idea of their difficulties because they were seen at home and only 12% would have preferred to have been seen in the out-patient clinic or a GP's surgery. If, as a result of a home assessment the patient feels that their difficulties have been understood they are more likely to trust the professional involved and co-operate in the management plan. The personal aspect of being allowed to observe the patient's home and subtle aspects of their personality demonstrated in their choice of belongings, interests and type of environment can facilitate a closer rapport as well as contributing to the assessment.

Urgent home assessments will not be viewed so positively if the referral is not initiated by the patient asking for help or where the patient does not accept that they have a mental health problem. In such circumstances a home visit may seem intrusive and threatening. This is particularly the case when the assessment is for compulsory admission under the 1983 Mental Health Act. One of the reasons most commonly stated by patients for preferring to be seen in their GP's surgery, away from the hospital, is that this reduces stigma (Tyrer, 1984). However, the reverse may be the case in crisis assessments where the presence of mental health professionals, sometimes accompanied by the police, may draw local attention to the patient involved and can be potentially more stigmatising in the long-term unless handled discretely. Assessments for a compulsory admission under the Mental Health Act may have been the only reason a patient received a home visit in a hospital-based service, and the introduction of additional visits from a community psychiatric nurse (CPN) or multidisciplinary team may be initially viewed with reasonable suspicion.

Community assessment strategy

The form of the assessment of psychiatric disorder in a crisis is essentially unchanged by the move from the hospital to the community, but the emphasis of the assessment changes from a narrow focus on the patient's diagnosis to a wider assessment of the functioning of the individual in his or her social context. Our discussion of a community assessment strategy is therefore based on those aspects where the change in environment is particularly relevant. For a general guide to carrying out a psychiatric interview we would refer readers to a standard psychiatric text (Departments of Psychiatry and Child Psychiatry, 1987).

Preparation

Information gathering

In preparing to make a visit for a community assessment it is important to gather as much background information as possible so that the single assessment visit can be seen in context and details of the history verified. The referral may have been received from the GP, other professionals, carers or relatives, or directly from the patient. Where possible, at least one of those involved in the referral should be contacted directly or invited to be present at the assessment. It is useful to clarify the nature, severity and duration of the current problem, any details of similar problems and treatment in the past, the effect of the problem on the functioning both of the patient and their family or immediate community. It is also important to clarify what is being sought from the referral. The referrers are more likely to be satisfied with the outcome if it is known at the outset whether an opinion and advice on an aspect of management is all that is required, or a comprehensive assessment with a management plan implemented by the psychiatric services. It is also important to obtain details of episodes of violence in the past, both to determine the appropriate levels of back-up required at the assessment, and to assist in the assessment of future risk.

Arranging where the interview is to take place and who is to be present

The choice of interview venue is not confined to hospital or home. Those who attend day centres, or voluntary sector organisations, can sometimes be interviewed there; the GP's surgery is another possibility. Assessments carried out in this way may be safer for the assessor, less threatening to some patients, and provides access to people who may know the patient. The practice of arranging assessments in voluntary sector settings is particularly encouraged by black and ethnic minority voluntary groups (Goldberg *et al.*, 1993) as a way of overcoming the mistrust of statutory services dominated by white staff (Mercer, 1984).

It is important to consider whether to invite the GP or those closely involved in the patient's care without overwhelming the patient with excessive numbers. Where the patient has an established history of mental illness they may have a friend or advocate (Binder 1985; Freddolino *et al.*, 1989) whom they might wish to be invited. An interpreter will be required if the patient is not fluent in English. The use of a family member as an interpreter is not ideal as they may unintentionally inhibit the patient from expressing 'unacceptable feelings' or suicidal thoughts (Steinberg, 1991). An interpreter should have experience of the type of psychiatric symptoms that occur, to ensure that they do not paraphrase or rationalise abnormal phenomena. Despite the potential problems, patients interviewed with an interpreter report feeling more understood, more satisfied with the help provided and more likely to return for further treatment than patients who know some English and are seen without an interpreter (Kline *et al.*, 1980).

Arranging an appropriate level of back-up for safe working practices

Concern is often expressed about the vulnerability of mental health workers making home assessments without immediate back-up. However, the Health Services Advisory Committee survey of the NHS (1987) indicated that the working environments where major physical injuries were most common were psychiatric hospitals, mental handicap settings and accident and emergency departments despite the numbers of staff available. Staff working in the community had experienced relatively low levels of physical assault but high levels of verbal aggression. A number of studies have reported a progressive increase in in-patient violence (Haller & Deluty, 1988; Noble & Rodger, 1989). The reasons are unclear, but may include the movement of more able patients to the community leaving a higher concentration of severely disturbed patients in hospital.

A community assessment in a familiar and less threatening setting may reduce the frequency of physical violence, although when it does occur the potential risk is greater. As a precaution, team guidelines on safe working practices should be agreed and consistently applied.

These may involve allocating a team member who will be informed of the details of: where the visit will be, who is being seen, the expected time of return and procedure to be followed if the team is not contacted by an agreed time. An example of guidelines developed for the use of a team working in an inner city area is given in Table 8.1. Where there is a past history of violence or likely to be other risk factors for violence (see Table 8.3), assessments should not be made alone but with another professional or possibly accompanied by the police.

History taking

History from patient

Referrals are often initiated by a family member or neighbour when the patient is unwilling to accept that they have a problem or to seek help in the conventional way. Such referrals, made without the patient's agreement and sometimes without their knowledge, can create great difficulties in establishing a therapeutic alliance and common aims. In such circumstances the assessor needs to be seen to be neutral and additional history should, where possible, be obtained from a family member not initiating the referral (Viaro & Peruzzi, 1983). One should usually offer to see the patient alone before seeing them with the family or other informant.

History from carer/family

The immediate carers may be the patient's family or staff of a residential home. The patient who lives alone may have a network of caring supportive relationships with neighbours, friends or regular visitors such as their home help, 'befriender' or church visitor. The carers can provide valuable background information on the current episode, the patient's normal functioning and their level of dependence. Assessments of the symptoms and behaviour problems of long-term psychiatric patients living in the community using interviews with families or residential staff reveal much higher levels of problems than interviews either with the patient alone or with staff only in contact with the patient during the day (Brewin *et al.*, 1990). Families may also be a source of information on signs of early relapse (Birchwood *et al.*, 1989), particularly if the patient and their family are already known to the service and preliminary work has been carried out to

Table 8.1 *Safety guidelines for community interviewing*

Prior to every interview
- Check patient details for any history of violence or threatening behaviour. If there is any known or suspected history **DO NOT GO ALONE**. Discuss with staff who know patient, and if it felt to be safe, arrange joint interview.
- Check patient's address, and that you know exactly where to go.
- Tell someone where you are going, who you are going to see and when you expect to be back.
- Remember to carry your identification.

Going to the interview
- Carry as little as possible, leaving unnecessary valuables and cash behind.
- Walk purposefully towards your destination, avoid walking through groups of young people, and avoid eye contact with anyone who is thought to be potentially threatening.
- If anyone does snatch at a bag, let it go: personal safety is paramount.
- In 'dodgy' or unknown areas, first visits should be made in daylight.
- When meeting a person for the first time on their doorstep, if you are worried for any reason, arrange to come back another day with someone else.

During the interview
- If you are uneasy, or in danger **LEAVE**. You can always come back with someone else another day.
- Be aware of exit routes, and position yourself so that the interviewee is not between you and the exit.

After the interview
- Inform the team of your return.
- If you had any concerns at all during the interview, discuss them with the rest of your team, and make sure that it is recorded.

provide education and involve the family in the planning of management (Intagliata *et al.*, 1986; Smith & Birchwood, 1990).

Examination

Mental state and home environment

The formal mental state examination can be assisted by observation of the patient's living space for evidence of the patient's level of self care and cues that may indicate abnormal beliefs, deficits in cognitive function, and the presence or level of substance abuse. Specific items can be incorporated into a discrete assessment of cognitive function, for example asking the patient to name people in photographs. Abnormal beliefs which are otherwise difficult to elicit can become evident from questions about what appear to be unusual or symbolic arrangements of objects or furnishings. Aspects of the patient's personality such as obsessional traits may be demonstrated in a meticulously ordered environment. Cues to more subtle aspects of their character, interests and social group may be recognised from photographs, pictures or books. An assessment in the home and in the company of relatives or carers provides a unique opportunity to observe relationships and patterns of interaction and one may make an informal assessment of the level of 'expressed emotion' (Vaughan & Leff, 1976). Although access to lethal methods of self-harm such as inhalation of exhaust fumes or self-poisoning are almost universally available, during an assessment in the home the unusual availability of methods of self-harm such as firearms or high rise accommodation can be taken into account (Salmons 1984; Marzuk *et al.*, 1992).

Social state

One aspect of the medical assessment that tends to receive inadequate attention in the hospital setting is the section that describes the social circumstances of the patient. In the hospital setting this is usually based solely on information from the patient, whereas in the home this can be verified. The social resources of the patient can be recorded under the five headings of: accommodation, finances, home activities, outside activities, and details of formal and informal carers (Campbell & Szmukler, 1993). A description of the accommodation should include the type of home, quality of the environment, access and security. Financial assessment would include the source of income, ability to budget, any debts and whether the illness results in excessive expenditure. An assessment under the heading of home activities would include an assessment of the patient's ability to carry out daily living skills, how they spend a typical day and relationships with immediate neighbours. Outside activities should describe a person's occupation, social contacts and the ease and frequency with which they shop, travel or attend social functions (e.g. pub, cinema). Issues such as the difference in age and sex between carer and patient, their other commitments or employment, proximity to the home, physical and mental health, and the nature and quality of their relationships should be noted. Details of formal carers such as NHS, social service or voluntary sector staff, should be recorded. Obtaining information on other services that are involved is important to avoid duplication of effort and to improve liaison between multiple agencies.

All such information is more easily obtained during an assessment in the home either directly from observation, by recognising which questions or problems are most likely to be relevant, or because of the opportunity to ask others. Such questions are more likely to be acceptable to the patient as normal social enquiry in contrast to such questions posed in a hospital setting.

Assessing the feasibility and appropriateness of home based treatment

A series of studies over the past 15 years have indicated that where a comprehensive community service is available, most people with acute psychiatric illness can be treated at home for the majority of their illness (Dedman, 1993). No studies have found hospital care to provide a better outcome than home care. Community services are preferred by patients and relatives and are also more effective in keeping patients in long-term follow-up (Dean *et al.*, 1993). However, it is likely that there will remain a proportion of patients with high dependency needs who require the safe environment and 24-hour staffing of a hospital.

The factors associated with admission to hospital as an outcome of an emergency psychiatric assessment have been reviewed by Gerson and Bassuk (1980) and more recently by Marson, *et al.* (1988). From their review Gerson and Bassuk concluded that a model that focused on the 'patient's and the community's adaptive resources and competence' and minimised subtle diagnostic considerations would be of more practical value in assessment than the current hospital orientated 'severity and symptom based model'. Their proposed model considered the following factors: (i) the nature and availability of the support system and the capacity of the patient to use it, (ii) dangerousness, (iii) psychiatric history and current status, (iv) ability to self care, (v) motivation and capacity to participate in the treatment process, (vi) the requests of patient and family and (vii) medical status. The social characteristics of the patient and referral have been found to be more likely than illness factors (such as diagnosis) to determine which patients can be treated at home (Dean & Gadd, 1990).

A small number of studies have sought to develop rating instruments to assist in the decision whether to admit a patient in a psychiatric emergency (Warner, 1961; Whittington, 1966; Flynn & Henisz, 1975), but none of these early scales have so far been evaluated prospectively. Bengelsdorf *et al.* (1984) developed a brief crisis triage rating scale (CTRS) for use by a mobile multidisciplinary crisis intervention team based on three dimensions of: dangerousness, support system and ability or motivation to co-operate in a management plan. This study reported that the decisions based on the CTRS were concordant with clinical decisions to admit in 97% of cases. But in this first study, clinical decisions were influenced by the CTRS scores. A later replication using the scale in a hospital emergency department where independent assessments were made, found a concordance rate of 75% when the cut-off score was adjusted for the different environment (Turner & Turner, 1991). Stepwise discriminant analysis indicated that dangerousness was the most influential factor in the decision to admit, followed by the availability of family, friends and community support. The patient's motivation and capacity to co-operate contributed least, but gave an indication of their ability to avoid hospitalisation by attendance at out-patients. Following a similar model to Gerson and Bassuk and the CTRS, we will first discuss whether home-care is feasible, and secondly whether home care is appropriate. The feasibility of home-based care is determined by considering the following two factors:

- The risk of self and others as a result of the patient's illness.
- The available community support, supervision and the degree of risk that is acceptable to the family and immediate environment.

The risk to self and others as a result of the patient's illness

There has been concern that for a number of reasons, failures in the planning of community care may contribute to an increased risk of suicide for the mentally ill. These include: fragmentation of services, hostility to the medical model, difficulties in monitoring and evaluation, and premature discharge of patients from under-resourced in-patient facilities (Morgan & Priest, 1991; Morgan, 1992). It is therefore particularly important that a careful assessment of suicide risk is made, and that continuity of care and follow-up in the community is provided for individuals identified as vulnerable.

Although suicide is a rare event in the general population, the risk of suicide in the year following an attempt is approximately 1%. As a result, there have been numerous attempts to develop rating scales to identify risk factors for suicide of which two of the best known and most validated are those of Tuckman and Youngman (1968) and the Suicide Intent Scale developed by Beck *et al.* (1974). Suicide risk factors are useful in identifying high risk groups of individuals and planning service interventions, but cannot be relied upon to predict risk in the individual patient due to the rarity of the predicted event and the low sensitivity and specificity of such scales (Pokorny, 1983; Pallis *et al.*, 1984; Hawton, 1987). Another limitation is that most scales have been developed for the assessment of long-term risk. Few have addressed short-term risk to assist the clinician in planning immediate management (Fawcett *et al.*, 1990). A summary of the main factors that need to be considered when making an assessment of suicide risk following a prior attempt is given in Table 8.2. For a more detailed account of suicide assessment see Hawton and Catalan (1987). Whether there is a history of a prior attempt or not, the patient should always be asked directly about suicidal ideas or intent. Although fleeting suicidal ideas are common in the general population, a statement of intent or suicidal plans should be taken seriously.

The prediction of violence and assessments of dangerousness are generally accepted to be difficult and at best an inexact science (Chiswick, 1988; Whittington & Wykes, 1994). The most reliable predictor of violent behaviour is previous violent behaviour and this underlines the importance of gaining background information (including any forensic history) prior to assessment, plus high standards of communication and clinical recording (Noble & Rogers, 1989). The likelihood of violent behaviour may be predicted from identifying circumstances in which violence has occurred in the past, and assessing whether similar circumstances are likely to occur again, for example when a person who has been violent due to morbid jealousy starts a new relationship. Violence closely associated with acute episodes of a long-term mental illness can be anticipated when relapses are likely due to stopping maintenance medication. In a large community survey in the United States, Swanson *et al.* (1990) concluded that the presence of a diagnosis of a major mental disorder raised the risk of violence above that of the general population. However, much higher levels of violence were reported by those patients with a diagnosis of alcohol or drug abuse (Table 8.3), and the levels of violence increased further when drug or alcohol misuse co-existed with a major mental disorder or when the patient had multiple psychiatric diagnoses.

Table 8.2 *Factors associated with a risk of completed suicide following a previous attempt*

Sociodemographic
- Age 45 or older
- Sex male
- Ethnicity white
- Marital status separated, divorced, widowed
- Living alone
- Unemployed or retired

Recent sociodemographic 'at risk' groups
- Young Asian females
- Young males

Medical and psychiatric history
- Affective disorder (risk early in disorder)
- Schizophrenia (risk early in disorder)
- Alcohol abuse (risk later in disorder)
- Anorexia nervosa
- Poor physical health
- Medical care in previous six months

Family history
- Family history of completed suicide

Precipitants
- Bereavement; particularly if a previous psychiatric history and a lack of family support

Method
- Violent methods: hanging, firearms, jumping or drowning
- Dangerousness of the attempt in self-poisoning not a good indicator unless the patient has specialist knowledge

Circumstances of the attempt
- Season (April–September)
- Time of day (6 a.m.–6 p.m.)
- Attempt made at own or someone else's home
- Suicide note

Suicidal intent
- Precautions made against discovery
- Seeking help during, or after, the attempt
- Actions in anticipation of death
- Degree or planning for the attempt

Accidental self-harm is most likely to occur in patients suffering from a functional or organic psychotic illness and may arise from poor concentration, apathy, memory impairment, psychotic experiences, disinhibition or distractibility. The types of risks that should be considered are those of the patient: being a fire hazard either from

Table 8.3. *Factors associated with a risk of violence*

Sociodemographic
- Age under 45
- Sex male
- Low socio-economic status

Medical and psychiatric history
- A history of violence, especially recent violence
- Drug or alcohol abuse
- Major mental disorder, especially if thought disordered or hallucinated
- Co-morbidity (two or more diagnoses)
- Experiencing pain

Family history
- Violence in the family of origin

Behaviour
- Verbally abusive and/or issuing threats,
- Speaking in a loud voice or is suddenly silent
- Overactive and aroused or suddenly stops moving
- Suspicious

Interactions where someone has to:
- Enforce rules or deny privileges
- Demand activity from the patient
- Intrude on and/or touch the patient

smoking or leaving electrical appliances on (Phelan & Fisher, 1993), leaving the front door open, wandering at night or taking an accidental overdose. Self-neglect resulting in failure to eat or drink adequately may be acute and severe and potentially life threatening in a major depressive episode, or may result in a slow deterioration in health and nutritional status. In the long-term mentally ill the possibility of such a slow decline may not be recognised until the patient is assessed in his or her own home and the lack of provisions, or facilities becomes apparent. Patients with mental illness have higher than average rates of physical illness, which are often untreated (Brugha *et al.*, 1989). Close liaison with the GP and primary care team will assist in obtaining appropriate physical care for patients who are to be treated in the community (Honig *et al.*, 1992). Where there are indications that the patient may be suffering from an acute physical illness, particularly where this may be a cause of the psychiatric crisis (e.g. acute confusional states in the elderly), an urgent medical assessment should be arranged and, if necessary, treatment on a medical ward.

When the patient is the only active adult in the household, the risk of neglect of children or an elderly or infirm relative needs to be considered. The patient must be willing to accept assistance in the home or the child or relative should be temporarily transferred to an alternative caring environment (social services, hospital or relatives). Where possible, the assessment should include both a short- and long-term assessment of risk rather than being a snapshot of behaviour. Further deterioration may be predictable in circumstances where compliance with medication is reduced or refused, and an assessment and management plan should take this into account.

The available community support, supervision and the degree of risk that is acceptable

The level of support and supervision available from the family or other informal carers depends on whether the carer shares the home with the patient, whether they have other commitments (such as a part-time job), whether they have other dependants (such as children or elderly relatives), and whether their own physical or mental health is good. Lesser degrees of support and supervision may be provided by neighbours or friends who may be willing and able to visit on a regular basis. If the patient is socially isolated, alternative sources of support may be available through the voluntary sector in the form of befriending schemes, church visiting schemes or other voluntary sector initiatives.

If support is to come from informal carers the patient needs to be willing for some information to be shared with them (Petrila & Sadoff, 1992). They need to be provided with contact numbers so that they can inform a key worker or team member and obtain further assistance should acute difficulties arise. One strategy is to involve the patient and carer in formulating a written management plan (Falloon & Fadden, 1993), copies of which will be provided for the patient, the identified carer, the psychiatric team and GP. This plan may include an agreement for medication intake to be regularly monitored by a carer, the named keyworker for the patient and their contact number or address, details of the GP's involvement and information on who to contact in a crisis 24-hours a day, as well as information about available support for the carer. An assessment needs to be made of whether these carers are able to understand any risks involved, whether they are able to monitor or manage such situations appropriately, judge when further assistance is required, accept a management plan which involves them and find the potential level of risk acceptable and manageable.

If the patient lives alone, practical issues need to be considered such as whether they are able to cope with the demands of daily living (attending to cooking, self-hygiene, managing the home and finances) whilst acutely unwell. Where the patient is not able to cope, are informal carers able to provide sufficient help or can social services provide adequate temporary support in the form of home help, meals on wheels or a luncheon club? Formal care in the community may be available from a multidisciplinary team that provides home treatment visits. Alternatively, day care may be provided from a day hospital that is able to accept urgent referrals, social services or voluntary sector day centres.

If home care is considered to be viable, the next decision is whether home care is appropriate. This is determined by:

- The advantages and disadvantages of home care for the patient.
- The advantages and disadvantages of home care for the family and immediate environment.

The advantages and disadvantages of home care for the patient

Home treatment is generally preferred by patients as this avoids the demoralisation and stigma associated with admission to hospital. For patients who do not have a formal mental illness but personality disorders, adjustment difficulties or situational crises, an admission to hospital may risk undermining existing coping mechanisms, fostering dependence and reinforcing the sick role. These are the patients for whom Caplan's model of crisis theory is most applicable (Caplan, 1964). A community intervention aimed at strengthening existing appropriate coping mechanisms and reducing inappropriate strategies can have an educational function that may reduce the risk of decompensation and crises in similar circumstances in the future (Caplan, 1964; Szmukler, 1987).

For patients with a history of schizophrenia, an environment of high expressed emotion or frequent criticism is associated with a higher rate of relapse (Vaughan & Leff, 1976; Kavanagh, 1992). Recent evidence suggests that expressed emotion may emerge as a more generalised risk factor for relapse, with reports that expressed emotion predicts relapse in bipolar disorder (Miklowitz *et al.*, 1986, 1988; Priebe *et al.*, 1989) and depression (Hooley *et al.*, 1986; Hooley

& Teasdale, 1989). Management has focused on reducing contact with relatives prone to high levels of expressed emotion, on providing psycho-educational family interventions, or on social skills training for the patient to reduce conflict in the family. Whilst education and training interventions can reduce expressed emotion in the long-term, in an acute relapse it is not known whether an attempt to provide treatment in a high expressed emotion home hampers recovery. However, in situations that have deteriorated towards overt hostility, it is more likely that the patient will be treated successfully in a different environment and admission to an in-patient unit or day hospital may be more appropriate. Although originally described in families, high expressed emotion may equally be demonstrated by staff involved in the long-term care of mentally ill patients in hostels or day hospitals (Moore *et al.*, 1992).

The advantages and disadvantages of home care for the family and local environment

It is important to consider the needs of the carer and their ability to cope (Fadden *et al.*, 1987). The move towards community care had been criticised for transferring the responsibility and burden of care from institutions to families. This burden is particularly great at times of crisis, and carers report that their difficulties could be alleviated by the provision of 24-hour emergency care, more information and communication from mental health professionals and greater consultation with families with regard to treatment planning (Francell *et al.*, 1988).

In the first episode of an illness, the family or other carers may find the possibility of a relative suffering from a mental illness hard to comprehend or accept. They may have frightening ideas about mental illness, and react by either becoming overprotective or partially denying the extent of the problem and underestimating the severity. By explaining the nature of the illness, its management and likely prognosis, and by allowing them to participate in the management of the problem in the home, the family or carers can be helped to have a more realistic understanding, to develop specific coping skills and to increase their confidence. The effect of mental health professionals visiting the home can be a useful modelling experience for carers and an opportunity to alter or prevent the development of patterns of family interaction (such as high expressed emotion) that may be maintaining a disorder or predispose to further relapse.

The level of 'burden' for the carer depends mainly on the level of functioning of the patient and the coping skills of the carer. However, some families may be highly motivated and skilled in providing help but exhausted with the often long-term commitment this involves and in need of some respite from the caring role. The patient may also have persecutory beliefs involving a family member, and may therefore be unable to trust and accept their care or even their presence, whilst acutely ill. In such situations support can be appropriately provided in the form of an admission for respite. A history of frequent psychiatric crises may itself be an indication of how a family needs more long-term support and education to help them cope with a member suffering from a mental illness. Kuipers *et al.* (1992) recommend the following simple criteria for offering family intervention when patients suffer from schizophrenia:

- Relatives living with patients who relapse more often than once a year despite being compliant with maintenance neuroleptics.
- Relatives who frequently contact staff for reassurance or help.
- Families in which there are repeated arguments leading to verbal or physical violence and any family that calls in the police.
- A single relative, usually the mother, looking after a schizophrenic patient on her own.

Another important factor is the effect of the patient on the local community (Bhugra, 1989; Brockington *et al.*, 1993). Where a patient exhibits problem behaviour, it is not only the tolerance of the family that may be exceeded but that of the neighbours, landlord, local shopkeepers, publicans and friends. Obviously our primary responsibility is towards the best interests of the patient. But their best interests will not be served if the result of attempting to manage a patient with disruptive behaviour in the community during an acute episode, results in resentment, eviction, being banned from shops or pubs, or at the worst, retaliation and victimisation.

Ethical issues

One of the main influences behind the move to de-institutionalisation was the civil libertarian lobby (Bachrach, 1978). Through asserting the patient's right to autonomy whatever their situation or mental illness, organisations such as MIND were instrumental in bringing about changes such as the 1983 Mental Health Act, limiting involuntary hospitalisation to those where there was evidence of danger to self or others. In contrast to the civil libertarian perspective where principles of liberty or autonomy dominate, the medical model has traditionally been described as being more paternalistic or utilitarian, being based on the belief that the morality of acts or management decisions are determined by the extent to which these acts serve the good of the individual or society (Chodoff, 1984).

During the 1980s the formation of the National Schizophrenia Fellowship (NSF), and SANE, representing primarily the families of patients, in combination with increasing public concern over the welfare of the mentally ill in the community, has lead to a re-evaluation of the current balance between these two models. The public's experience of more mentally ill people living in the community has initiated calls for a greater degree of paternalism and a utilitarian approach that takes into account the rights and needs of families and the wider community. Criticisms have frequently been made of the situation where a patient with a history of mental illness who refuses treatment may suffer from self-neglect but cannot be treated unless they deteriorate to a point that they are so severely ill that they constitute a danger to themselves or others. Critics have pointed out that, in addition to the right of autonomy, patients have a right to treatment, health and welfare (Miller, 1991; Haslam, 1993). Such criticisms have now lead to a revision of the interpretation of the 1983 Mental Health Act. New guidelines emphasise that the Act provides for compulsory admission in the interests of the patient's health and not just on the basis of safety (Code of Practice, DoH and Welsh Office, 1993).

Two other ways in which this debate affects the practice of community psychiatry are: issues of confidentiality and the degree of assertiveness of follow-up in the community. At present, the provision of confidential psychiatric information is strictly regulated by professional ethical standards to protect the rights of the individual. Information can generally only be provided with the consent of the patient (Joseph & Onek, 1991). In the provision of community psychiatric care a constant informal flow of current information is frequently required to enable relevant agencies to work together in the interests of the patient. In the absence of consent, the patient may be severely disadvantaged in terms of access to services such as housing. Families have expressed concerns that, whilst they may be expected to take on the responsibility of care-giver, they may be excluded from information that would assist them in this task (Francell *et al.*, 1988). Concern about confidentiality can also interfere with staff efforts to provide a service to other residents in the community who request help in dealing with the patient's behaviour (Diamond & Wikler, 1985). Where patients have a history of bizarre behaviour in public places it may be well known locally that the patient has a history of mental illness and receives treatment but staff are formally restricted from providing a degree of explanation that may facilitate understanding and tolerance.

When patients with a long-term mental illness are being followed-up in the community, a missed appointment or refusal of medication is often considered a signal that additional efforts should be made to contact them and continue treatment if possible. Their withdrawal and suspicion about their medication may be an indication that they are already relapsing, or they may be at risk of a relapse unless follow-up and treatment is continued. Efforts to maintain contact by staff repeatedly visiting the patient's home may be made despite clear statements from the patient that they do not want to be seen. Although treatment is not being given involuntarily, in these situations the patient's decision is not being considered a competent exercise of their right to refuse follow-up, but a part of their illness (Hirsch & Harris, 1988). Staff have a choice between continuing this essentially paternalistic approach despite the feeling of intrusion and occasional hostility from the patient, or taking a civil-libertarian approach and stopping follow-up until further contact is made either by the patient, or (unfortunately, more frequently) by the GP or police requesting an assessment for involuntary admission to hospital.

Calls for a compulsory supervision order in the community have been made in recognition of the problem of the 'revolving door' patient who responds to treatment but regularly defaults from community follow-up (Royal College of Psychiatrists, 1993; Bluglass, 1993a). However, proposals for a community supervision order have been rejected by the government (Department of Health, 1993; Bluglass, 1993b), due at least partially to the likelihood that the current proposals would be judged unlawful by the European Court of Human Rights (Eastman, 1994). As an alternative, the Department of Health has proposed a new supervised discharge order and greater use of guardianship orders, but neither proposal provides any legal right to enforce management plans in the community. The 1983 Mental Health Act was designed for a service model where treatment was provided mainly in hospital, but there now seems to be some consensus that reform is required to provide for care both in the hospital and in the community. However, particularly in view of the patchy development of community services in some areas, reform should be based on the principle of reciprocity; that restriction or removal of civil liberties for the purpose of care should be accepted only when matched by the provision of adequate resources and quality of services (Eastman, 1994).

References

Bachrach, L. (1978). A conceptual approach to deinstitutionalisation. *Hospital and Community Psychiatry*, **29**(9), 573–8.

Beck, A. T., Schuyler, H. & Herman, J. (1974). Development of suicidal intent scales. In *The Prediction of Suicide*, ed. A. T. Beck, H. L. P. Resruk & D. J. Lettieri. Maryland, Charles Press.

Bengelsdorf, H., Levy, L. E., Emerson, R. L. & Barile, F. A. (1984). A crisis triage rating scale. Brief dispositional assessment of patients at risk for hospitalisation. *Journal of Nervous and Mental Disease*, **172**(7), 424–30.

Bhugra, D. (1989). Attitudes towards mental illness. A review of the literature. *Acta Psychiatrica Scandinavica*, **80**, 1–12.

Binder, R. L. (1985). Patients' rights advocates in San Francisco. *Bulletin American Academy of Psychiatry and Law*, **13**(4), 325–36.

Birchwood, M., Smith, J., Macmillan, F., Hogg, B., Prasad, R., Harvey, C. & Bering, S. (1989). Predicting relapse in schizophrenia: the development and implementation of an early signs monitoring system using patients and families as observers. *Psychological Medicine*, **19**, 649–56.

Bluglass, R. (1993a). Maintaining the treatment of mentally ill people in the community. *British Medical Journal*, **306**, 159–60.

Bluglass, R. (1993b). New powers of supervised discharge of mentally ill people. *British Medical Journal*, **307**, 1660.

Brewin, C. R., Veltro, F., Wing, J. K., MacCarthy, B. & Brugha, T. S. (1990). The assessment of psychiatric disability in the community: a comparison of clinical, staff, and family interviews. *British Journal of Psychiatry*, **157**, 671–4.

Brockington, I. F., Hall, P., Levings, J. & Murphy, C. (1993). Tolerance of the mentally ill. *British Journal of Psychiatry*, **162**, 93–9.

Brugha, T. S., Wing, J. K. & Smith, B. L. (1989). Physical health of the long-term mentally ill in the community. Is there unmet need? *British Journal of Psychiatry*, **155**, 777–81.

Burns, T., Rafferty, J., Beadsmoore, A., McGuigan, S. & Dickson, M. (1993). A controlled trial of home-based acute psychiatric services. II: Treatment patterns and costs. *British Journal of Psychiatry*, **163**, 55–61.
Campbell, P. G. & Szmukler, G. I. (1993). The Social State; a proposed new element in the standard psychiatric assessment. *Psychiatric Bulletin*, **17**, 4–7.
Caplan, G. (1964). *Principles of Preventative Psychiatry*. London, Tavistock.
Chiswick, D. (1988). Forensic psychiatry. In *Companion to Psychiatric Studies*, 4th edn. ed. R. E. Kendel & A. K. Zealley. London, Churchill Livingstone.
Chodoff, P. (1984). Involuntary hospitalisation of the mentally ill as a moral issue. *American Journal of Psychiatry*, **141**(3), 384–9.
Coles, R. J., von Abendorff, R. & Herzberg, J. L. (1991). The impact of a new community health team on an inner city psychogeriatric services. *International Journal of Geriatric Psychiatry*, **6**, 31–9.
Colligan, G., Macdonald, A., Herzberg, J., Philpot, M. & Lindesay, J. (1993). An evaluation of the multidisciplinary approach to psychiatric diagnosis in elderly people. *British Medical Journal*, **306**, 821–4.
Dean, C. & Gadd, E. M. (1990). Home treatment for acute psychiatric illness. *British Medical Journal*, **301**, 1021–3.
Dean, C., Philips, J., Gadd, E. M., Joseph, M. & England, S. (1993). Comparison of community based service with hospital based service for people with acute, severe psychiatric illness. *British Medical Journal*, **307**, 473–6.
Dedman, P. (1993). Home treatment for acute psychiatric disorder. *British Medical Journal*, **306**, 1359–60.
Dening, T. (1992). Community psychiatry of old age: a UK perspective. *International Journal of Geriatric Psychiatry*, **7**, 757–66.
Department of Health (1993). *Legal Powers on the Care of the Mentally Ill in the Community. Report of the Internal Review*. London, DoH.
Department of Health and Welsh Office (1993). *Code of Practice; Mental Health Act 1983*. London, HMSO.
Departments of Psychiatry and Child Psychiatry, the Institute of Psychiatry and Maudsley Hospital (1987). *Psychiatric Examination; Notes on Eliciting and Recording Clinical Information in Psychiatric Patients*. Oxford University Press.
Diamond, R. J. & Wikler, D. I. (1985) Ethical problems in community treatment of the chronically mentally ill. In *The Training in Community Living Model: A Decade of Experience. New Directions for Mental Health Services*, No. 26, ed. L. I. Stein & M. A. Test. San Francisco, Jossey-Bass.
Donaldson, L. J. & Hill, P. M. (1991). The domiciliary consultation service: time to take stock. *British Medical Journal*, **302**, 449–51.
Eastman, N. (1994). Mental health law: civil liberties and the principle of reciprocity. *British Medical Journal*, **308**, 43–5.
Fadden, G., Bebbington, P. & Kuipers, L. (1987). The burden of care: the impact of functional psychiatric illness on the patient's family. *British Journal of Psychiatry*, **150**, 285–92.

Falloon, I. R. H. & Fadden, G. (1993). *Integrated Mental Health Care*. Cambridge, Cambridge University Press.

Fawcett, J., Scheftner, W. A., Fogg, L., Clark, D. C., Young, M. A., Hedeker, D. & Gibbons, R. (1990). Time-related predictors of suicide in major affective disorder. *American Journal of Psychiatry*, **147**(9), 1189–94.

Flynn, H. R. & Henisz, J. E. (1975). Criteria for psychiatric hospitalisation: experience with a checklist for chart review. *American Journal of Psychiatry*, **132**(8), 847–50.

Francell, G. G., Conn, V. S. & Gray, D. P. (1988). Families' perceptions of burden of care for chronic mentally ill relatives. *Hospital and Community Psychiatry*, **39**(12), 1296–300.

Freddolino, P. P., Moxley, D. P. & Fleischman, J. A. (1989). An advocacy model for people with long-term psychiatric disabilities. *Hospital and Community Psychiatry*, **40**(11), 1169–74.

Gerson, S. & Bassuk, E. (1980). Psychiatric emergencies: an overview. *American Journal of Psychiatry*, **137**(1), 1–11.

Goldberg, D., Mann, A., Pilgrim, D., Rogers, A., Sharp, D., Sutherby, K., Strathdee, G., Thornicroft, G. & Wykes, T. (1993). *Developing a Strategy for a Primary Care Focus for Mental Health Services*. Report commissioned by the South East London Health Authority and Lambeth, Southwark and Lewisham FHSA, November.

Haller, R. M. & Deluty, R. H. (1988). Assaults on staff by psychiatric inpatients. A critical review. *British Journal of Psychiatry*, **152**, 174–9.

Haslam, M. T. (1993). Human rights: the right to receive treatment and care. *Medicine and Law*, **12**(3–5), 291–5.

Hawton, K. (1987). Assessment of suicide risk. *British Journal of Psychiatry*, **150**, 145–53.

Hawton, K. & Catalan, J. (1987). *Attempted Suicide: A Practical Guide to its Nature and Management*, 2nd edn. Oxford, Oxford University Press.

Health Services Advisory Committee (1987). *Violence to Staff in the Health Services*. London, HMSO.

Hirsch, S. R. & Harris, J. (1988). *Consent and the Incompetent Patient: Ethics, Law and Medicine*. London, Gaskell.

Hooley, J. M., Orley, J. & Teasdale, J. D. (1986). Levels of expressed emotion and relapse in depressed patients. *British Journal of Psychiatry*, **148**, 642–7.

Hooley, J. M. & Teasdale, J. D. (1989). Predictors of relapse in unipolar depressives: expressed emotion, marital distress, and perceived criticism. *Journal of Abnormal Psychology*, **98**, 229–35.

Honig, A., Pop, P., de Kemp, E., Philipson, H. & Romme, M. A. J. (1992). Physical illness in chronic psychiatric patients from a community psychiatric unit revisited. *British Journal of Psychiatry*, **161**, 80–3.

Intagliata, J., Willer, B. & Egri, G. (1986). Role of the family in case management of the mentally ill. *Schizophrenia Bulletin*, **12**(4), 699–708.

Johnson, S. & Thornicroft, G. (1991). *Psychiatric Emergency Services in England and Wales*. Report to the Department of Health. London, PRiSM, Institute of Psychiatry.

Jones, S.J., Turner, R.J. & Grant, J.E. (1987). Assessing patients in their homes. *Bulletin of the Royal College of Psychiatry*, **11**, 117–19.

Joseph, D. & Onek, J. (1991). Confidentially in psychiatry. In *Psychiatric Ethics*, 2nd edn., ed. S. Bloch & P. Chodoff. Oxford, Oxford University Press.

Kavanagh, D.J. (1992). Recent developments in expressed emotion and schizophrenia. *British Journal of Psychiatry*, **160**, 601–20.

Kline, F., Acosta, F.X., Austin, W. & Johnson, R.G. (1980). The misunderstood Spanish-speaking patient. *American Journal of Psychiatry*, **137**(12), 1530–3.

Kuipers, L., Leff, J. & Lam, D. (1992). *Family Work for Schizophrenia; A Practical Guide*. London, Gaskell.

Littlejohns, P.C. (1986). Domiciliary consultations – who benefits? *Journal of the Royal College of General Practitioners*, **36**, 313–15.

Marson, D.C., McGovern, M.P. & Pomp, H.C. (1988). Psychiatric decision making in the emergency room: a research overview. *American Journal of Psychiatry*, **145**(8), 918–25.

Marzuk, P.M., Leon, A.C., Tardif, K., Morgan, E.B., Stajic, M. & Mann, J.J. (1992). The effect of access to lethal methods of injury on suicidal rates. *Archives of General Psychiatry*, **49**, 451–8.

Mercer, K. (1984). Black communities' experience of psychiatric services. *International Journal of Social Psychiatry*, **30**(1 & 2), 22–7.

Miklowitz, D.J., Goldstein, M.J., Nuechterlein, K.H., Snyder, K.S. & Doane, J.A. (1986). Expressed emotion, affective style, lithium compliance and relapse in recent onset mania. *Psychopharmacology Bulletin*, **22**, 628–32.

Miklowitz, D.J., Goldstein, M.J., Nuechterlein, K.H., Snyder, K.S. & Mintz, J. (1988). Family factors and the course of bipolar affective disorder. *Archives of General Psychiatry*, **45**, 225–31.

Miller, R. (1991). The ethics of involuntary commitment to mental health treatment. In *Psychiatric Ethics*, 2nd edn., ed. S. Bloch & P. Chodoff. Oxford, Oxford University Press.

Moore, E., Ball, R.A. & Kuipers, L. (1992). Expressed emotion in staff working with the long term adult mentally ill. *British Journal of Psychiatry*, **161**, 802–8.

Morgan, H.G. (1992). Suicide prevention, hazards on the fast lane to community care. *British Journal of Psychiatry*, **160**, 1149–53.

Morgan, H.G. & Priest, P. (1991). Suicide and other unexpected deaths amongst psychiatric inpatients. *British Journal of Psychiatry*, **158**, 368–74.

Noble, P. & Rodgers, S. (1989). Violence by psychiatric inpatients. *British Journal of Psychiatry*, **155**, 384–90.

Pallis, D.J., Gibbons, J.S. & Pierce, D.W. (1984). Estimating suicide risk among attempted suicides. II Efficiency of predictive scales after the attempt. *British Journal of Psychiatry*, **144**, 139–48.

Petrila, J.P. & Sadoff, R.L. (1992). Confidentiality and the family as caregiver. *Hospital and Community Psychiatry*, **43**(2), 136–9.

Phelan, M. & Fisher, N. (1993). Fire risk: assessment and management in long-term psychiatric patients. *Psychiatric Bulletin*, **17**, 86–8.
Pokorny, A. D. (1983). Prediction of suicide in psychiatric patients. *Archives of General Psychiatry*, **40**, 249–57.
Priebe, S., Wildgrube, C. & Muller-Oerlinghausen, B. (1989). Lithium prophylaxis and expressed emotion. *British Journal of Psychiatry*, **154**, 396–9.
Rassaby, E. & Rogers, A. (1987). Psychiatric referrals from the police; variations in disposal at different places of safety. *Bulletin of the Royal College of Psychiatrists*, **11**, 78–81.
Royal College of Psychiatrists (1993). *Community Supervision Orders*. London, Royal College of Psychiatry.
Salmons, P. H. (1984). Suicide in high buildings. *British Journal of Psychiatry*, **145**, 469–72.
Smith, J. & Birchwood, M. (1990). Relatives and patients as partners in the management of schizophrenia. The development of a service model. *British Journal of Psychiatary*, **156**, 654–60.
Smith, M. V. & Blythe, J. D. (1971). Domiciliary consultations. *Update Plus*, **1**, 135–49.
Steinberg, A. (1991). Issues in providing mental health services to hearing impaired persons. *Hospital and Community Psychiatry*, **42**(4), 380–9.
Sutherby, K., Srinath, S. & Strathdee, G. (1992). The domiciliary consultation service: outdated anachronism or essential part of community psychiatric outreach? *Health Trends*, **24**(3), 103–5.
Swanson, J. W., Holzer, C. E., Ganju, V. K. & Tsutomu Jono, R. (1990). Violence and psychiatric disorder in the community: evidence from the epidemiologic catchment area surveys. *Hospital and Community Psychiatry*, **41**, 761–70.
Szmukler, G. I. (1987). The place of crisis intervention in psychiatry. *Australian and New Zealand Journal of Psychiatry*, **21**, 24–34.
Tuckman, J. & Youngman, W. F. (1968). A scale for assessing suicide risk of attempted suicides. *Journal of Clinical Psychology*, **24**, 17–19.
Turner, P. M. & Turner, T. J. (1991). Validation of the crisis triage rating scale for psychiatric emergencies. *Canadian Journal of Psychiatry*, **36**(9), 651–4.
Tyrer, P. (1984). Psychiatric clinics in general practice: an extension of community care. *British Journal of Psychiatry*, **145**, 9–14.
Vaughan, C. & Leff, J. (1976). The influence of family and social factors on the course of psychiatric illness: a comparison of schizophrenic and depressed neurotic patients. *British Journal of Psychiatry*, **129**, 125–37.
Viaro, M. & Peruzzi, P. (1983). Home visits in crisis situations – analysis of context and suggestions for intervention. *Australian Journal of Family Therapy*, **4**(4), 209–15.
Warner, S. L. (1961). Criteria for involuntary hospitalization of psychiatric patients in a public psychiatric hospital. *Mental Hygiene*, **45**, 122–8.
Whittington, H. G. (1966). *Psychiatry in the American Community*. New York, International Universities Press.

Whittington, R. & Wykes, T. (1994). The prediction of violence in a health care setting. In *Violence and Health Care Professionals*, ed. T. Wykes. London, Chapman & Hall.

CHALLENGE OF IMPLEMENTATION

Introduction

We now have substantial evidence from policy makers and researchers to guide clinical practice, yet real services often lag far behind best practice. The second section of this book addresses the challenge of implementation. Drs Geraldine Strathdee and colleagues sketch a framework within which a community orientated mental health service can be developed, and indicate that emergency services are only one component of this wider array of provision. While making large scale changes to move a service from a hospital to a community orientation is a major organisational challenge, the key issue is whether such a more local and disseminated service can gel to provide a better quality of care for patients in the long term. Professor Peter Tyrer draws upon his own experience to demonstrate the difficulties and successes of the Early Intervention Service in West London in this crucial consolidation phase. In practice, especially out of office hours, many such assessments take place in accident and emergency or emergency room facilities, and Drs Sonia Johnson and Howard Baderman address the special difficulties of undertaking a proper assessment in a general medical department.

Although traditionally hospitals have usually only been able to offer admission to in-patient beds, other models of care are now being developed, and Professor William Sledge and his colleagues from Yale University, USA, have pioneered the use of the crisis-respite house, and its comprehensive evaluation. Similarly, the placement of patients with other families while in crisis, on a short-term fostering basis is now under development, and Dr Bennett from Madison, USA, indicates that such schemes may be extremely therapeutic for some patients in this situation. Another treatment option is high intensity home-based care, and the service described by Professors Lorenzo Burti and Michele Tansella in South Verona, Italy, has offered such a service for over 15 years. For some patients, the best option may be acute day hospital treatment and Professor Francis Creed draws upon his extensive experience in this field to summarise the effectiveness of these facilities. Despite this range of alternative facilities, in many cases admission to an acute general adult psychiatric ward is appropriate, and it is striking that such facilities have been paid little research or clinical attention. Drs Tom Sensky and Jan Scott indicate how ward-based treatment can be optimised. The second section of the book therefore attempts to show how theoretical and policy ideas can be put to practical use to help patients.

9

Establishing a local emergency service

GERALDINE STRATHDEE, MICHAEL PHELAN AND ANN WATTS

Introduction

This book covers a wide range of different approaches to providing emergency mental health care, and describes specific approaches that have worked in different settings. In this chapter, the focus will be on the major issues facing anyone who has the responsibility of establishing a community-based emergency mental health service for a specific geographical area. The emphasis is on the strategic planning which is vital for the development of an effective and comprehensive service.

We have approached the task from the perspective of clinicians and managers involved in the development of a comprehensive community mental health service, of which an emergency service forms an integral component. The resources and facilities of mental health services are all too often dependent on historical and haphazard planning, and are therefore unresponsive to the current needs of the local population. For example, emergency services have been centred around hospital bases even when these are inaccessible or unsuitable. Emergency services are often considered in terms of the specific facilities that are available or planned. As different facilities can fulfil the same functions, it is a useful exercise to explore the numerous functions that a service can be expected to fulfil, before deciding on specific service components. The rational first step in developing any service is to collect information so that your service can be tailored to local need. The difficulties and issues involved in changing a service are illustrated in this chapter with a description of our experiences of bed reduction and the introduction of a community team and crisis house to a sector service. The chapter concludes by outlining the value and difficulties of evaluating an emergency service. A theme running through the whole chapter will be the importance of establishing common goals amongst the numerous people involved in service development, as well encouraging the involvement of the users of the service and community staff, such as general practitioners (GPs).

The chapter is based on our experience of establishing a community service in Nunhead, an area of South London, with a population of around 40,000. The local area ranks as the sixth most socially deprived in England and Wales, as measured by Jarmen's indices (Jarmen, 1983). Unemployment, single parenting and a lack of basic amenities are the central local problems. In three of the five electoral wards, people from ethnic minorities, particularly from African and Caribbean countries form 20–30% of the population.

Crisis services as a core component of a comprehensive mental health service

The development of community services have had two consistent themes: that services should be directed to meeting individual needs and that the traditional inherited service systems dominated by large institutions should be replaced with a more balanced and flexible range of alternative services (Hunter & Wistow, 1987). Ten core components of community services are listed in Table 9.1 (Strathdee & Thornicroft, 1995). These categories are not mutually exclusive, and in any particular local setting the organisation and form of services should always be built on local information and circumstances. However, crisis services should always be viewed as an essential core component and their development must be seen as an integral part of the whole service.

Functions of an emergency service

Emergency services are often considered in terms of the facilities available, rather than the actual type of service that is offered. For example, a frequently used measure of an acute service is the number of in-patient beds. Such figures can be easily obtained, and directly compared with other services. However, such comparisons can be deceptive, when similar facilities are being used for different functions.

Table 9.1. *Ten core components of a comprehensive mental health service*

1. Care registers and identification
2. Crisis intervention
3. Hospital and community places
4. Assertive outreach and care management
5. Day care
6. Assessment and consultation services
7. Carer and community education and support
8. Primary care liaison
9. Physical and dental care
10. User advocacy and community alliances

(Strathdee & Thornicroft, 1995.)

The functions of similar sized wards may be profoundly different, and difficult to measure. Even between members of the same multidisciplinary team there can be marked differences of opinion about the purpose of a specific facility. For example, ward staff may try to resolve patients' problems through long admissions when necessary. In contrast, staff working away from the hospital may view the ward as a brief stepping stone on a path to recovery, and feel that it is unrealistic to hope that problems can be resolved away from the patient's environment. If staff do not share views on what they are trying to achieve, disagreements and disputes are inevitable.

New services can be established, or current services left in place without anyone stepping back and considering what the functions of the service are. The result is a haphazard service, with provision largely dependent on the demands put upon the service, the views and approaches of individual staff and the availability of alternative help from other local organisations. Only when the functions of the service have been agreed upon is it possible to try and arrange for the most efficient provision.

There are three major functions that any service should fulfil: assessment, management and the provision of information (Table 9.2). For clarity, these three areas will be examined separately, although in practice there will clearly be an overlap between them.

Assessment

The assessment of people in crisis is an everyday function for emergency staff. They are called upon to see people who are acutely

Table 9.2. *The functions of an emergency service*

Assessment
- Source of referrals
- Time
- Response time
- Setting
- Staff
- Outcome

Management
- Setting
- Priorities
- Collaboration
- Intervention
- Discharge

Information
- About the service
- Alternative help
- Training

psychotic, confused, suicidal, intoxicated, depressed, homeless or simply desperate. Assessment can be examined along six dimensions.

Source of referrals

Requests for assessments may be received from GPs, hospital doctors, social services, the courts, police, voluntary organisations, informal carers and patients themselves. Encouraging referrals from a wide range of sources may increase the number of requests for help, but makes the service more accessible to people who may be unable to follow more traditional paths. This will be particularly true for people with special needs, such as the homeless and members of ethnic minorities, who may not be registered with a GP and are wary of statutory agencies. Our experience is that inappropriate referrals are no more common from non-medical sources.

Time

Assessments will be requested at times other than normal office hours. The level of service available during the evenings, at night and at weekends needs to be clarified. It is at these times that other services will be less available, and a greater degree of support and help may be required. This has to be matched against the needs of the staff, and the cost of out-of-hours working.

Response time

Speed of response should ideally be dependent on need, but this is not always apparent until the assessment has been conducted. When referrers are personally known by members of the team it may be easier for them to respond appropriately to specific requests. It may well be that some referrals can be delayed, if the referrer knows that he/she can contact the team again for an immediate assessment if the situation deteriorates.

Setting

Different settings are possible for assessments, and the extent to which these are available needs to be decided. The advantages and disadvantages of home assessments are discussed in chapter 8. No setting is suitable for all situations, and there is a need to be flexible.

Staff

A range of staff can potentially conduct assessments. Traditionally acute mental health assessments have been the domain of psychiatrists, however, it will often be advantageous for other professionals to be involved, either alone or working alongside a doctor. This encourages a broad approach to the person's problems from the outset, facilitates true multidisciplinary team working and training.

Outcome

One of the most vital aspects of an assessment is how the results are communicated back to the referrer. There will always be a place for formal letters, which offer a permanent and precise record of the assessment. But faster communication is also required. The increasing use of fax machines, e-mail and mobile telephones means that referrers should be able to be informed immediately about the outcome of an assessment, without staff wasting time trying to contact someone.

Management

After conducting assessments the other clear role of any emergency service is the subsequent management of emergency situations. Again this can be helpful examined along different dimensions.

Setting

The psychiatric ward has, for a long time, been the bedrock of the management of psychiatric emergencies, however, as this book demonstrates, the last 20 years have seen an increasing recognition of the limitations of a hospital for many people in crisis. As with long-term supported accommodation, a range of options is needed, if the best solution is to be found for each patient. There will always be a need for the high level of care which can be provided in hospitals, but the need for hospital beds will largely be determined by the alternatives available. Currently, the options usually available in any one area are extremely limited.

Priorities

Crises and emotional distress are normal and common experiences; no service can, or should, hope to help everyone in such a position. However, saying 'no' to people looking for help is difficult for staff, can upset referrers and may cause tension within a team. The need for priority setting must be understood by the team, if conflicts are to be avoided. Table 9.3 is one example of how referrals can be prioritised. No such list will cover all eventualities, and exceptions will always have to be made. If it is felt that a patient is not an appropriate referral the reasons why must be explained to the referrer, and alternative sources of help suggested.

Collaboration

It may be appropriate for the specialist mental health care team to take over a person's care completely, during a crisis. At the other extreme mental health staff may just give advice to the main carer be it a relative, GP or other professional. Active collaboration with the patient can ultimately only be achieved by staff who are willing to listen and respond to what the patient wants. This can be helped by the introduction of crisis cards, and close involvement with advocates.

Intervention

It is beyond the scope of this text to detail the wide range of physical, pharmacological and psychological interventions that may be required for various emergency situations. It is clearly essential for the team to

Table 9.3. *Prioritising emergency care*

High priority

Patients who suffer from a serious mental illness, resulting in severe social and psychological disability. In particular those who:

- are in current danger to themselves or others;
- have a history of poor engagement with services;
- are homeless, or have other special needs.

Medium priority

Patients who have a lesser degree of social dysfunction, e.g. those who are able to maintain an enduring relationship or to work at least part-time, including:

- those receiving appropriate help from other sources;
- present no immediate danger to themselves or others.

Low priority

Patients who do not have an identifiable mental illness, and whose problems appear predominantly to be related to long-term social factors, including:

- those whose problems are not interfering with daily activities;
- those who are unlikely to benefit from the help offered, and who can be offered help elsewhere.

(Adapted from Strathdee & Thornicroft, 1995.)

ensure that they have access to such treatments, as well as the necessary skills for effective and safe administration.

Discharge

Crises usually occur in people who have a long-standing predisposition to psychotic relapse, a vulnerable personality or poor social support. An integral part of crisis management is the planning of care after the immediate emergency, and in particular the development of strategies to avoid further crises. If a team is to continue to take new referrals, some patients must be discharged or transferred. This should be an active process, otherwise staff will become overloaded and the care of the less demanding, but not necessarily less needy patients will be the first to suffer. If patients are discharged inappropriately, they are more likely to relapse and much hard work will have been wasted.

Information

A third function of an emergency service, which is not as immediately obvious as assessment and management, is the provision of information.

To be effective, an emergency service must be known about by any potential referrers. The information that is required includes a contact person and the types of service that are and are not offered. Ideally, staff should get to know individual referrers, such as GPs. This will help to encourage appropriate referrals, and make the discharge and transfer of patients easier and safer. The provision of regular information is particularly important when the service is in a state of flux, and referral procedures may be changing every few months. In this situation a regular newsletter keeping local GPs and other relevant staff informed of the changes can be effective.

An emergency service can also reduce the number of inappropriate referrals by disseminating information about alternative services, such as counselling agencies and non-medical alcohol services. Finally, an emergency service may want to extend its role to educating others about the assessment and management of crises. Accident and emergency (A & E) doctors, GPs, social service staff, housing officers, hostel workers, user's, relatives and the police can all potentially benefit from such training. This will have the added benefit of developing closer links with all these other agencies.

The range of emergency service components

In Britain, during the last 30 years, emergency mental health services have developed in parallel with other medical specialities. Emergency assessments are usually conducted by junior doctors, sometimes psychiatrists in the accident and emergency departments of general hospitals, or by consultant psychiatrists doing requested domicillary visits. The management of patients in crisis has mainly been restricted to in-patient wards. Out-of-hours working has been limited to medical staff, ward-based nursing staff and duty social workers involved in compulsory detentions. Other professional groups have not appeared eager to have a greater involvement, possibly reflecting a reluctance to become committed to more out-of-hours working. Overall, psychiatrists have tended to accept a way of working which follows standard practice in other medical disciplines.

Alternatives approaches are possible, but the extent to which innovative approaches are incorporated into any service is largely dependent on the imagination, energy and commitment of the staff. Table 9.4 lists the possible components of an emergency service. Local

Table 9.4. *Potential components of an emergency service*

Centralised	*Community*
Hospital beds:	Residential places:
psychiatric/general	crisis house
locked/open	staffed hostel
	family placement
Accident and Emergency Department	CMHC
Psychiatric emergency clinic	Drop-in centre/session
Urgent slots in out-patients	Domicillary visits
Day hospital	Home based care
Other	
Liaison/parasuicide team	
Telephone help lines	
Interpreting service	

CMHC: Community mental health centre.

community services frequently provide some degree of emergency cover during working hours, but out-of-hours emergency services tend to become centralised. Only with the development of crisis teams and crisis houses can care become more accessible. When a lack of staff make 24-hour cover impossible the introduction of shift work can extend the teams' hours into the evening, and some limited help can be provided by a 24-hour telephone service.

Planning an emergency service based on local needs

From the outset we were determined to provide a crisis service which effectively met local needs and was integrated with the other service components. We therefore needed an accurate picture of the service provision and needs of the population. A wide range of demographic and service factors predict the need and demand for emergency care in any specific area (see Table 9.5).

Some indication of the needs of the population can be obtained by the current utilisation of emergency services, along with data on any recent changes that have occurred. The information available will obviously be dependent on local record keeping. As an absolute minimum, data should be kept on the number, type and source of

Table 9.5. *Information to inform service planning*

Current service provision and utilisation
- Number and type of patients referred
- Source of referrals and pathways to care
- Time of presentation
- Proportion of patients in contact with services
- Range of problems presented
- Standards achieved
- Staff mix
- Availability of staff (e.g. Section 12 approved doctors, approved social workers)

Characteristics of population
- Age distribution
- Unemployment rates
- Levels of deprivation
- Ethnic mix
- Seasonal changes

Characteristics of the locality
- Transport routes
- Hospitals
- Prisons
- Universities
- Range of supported accommodation

Alternative agencies
- Counselling services
- User organisations
- Citizen Advice Bureau
- Social services

Needs of the population
- Users of the service
- Carers
- General practitioners
- Social services
- General hospital doctors
- Housing officers
- Police
- Courts and probation service

referrals and the outcome of each episode. However, this information will take no account of the extent to which needy people are staying away because the service is inappropriate, inaccessible or unacceptable to them. A disproportionate number of referrals from certain sources may indicate inappropriate referring, or else be indicative of a lack of knowledge about the service or dissatisfaction by other referrers. Changes in services may result in the emergence of need which had previously been hidden.

For our own service we conducted a number of specific studies in the local area, and were fortunate to have access to the results of other research conducted in the same area, before introducing any service changes. Some of the findings that influenced the final pattern of our service are given below:

Use of acute in-patient beds

A three-month bed audit at the Maudsley hospital, in London (where all patients from the sector are admitted) was conducted. One-third of the 136 admitted patients had received in-patient care of some sort in the month prior to admission, and 70% were already known to the service. Twenty-three per cent of the patients were detained compulsorily, and at the time of admission, nearly all of the patients were judged to be in need of a high level of supervision; for two-thirds of the patients it was felt that this could have been provided by a 'high supervision hostel with good staffing levels'. Ninety per cent of the admissions were decided upon by a junior psychiatrist, and most of the patients appeared to have had some form of prodrome when early intervention would have been appropriate. Overall, it appeared as if the hospital was admitting patients with long-term severe mental illness, during repeated crises. The authors concluded by suggesting that improved out-patient management might reduce admission rates by diminishing the risk of crisis (Bebbington *et al.*, 1993).

Pathways into care

A further local study examined the routes into in-patient care taken by patients. Those under the age of 30 years were usually brought to the hospital by the police, or else presented directly to the psychiatric services. Older patients typically came via general hospital services, after domicillary visits requested by the GP or from psychiatric out-patients. The lack of any consistency in the routes, the high level of police involvement and the fact that many of the patients were by-passing primary care, led the investigators to suggest that there was a need for specialist outreach services and that the key to providing effective services in the area, especially for younger patients, was to ensure that services were both accessible and readily available (Moodley & Perkins, 1991).

Users' and carers' needs for crisis services

Using a methodology developed by Pilgrim and Rogers (1993) we conducted a study of users and carers in our local area in a number of settings. The users of our services expressed views which concorded with those expressed in similar work elsewhere (see chapter 3). Firstly, they valued rapid response in crisis situations, and asked for continuity of care by known and experienced health workers. Secondly, they were highly critical of the unsuitable environment and attitudes, experience, and management offered by A & E doctors in the general hospital setting. Thirdly, they were increasingly keen to have access to alternatives to acute hospital wards, such as crisis houses in the community, crisis flats and user-run sanctuaries. Finally, for women users there was growing concern about the safety aspects of admission to mixed-sex wards and a call for women only facilities, preferably with access to child care.

General practitioners

Britain is unique in the extent of its primary care infrastructure. Ninety-eight per cent of the population is registered with a GP and 90% of these patients will see their doctor in any three-year period (Sharp & Morrell, 1989). They act as the primary gatekeeper for entry to specialist services, including emergency mental health services. Even when patients are in contact with the secondary care services, the GP is often the point of first contact in crisis. In their follow-up study of patients with schizophrenia living in the community, Murray Parkes *et al.* (1962) concluded that 'while the hospitals and out-patient clinics were responsible for initiating most of the treatment required for maintaining the patients' health, it was the general practitioners who played the major role in dealing with the crises and relapses that occurred in over half the cases.' Thirty years later, in a study of the needs of GPs in caring for the mentally ill, 80% of the GPs asserted that often patients with long-term mental health problems only came to their attention when a crisis arose (Kendrick *et al.*, 1991).

In our area the findings from a survey of 184 GPs (Strathdee, 1990) were remarkably consistent with similar work done elsewhere (Ferguson, 1990). GPs stated that as a community agency they valued: rapid response on a 24-hour, seven-day basis by crisis intervention outreach teams, assessment by experienced staff, outreach assessment and treatment of suicidal and parasuicidal patients, and easily accessible Approved Social Worker services.

Community agencies

In a series of meetings with local social services, police and housing departments, we identified their needs for crisis services and these have subsequently formed the basis of pilot service level agreements and contracts with them. As with the GPs they wanted an exprienced opinion within 2–24 hours, and training in mutual issues of concern.

Together these studies pointed to an inflexible service which was reactively responding to successive crisis episodes, with little pro-active work to prevent further crises. There was little communication with other agencies, and the lack of early intervention and after care appeared to be contributing to frequent re-admissions. The service was meeting few of the demands or needs of the users of the service. There appeared to be a number of strategies which would improve the quality of the service and reduce the use of hospital beds: the establishment of a service that facilitated early intervention and which was more acceptable to the users; greater involvement of experienced and senior staff to help avoid unnecessary admissions and improve the continuity of care; the provision of short-term alternatives to hospital admission; and maintaining contact with patients after crises by establishing closer inter-agency working.

Developing a 24-hour emergency service

In order to illustrate some of the challenges and difficulties involved in changing services we will describe our experiences of reducing an in-patient ward from 25 to 12 beds, and simultaneously establishing a crisis team and crisis house in the community. Managing any type of change is widely recognised to be difficult. In order to make the process as painless as possible we sought out allies, at an early stage, who supported our ideas, and tried to establish the organisational power necessary to see the changes through. We spent a great deal of time explaining the reasons for introducing the changes, and the anticipated benefits, but at the same time tried to listen to the concerns and comments of others. Although we altered proposals in the light of certain and unavoidable restrictions, we believed it to be vital to maintain a broad, but consistent vision of how things were to be developed.

Bed reduction

Ideally bed reduction should only be considered after the establishment of alternative community resources and the establishment of a fully functioning community crisis team. However, this requires substantial transitional funding, which is rarely available. We were in the position of having to cut bed numbers and simultaneously develop the community resources – a stressful and potentially dangerous process. The key to bed reduction is strict bed management. Tyrer *et al.* (1989) demonstrated that the introduction of sectorisation in Nottingham, resulted in a reduction in bed usage. Burns *et al.* (1993) describe a 50% reduction in hospital admissions following the introduction of home assessments, rather than hospital out-patients. The experience of The Daily Living Programme (a community team established to evaluate the effectiveness of acute home-based care), was that when they no longer had control over admissions, there was a three-fold increase in length of stay (Marks *et al.*, 1994). Based on these findings, and our own experience, we introduced a range of strategies (Table 9.6).

Initially we closed three beds, and this allowed two of the 23 ward-based staff to begin working away from the hospital. These two staff initially focused their attention on around 25 patients, who had been identified as being frequently re-admitted to the ward. They concentrated on helping them to recognise their signs of relapse and to develop appropriate and effective coping strategies. They also ensured that they had someone to contact in a crisis. Within three weeks it was possible to close another three beds, down to 19. We stayed at this level for six months while staff gained experience of maintaining people outside hospital. We were then able to make a further reduction to 16 beds and create a fully functioning crisis team with eight staff. During this stage, limited transitional funding allowed us to employ two extra nursing staff temporarily. After another eight months the ward was reduced to 12 beds.

Most of the staff for the crisis team were recruited from the ward, but some were external appointments which was helpful in broadening the team's experience. Throughout these changes we worked closely

Table 9.6. *Strategies for successful bed management*

- Home assessments
- Senior gatekeeping
- Experienced nurse with triage function
- Immediate discharge planning on admission
- Intensive follow-up care, immediately after discharge
- Urgent out-patient appointments
- Community teams having control over beds

with the hospital personnel department and the unions to try and ensure that staff did not feel insecure. As the beds were reduced the intensity of the ward work increased, and as the ward staff reduced in number we ensured that the proportion of trained and experienced staff on the ward increased, reflecting the increasing demands put upon them.

Both ward and community staff were described as working for the PACE team, helping to create a sense of unity. A 24-hour day–night rota was introduced on the ward to prevent night staff from being isolated. We established a scheme for ward and community staff to rotate positions for three months, to improve understanding about the different roles and increase awareness of the difficulties faced by each other. We are also beginning to pair-up ward and community staff, again to improve communication and to broaden experience.

The team now provides a comprehensive service from 8 a.m. to 8 p.m., and a limited call-out service over night. If staff have to make calls at night there is a reciprocal arrangement that they will go with the duty nurse from the PACT team, the parallel continuing care team in the sector.

Establishment of a crisis house

Experience of community crisis houses in Britain is still very limited. From the outset we believed it was essential to be very clear about what exactly the house was for and for whom. Table 9.7 lists some of the criteria for admission to the house. Any potential resident has to have a permanent address within the sector, and to be already known to the team. Before going to the house a detailed care plan is drawn up with the care co-ordinator incorporating the reason and aims of the admission, the planned length of stay, criteria to be met for discharge/transfer and treament plan including activities, medication

Table 9.7. *Suggested criteria for admission to crisis house*

Inclusion

- Patients who have had a period of in-patient care, but who are not ready to return to their permanent accommodation, or who cannot return because of practical difficulties such as a lack of electricity.
- Patients who require a short period of respite away from their home, but who do not require 24-hour nursing care.
- Patients who require a period of assessment, but who cannot be assessed at home.
- As part of an on-going treatment plan for patients with rapid cyclical disorders.
- For patients whose treatment is being sabotaged by co-habitees, or who are at risk of self-neglect.

Exclusion

- High degree of danger to self or others, which cannot be managed without high levels of support, containment and supervision.
- Poor physical health which may require urgent specialist intervention.
- Unacceptable fire risk.

and support. Before admission, residents are asked to sign a contract agreeing to the rules of the house. Usually admissions are between a day and three weeks, but at times admissions have stretched to three months.

There are no staff dedicated specifically to the crisis house, so staffing has to be provided from within the team resources, and fluctuates depending on need. Staff will visit up to three times a day, but the lack of 24-hour staffing has limited the use of the house. For instance, so far we have not admitted men and women to the house at the same time. One important safety measure is a large poster above the telephone with instructions on how to contact the duty team member urgently.

There are extensive management implications of running such a property. Health and safety guidelines have to be met. Contracts for housekeeping duties and maintenance have to be arranged. The decisions about informing local residents and the police are delicate, and have to be balanced against issues of privacy. Theft and burglary are a constant threat. Keys frequently get lost, and locks have to be changed. However, despite the difficulties our experience is that it is an appreciated resource, and for some patients offers marked advantages over an in-patient admission.

Evaluation

All health services are under increasing pressure to demonstrate their effectiveness. Governments, desperate to control the exponential rise in health care costs are demanding that services demonstrate their effectiveness. Mental health services are a major source of expenditure (Department of Health, 1991), and along with other specialities need to demonstrate that the money is being well spent. A degree of evaluation must be incorporated into any emergency service. Although new approaches to providing emergency care appear to have advantages the jury is still out. There is a desperate need for high quality evaluative research to determine what works well, why it works and in what locally acceptable form it might be implemented. Only in this way can future developments be based on proven good practice. There is a need for routine services to be fully evaluated, as well as innovative projects.

The evaluation of any mental health service presents difficulties. The aims of services are frequently broad, and often overlap with social and voluntary services. Care is frequently aimed at maintaining patients in a stable condition, without discrete episodes of illness and definite end-points. Approaches to care are often individualistic, and difficult to define. There are few hard outcome measures in mental health. Research has to be largely based on questionnaires administered to patients, staff and carers. It is time consuming and dependent on having co-operation from all involved.

The attraction to evaluating emergency services is that the potential change in patients is large, compared to continuing care teams. Here is an excellent opportunity to demonstrate the effectiveness of mental health care. Although time consuming, if staff can be involved in evaluation, and be fully informed of the results of any research, then it can improve morale and encourage service improvements.

However, there are some specific difficulties in trying to evaluate emergency services, compared to a continuing care service with a stable patient base. A significant proportion of patients seen by an emergency service will only be in contact for a short time. Some may be transferred to other services, others will have quickly resolved problems and others will lose contact. There will inevitably be difficulties in trying to follow everyone up after their initial presentations.

The work level will always be unpredictable and variable, and at busy times staff will be tempted to cut out any extra work which is not immediately related to direct patient care. As much of the work is out-of-hours, specific research staff may not be present all the time. Obtaining informed consent from patients in crisis who are not known to the staff can be difficult, and ethically dubious in those who are severely psychotic. For all these reasons, any research must be realistic in its expectations and flexible in its approach.

Routinely collected socio-demographic, diagnostic and service utilisation data is an essential starting point for any evaluative research. This data can be used for a variety of purposes. Staff can compare workloads. Changes over time can be monitored, and reports prepared with relative ease for business plans and purchasing contracts. The routine collection of data is increasingly being aided by computer systems specifically designed for use by mental health services (Lelliott *et al.*, 1993). Such systems offer clear advantages, but do require significant capital expenditure and investment in staff training if they are to be effective. More detailed evaluation will entail the collection of extra data, usually in the form of specific questionnaires. Areas which are of particular relevance to emergency services are listed in Table 9.8. Specific examples of this type of evaluative research are described in other chapters.

Future plans

To move from a centralised hospital-based emergency service, and to develop alternative provision, has required a great deal of hard work and commitment from all involved. Our early experience is in line with research findings from experimental services, i.e. that patients prefer community-based emergency care and that there are advantages for patients from such alternative forms of care. We hope to confirm this with detailed evaluative research that is currently under way.

For the future we have two main aims. Firstly, we want to move towards having closer liaison with social workers, so that we can offer integrated health and social crisis care. Secondly, we have become increasingly convinced that strategies which aim to maximise 'engagement' with patients, rather than achieve 'compliance' are what we should strive for. We are therefore continuing to develop

Table 9.8. *Key areas of evaluation of emergency services*

- Assessment of needs
- Service utilisation (including rates of compulsory treatment)
- Mental state
- Physical health
- Patient and carer satisfaction with services
- Impact on carers
- Quality of life
- Global functioning
- Costs

psycho-educational interventions for patients and to work with their carers and GPs in developing crisis intervention contracts.

References

Bebbington, P., Fennel, S. & Flanging, C. (1993). Auditing the use of psychiatric beds. In *Measuring Mental Health Needs*, ed. G. Thornicroft, C. Brewin & J. Wing. London, Royal College of Psychiatrists, Gaskell Press.

Burns, T., Raftery, J., Beadsmoore, A., *et al.* (1993). A controlled trial of home-based acute psychiatric services. II: Treatment patterns and costs. *British Journal of Psychiatry*, **163**, 55–61.

Department of Health (1991). *The Health of the Nation*. London, HMSO.

Ferguson, B. (1990). Clinical audit – a proposal. *Psychiatric Bulletin*, **14**, 275–7.

Hunter, D. & Wistow, G. (1987). Mapping the organisational context. 1. Central departments, boundaries and responsibilities. In *Community Care in Britain: Variations on a Theme*, ed. D. Hunter & G. Wistow, London, King Edward's Hospital Fund for London.

Jarmen, B. (1983). Identification of underprivileged areas. *British Medical Journal*, **286**, 1705–9.

Kendrick, T., Sibbald, B., Burns, T. & Freeling, P. (1991). Role of general practitioners in care of long-term mentally ill patients. *British Medical Journal*, **302**, 508–10.

Lelliot, P., Flannigan, C. & Shanks, S. (1993). A review of seven mental health information systems: a functional perspective. London, Gaskell/Royal College of Psychiatrists.

Marks, I. M., Connolly, J., Muijen, M., Audini, B. McNamee, G. & Lawrence, R. E. (1994). Home-based versus hospital-based care for people with serious mental illness. *British Journal of Psychiatry*, **165**, 179–94.

Moodley, P. & Perkins, R. (1991). Routes to psychiatric care in an inner London borough. *Social Psychiatry and Psychiatric Epidemiology*, **26**, 47–51.

Murray Parks, C., Brown, G. W. & Monck, E. M. (1962). The general practitioner and the schizophrenic patient. *British Medical Journal*, **1**, 972–6.

Pilgrim, D. & Rogers, A. (1993). Mental health service users' views of medical practitioners. *Journal of Interprofessional Care*, **7**, 167–76.

Sharp, D. & Morrell, D. (1989). The psychiatry of general practice. In *Scientific Approaches on Epidemiological and Social Psychiatry. Essays in Honour of Michael Shepherd*, ed. P. Williams, G. Wilkinson & K. Rawnsley. London, Routledge.

Strathdee, G. (1990). The delivery of psychiatric care. *Journal of the Royal Society of Medicine*, **83**, 222–5.

Strathdee, G. & Thornicroft, G. (1995). Community psychiatry and service evaluation. In *Essentials of Postgraduate Psychiatry*, 3rd edn., ed. R. Murray, P. Hill & P. McGuffin. London, Academic Press. (In press.)

Tyrer, P., Turner, R. & Johnson, A. (1989). Integrated hospital and community psychiatric services and the use of inpatient beds. *British Medical Journal*, **299**, 298–300.

10

Maintaining an emergency service

PETER TYRER

Although there is now overwheliming evidence that psychiatric services concentrating on rapid response in community settings are superior to more conventional services (Stein & Test, 1980; Dean & Gadd, 1990; Merson *et al.*, 1992; Burns *et al.*, 1993) there is still scepticism about the feasibility of organising rapid services nationally. Much of this concern appears to focus on the phenomenon of burn-out; teams work well for a time (usually when research is being undertaken on the service), but then a state of despondency and poor morale develops, the team breaks up and enthusiasm is lost (Dedman, 1993). If this was indeed a common state of affairs it would nullify a large part of the research evidence to date. Above all, service research has to be applicable to practice, and if the findings are only applicable under certain circumstances we need to know exactly what these circumstances are. In this chapter I will argue that burn-out is an unsatisfactory term used to describe a range of difficulties experienced by psychiatric teams involved in caring for those with severe mental illness, of which the strain imposed by direct patient care is only one. Many of the others can be overcome.

Most of my recent experience is based on working in the Early Intervention Service (EIS), a community-based service set up as a demonstration project by the Department of Health in 1987 to provide a rapid response service for patients with severe mental illness. It is now integrated into the mental health services for the area. The service sees patients in their homes or at other appropriate settings, including general practices, the community team base, day centres or, relatively rarely, hospitals. Most patients are seen at home first, but as this focus is dealt with by Professors Lorenzo Burti and Michael Tansella in a later chapter it will not be described in detail here.

Before taking up my post with the EIS, I was working in mainstream hospital psychiatric service in Nottingham, where I and my colleagues were involved in expanding the services outwards into primary and home-based care. Although there are many contrasts between these experiences, one starting with a hospital service and moving it outwards and the other starting with a community service and moving it inwards (i.e. by making changes which alter hospital practice), there are common issues in running and maintaining both types of service. However, most of this chapter will be concerned with my recent experience with the EIS because this is in an area where the problems of operating a service tend to be greater than elsewhere. This will be tempered and reinforced by my earlier experiences in Nottingham, where appropriate.

Demographic characteristics of the catchment area

The EIS was established in 1987 in Paddington and North Kensington in the western part of central London. This district, now subsumed into the Kensington, Chelsea and Westminster purchasing authority, was the fourth most deprived area in England using the Jarman scores for underprivileged areas derived from the 1981 UK census (Jarman, 1983, 1984). It is particularly noted for its large number of temporary residents, many of whom are placed in bed and breakfast hotels in the district, and it ranks second in the Jarman indices for mobility of population.

Until recently, central London psychiatric units had no clear catchment areas and were not therefore responsible for their local populations. Most in-patient psychiatric care in the catchment area was provided at mental hospitals in Surrey (20 miles distant) or the Tooting area of south London (10 miles distant) and so hospital–community links were difficult to establish. Some compensatory adjustments take place in such areas. In particular, local, mainly voluntary, agencies tend to grow more strongly than in other areas because there is an obvious need for the local population to have a community mental health resource.

The impetus for setting up the EIS was the need to develop a community arm of the existing hospital service, particularly the one based in Paddington. However, it was appreciated that many community services become involved with the less severely mentally ill, and as the area concerned was such a deprived one, it was felt that the numbers of patients with severe mental illness in the community were sufficiently high to accord their needs as a priority.

The community service

The EIS is an eight-strong multidisciplinary team of two community psychiatric nurses, two social workers, a clinical psychologist, occupational therapist, a senior psychiatrist (P.T.) and an administrator. Recently some of the staff have been working part-time and sessional senior registrar sessions have also been attached. Despite this, the team remains a small one with only the equivalent of 6.5 full-time members. The average case-load varies from 20 to 25. The EIS takes patients from a defined catchment area (Paddington and North Kensington) and has an open referral, rapid response system with assessment of all referrals, usually at the patient's home, within a few days; however, it is not a crisis intervention service and does not have 24-hour cover (Onyett *et al.*, 1990). A case manager system (although 'case management' in this context is quite different from the term used in the context of current guidelines from the Department of Health) is used with clinical decisions reached by consensus at regular team meetings and implemented by a named key worker who can be reinforced by other team members when needed. An operational policy was developed early in the history of the service by the first co-ordinator (Steve Onyett) and was regularly updated and refined. It is described elsewhere (Onyett, 1992) and its overall philosophy is to try and treat all mental disorders outside hospital in the first instance, with particular emphasis on joint working with other agencies, home treatment when necessary, and a collaborative approach to care that involves the patient as an active participant in all treatment decisions.

This is a more radical approach than that commonly employed in most psychiatric services and could be regarded as too idealistic. In my previous work in Nottingham the community 'arm' of the service was integrated closely with the hospital service and was orientated more to liaison with general practitioners (GPs) than to home treatment (Tyrer *et al.*, 1990). In theory, the EIS model could become badly unstuck when admission to hospital, particularly compulsory admission, is necessary, because it appears to contradict the tenets of the community-based treatment ethos of the service. In practice, however, this has not caused any serious difficulties, and the strong orientation of team members to community treatment wherever possible has cemented working relationships and has had some surprising gains. For example, whereas our service in Nottingham had little effect on the admissions of patients with schizophrenia (Tyrer *et al.*, 1989) the EIS has had great success with keeping these patients out of hospital, and this impact has been greater for this diagnosis than for any other (Tyrer, 1992).

Because it is appreciated that the EIS will be likely to receive a large number of referrals it was important not to have too great a case-load of continuing care. The early policy of the service was to see patients for no longer than six months and to concentrate on liaison with other services as part of its clinical work. The hope was that this liaison would enable patients to be transferred to an appropriate agency once acute work had been completed. In practice, and perhaps it could have been predicted, a significant number of patients have no appropriate agency to refer to because of the needs that still remain after early intervention. As a consequence some patients remain on the case list for the service for two years or more. Nevertheless, most of the patients can be referred to another agency and, as the EIS has a policy of taking re-referrals at any time, there is no reason why such patients cannot come back to the EIS at times of crisis or of deterioration in their conditions.

Management of the service

The EIS is a relatively cheap service with, for example, a total annual budget in 1992 of around £180,000. This is partly because management costs are kept to a minimum. Most decisions are reached by the team as a whole and this includes both clinical and business decisions. There is a team co-ordinator, currently a social worker, who represents the team in its negotiations with management and with other agencies. Line management for each of the disciplines within the team is maintained by senior professionals from the relevant disciplines, although in practice this occupies a very small amount of time and is largely concerned with career developments and other long-term aims because almost all clinical and professional support is given from within the team.

In this respect the EIS differs from many other services in which there is a clear management who gives the team direction and, at least to some extent, imposes control. The mistake is often made by those who visit the service in thinking that I, as the senior psychiatrist, am the team manager and the controlling influence. This misperception is resented by other members of the team, not least because I am a part-time member of the service, and such views give the impression that the team has much less autonomy than is indeed the case. However, I do have an important role in being able to link the EIS to other parts of the mental health services in the district. Initially, the service did not have direct access to beds and it was difficult to maintain continuity of care when patients were admitted. As a consequence of this the team now has acute beds in the psychiatric unit and so when patients are admitted, key workers in the EIS can continue to retain contact and are involved with planning discharge and after-care (and often retaining their role as a key worker throughout). These links to other parts of the service help to maintain the profile of the EIS and prevent it from becoming isolated at the periphery of the mental health services at a time of rapid reform.

The patients

Patients can be referred to the EIS from any source, including self-referral. The advantages of this approach are mentioned below. The disadvantage of such an approach is that any service which is seen to be successful in meeting need tends to get flooded with increasing numbers of patients from a wide variety of sources and is unable to cope with the demand.

The numbers of patients referred to the EIS since its inception are shown in Table 10.1. To some extent the fears of inundation have been realised in that more referrals have come to the service and we are now at a point of saturation at present levels of staffing. From time to time we have to remind our referrers, particularly GPs, that we remain a service that is concentrating on treating mental illness that is both severe and acute and that many patients referred do not meet the criteria for our service because their complaints are relatively minor or chronic. This has occasionally caused irritation, even though we give guidance on other possible sites for referral, and the management in our Mental Health Trust are sometimes a little concerned that, as GPs are major purchasers, if we do not agree to see

Table 10.1. *Numbers of patients seen by Early Intervention Service since its inception in 1987*

Year	Number of patients referred	Number of patients seen (% of referrals)	Number of team members (full-time equivalents)
1988	252	203 (80.5)	8
1989	275	234 (85.1)	8
1990	326	277 (85)	7
1991	391	316 (80.8)	6.5
1992	431	345 (80)	6.5

all their patients there could be repercussions with our contracts. By highlighting deficiencies in other areas of practice, however, we can serve as a useful pressure group and already we have been able to assist in the introduction of new services for counselling at the local branch of MIND.

There have been some alterations in the profile of referrals over the years of operation of the service but there has always been a rough separation into three diagnostic groups of equal size; mood disorders, adjustment and stress disorders, and schizophrenia. Although the team does not treat primary drug and alcohol problems, a small group of patients does have these problems to a significant extent.

Good diagnostic comparison has been possible because the EIS has from the beginning adopted the policy of giving a formal diagnosis to all patients taken on by the service using the ICD-10 notation. Comparison of referrals early in its history and those recently show relatively little change in the type of patient being taken on by the service and, in particular, the phenomenon of 'up-market drift' so often found with community mental health teams (Dowell & Ciario, 1983) has not been shown; our referrals are not getting any easier!

Patients are almost invariably seen as a joint assessment on the first occasion, at which attempts are made initially to carry out the assessment with the referrer. If this is not possible then two members of the EIS see the patient. Clinical review meetings are held twice weekly, in which all members of the team take part. The first part of these meetings involves allocation of new referrals and feed-back from assessments. In many cases it is possible after the end of the first assessment to plan further care but, if necessary, this decision is delayed until the next clinical review meeting in which the decision about the best form of further care is made and then communicated to the patient. Most patients (>80%) are seen at home in the first instance, although subsequently care may take place at any setting, including the team's base at the EIS, which has an interview room.

Maintaining expertise and morale: the skill-share model

The EIS operates a model of care that is somewhat unusual. It is often aspired to in theory but seldom achieved in practice. We call it the skill-share model. In this model of care all disciplines contribute to each other's skills through close working arrangements and open discussion at clinical review meetings. Every patient seen by the service is reviewed weekly at the two clinical review meetings. As the average case-load is around 140 this requires economy and efficiency and this is imposed by the Chair of the meeting (who rotates every two months). Team members are encouraged to contribute their specialist knowledge at all times so that the key worker for the patient is equipped to deal with all relevant aspects of the clinical problem. Where necessary, other members of the clinical team can be introduced for short periods to deal with specific issues, but the key worker retains responsibility for co-ordinating care.

The consequence of this is that, almost imperceptibly, each team member loses the professional label that was originally attached. Team members now find it somewhat embarrassing to be introduced to visitors with the epithet of their parent discipline because in their work with the service they are not really acting as a member of that discipline. Clearly some responsibilities remain restricted to certain disciplines (e.g. injections of drugs to medical and nursing staff; assessments for compulsory admission by social workers and doctors). Many others can be shared and, for example, one of our social workers is now our main cognitive therapist, both of our community psychiatric nurses have skills in family therapy, and an occupational therapist has become expert in monitoring drug treatment.

This crossover of skills is illustrated by the following patient currently in active care with the EIS.

A young Afro-Caribbean man was referred to the EIS by his GP because of concern from his family, particularly his mother, that he was neglecting himself in his flat and might be becoming ill. In the past he had been diagnosed as schizophrenic and been treated extensively in hospital but always refused to take medication on discharge. The original assessment was made by the psychiatrist (the author) and a social worker and it was felt that he probably had a diagnosis within the schizophrenia group, although he had no positive symptoms. Eventually a diagnosis of schizo-typal disorder was reached. Compulsory admission to hospital was considered when he refused to take medication but was rejected on the grounds that it would almost certainly lead to alienation from our service and not help the patient in the longer term as he was bound to refuse medication on discharge.

He continued to be seen by the social worker (case manager) who liaised with the family. The patient maintained a precarious position within society but maintained he was happy with his life and did not want further intervention. However, when he began to drink more heavily and take cannabis, and also was involved in petty theft from local shops, the police were involved who felt that further action was necessary.

After discussion at clinical review meetings I was involved again for further assessment and, as by now he had more confidence in members of the service, it was not difficult to persuade him to come into hospital for a short in-patient assessment (a ten-day period which was agreed in advance). During this period it was felt that he had sufficient symptoms to justify antipsychotic medication and he agreed to take this by depot injection (flupenthixol decanoate 40 mg every month).

After discharge from hospital he also agreed to have help in improving his daily living abilities and the occupational therapist in the team assessed him at home and subsequently arranged a short programme to improve his cooking skills.

Although this went well, after two and a half months his mother was greatly concerned by the appearance of some abnormal movements at his mouth and these were also noted by the occupational therapist. She had always had doubts about the value of medication for her son and partly blamed his past (high dosage) antipsychotic drug treatment for some of his problems. Because of this concern, the social worker and I saw the family and the patient together. It was clear that his abnormal movements represented the rotatory bucco-lingual movements of early tardive dyskinesia so it was agreed to stop treatment. At the next clinical review meeting it was decided to continue without drug therapy and to monitor progress with regard to social function and general activity as well as seeing his family regularly. The social worker continues to act as case manager.

This illustrates several important aspects of the skill-share model:

- The case manager can be of any discipline and responsibilities for co-ordinating care do not change when the patient is admitted to hospital or moves to other centres.
- The problems that are beyond the individual case manager's expertise are tackled within the team by joint working.
- The case manager takes on a much greater role than is normally expected of the relevant discipline.
- When consultation is sought from other disciplines it can be provided indirectly through a clinical review meeting or directly by involvement of additional members of the team. There is no armchair advice.

I have argued elsewhere that psychiatrists need to be much more open in sharing their skills with their non-medical colleagues and also need to be more active at the forefront of community care (Tyrer, 1993). This type of case illustrates the advantages of this approach and also shows that it is economical of medical time (involving a total of around eight hours of total time spent by me personally in this case to date), as well as helping to reinforce the clinical skills of other practitioners.

In this particular instance the early symptoms of tardive dyskinesia were recognised by the social worker and the occupational therapist, because they now have the necessary skills to identify these fairly straightforward physical signs.

The skill-share model: budget

Because all members of the team are clinically active the functioning of the service is economical. In strict terms there are no management charges apart from a small sum given to the team co-ordinator for additional responsibilities. Even the administrator, who might be expected to have a managerial role, is a clinician, at least in *forme fruste*. The job involves taking all referrals and as most of these come by telephone a suitable skill is needed to extract the relevant information suitable for allocation of initial assessors, to decide whether the case is appropriate for the team and also to determine the degree of urgency.

In the formal comparison of the EIS and the standard hospital service, described in more detail below, confirmation of the relatively low cost of the EIS was demonstrated. Despite the fact that each visit from the service cost £132, the total cost was 2.5 times greater in the hospital service when all aspects of health care were taken into account (Merson *et al.*, 1995).

Integration with psychiatric services

One of the major problems attending the introduction of community mental health centres in the United States was the relative isolation of staff, leading to a loss of morale and subsequently to a mass exodus of staff to other more attractive work settings. The EIS has always tried to maintain close contact with other services, although this has not always been easy. The EIS was introduced to a service where it was not particularly wanted. The introduction of a new service to remedy deficiencies in an existing one is hardly likely to promote plaudits all round. Initially the service was restricted in its access to referrers and there was also the suspicion that reduction in services elsewhere were a direct consequence of the introduction of the EIS. These difficulties have naturally been more marked with other community services and still there are some difficulties outstanding.

This has disadvantages but also has the bonus of helping the team fuse together more effectively than if it was welcomed with open arms. Members of the service often still feel they are on probation and have to prove their mettle in their work. Although this has disadvantages (the myth of the hero innovator) it does have the consequence of maintaining morale. The fact that the EIS is largely responsible for forging its own destiny (or in psychological terminology, has an internal locus of control) also helps. Helplessness promotes demoralisation, and the team has never been helpless.

One of the consequences of this is that staff turnover in the EIS has been remarkably low. Only six changes have occurred in five years; four of these have been promotions, and four staff have stayed in post since the inception of the service. One problem this has highlighted is the difficulty of establishing an adequate career structure in a multidisciplinary team. It is difficult for team members to leave for other posts where they can continue to act in the same way as in the EIS; to some extent all those who have left for promotions have had to become more restrictive in their clinical work. This problem can to some extent be redressed by the ability of providers to set their own pay scales so that clinical excellence can be rewarded.

As the EIS has become established close links have been established to important parts of the service. This includes the day hospital (where a former member of the EIS is now the clinical manager), in-patient wards (improved now the EIS has access to its own beds), general practices (particularly those with many practitioners who are also fundholders) and voluntary organisations such as MIND. The policy of joint working means that members of the service are always in contact with their colleagues from other parts of the psychiatric network.

Problems with a mobile population

One of the main problems of a mobile population is the difficulties that many people have in integrating into the local community services. These include, in particular, primary care and social support networks. The consequence of this is that many psychiatric problems bypass the filters that normally prevent preventable psychiatric admissions. In a typical case, a patient presents directly to a psychiatric specialist and is admitted without any other filter intervening. This is a common state of affairs in the United States, termed 'the American by-pass' by Goldberg and Huxley (1980).

An open referral system tends to obviate these problems. If referrals are accepted from patients themselves, their neighbours, voluntary agencies and other health professionals apart from doctors, then they are likely to be seen earlier than if they are seen in the sometimes bureaucratic statutory systems. In the EIS the policy of open referral has been operated from its beginning and has worked well. There is no evidence that those who are not medically qualified refer more inappropriate cases and in practice the more severely mentally ill patients are referred from non-medical sources.

Evaluation and audit, including comparison with other services

After the first year of its operation the EIS circulated all those agencies who had referred patients to ask their opinions. These were presented in the form of positive and negative statements about the service, to which respondents indicated whether they agreed or disagreed to varying levels of intensity. At this stage the EIS was still a demonstration project and its future was uncertain, so one of the statements referred to the possibility of permanent status in the area. Sixty-one per cent (62 of 102) of the referrers returned their forms and their results indicated a strong preference for the EIS procedures of joint working, visiting patients at their homes, referral arrangements and need for permanent status. Further audit of referrers has continued; although there is still general approval there has been concern expressed in the last year, particularly by GPs, about the priority we give to referrals of major mental illness, or to be more precise, the relative lower priority given to less severe illness. We have reminded referrers that requests for counselling and support for patients are seldom appropriate for the team, not least because other resources are available in the area. We have therefore rejected some of these referrals.

We also need to determine whether our service was different from others dealing with the same population. This was possible because the EIS, although dealing with a specified catchment area, was only one of several service providers.

A formal study was then set up to evaluate the EIS by comparing its efficacy, impact on patients' views and use of resources by comparison with the parallel hospital service. Using a randomized controlled design, patients presenting as emergencies to either the hospital doctors or psychiatric social work department (who could equally have been referred to the hospital service or the EIS) were allocated to their service by the referring doctor or social worker opening a sealed envelope.

Selection of treatment in both services was clinically determined without any restrictions imposed by the study design, but in practice more EIS patients received psychological intervention than in the hospital service. Most EIS referrals were seen at home initially, with referrals to the hospital service seen mainly in psychiatric out-patient clinics.

After randomisation, patients were assessed by a psychiatrist blind to service allocation, which included demographic and clinical information (symptoms, social function, premorbid personality). Further assessment and scoring of symptoms and social function were carried out 2, 4 and 12 weeks after randomisation, either at home or hospital depending upon patients' preference.

Table 10.2. *Summary of findings of randomised controlled trial of Early Intervention Service and standard hospital service in treatment of psychiatric emergencies over a period of 12 weeks*

	Early Intervention Service	Standard service
Number allocated	48	52
Number seen and engaged by services	47	37
% reduction in symptoms	36.4	16.9
In personality disorder	1.6	25.6
In non-personality disorder	34.0	17.2
% improvement in social function overall	15.4	18.8
Mean psychiatric bed days	1.2	9.3
% satisfied with care	83	54
Mean cost of care/patient	£1160	£2502

(Data derived from Merson *et al.*, 1992, 1995; Tyrer *et al.*, 1994.)

Of 100 patients consenting to inclusion in the study, 52 were randomly allocated to the control and 48 to the experimental group; 95 patients completed the research assessments at 12 weeks. The results (Merson *et al.*, 1992) are summarised in Table 10.2 and showed greater take-up of services with the EIS together with greater satisfaction with care, reduced in-patient bed use and greater reduction in symptoms but not social functioning.

Difficulties in developing skill-share services

Although we feel confident that we have identified an efficient and effective model of practice that reinforces practioners' skills and avoids burn-out we are well aware of the difficulties involved in implementing this approach elsewhere. These are listed in Table 10.3.

Until we have a consistent core of training for all mental health professionals we are bound to have continuing conflict in community psychiatric teams. The past arguments between professional groups, still unnecessarily rehearsed and repeated in formal teaching, build up the ammunition of resentment and antagonism ready to be exploded when trainees are released into clinical practice. As a consequence early conflict in community teams is the norm and many respond by retreating into unidisciplinary purdah, only venturing out to converse with other disciplines on formal occasions when rules

Table 10.3. *Problems to be overcome before skill-sharing can be implemented*

Contradictory training
Inter-professional rivalry
Understanding of clinical responsibility
Empowerment

of etiquette are strictly observed. This should not be allowed to develop and a period of common training would help greatly in its resolution (Goldberg & Huxley, 1992).

Inter-professional rivalry follows from inter-professional conflict and should also be reduced by common training. It never continues to amaze me that, for a professional group that is said to be expert in the art of communicating, we persistently fail to apply our skills when we interreact with colleagues. The skill-share approach removes rivalry and aids communication. Similarly, arguments over who is clinically responsible for patients should not be used as an excuse to create an unnecessary hierarchy in community teams. The doctor is medically responsible, the social worker is similarly responsible for specific social work tasks, and so on. Even medical students when attached to the team carry some responsibility for their behaviour and actions that can in no way be transferred to others. In the skill-share approach the clinical team becomes a responsible body in its own right and much of this unnecessary debate disappears.

'Empowerment' is an over-used word of the moment but is relevant in maintaining morale and enthusiasm in community teams. If each member of the team feels their particular skills and potential are being exercised and acknowledged this is an excellent reinforcer of self-esteem. This is particularly important for new team members. We can usually detect when such members have achieved the necessary empowerment for good functioning in the team; they have the confidence to express their disagreements with others openly! A strong team is one that can express its disagreements without rancour and when these are genuine ones involving opinions about difficult clinical decisions rather than the phoney exercise of pre-existing prejudices they ultimately improve the team's function. To end where I began this chapter, burn-out is not an explanation of difficulties in community psychiatric teams, it is an apology for an explanation. No one can pretend that the professional life of a committed team member is an easy one but when the rewards consistently exceed the handicaps, burn-out is nowhere to be seen.

References

Burns, T., Beadsmoore, A., Bhat, A. V., Oliver, A. & Mathers, C. (1993). A controlled trial of home-based acute psychiatric services. I. Clinical and social outcome. *British Journal of Psychiatry*, **163**, 49–54.

Dean, C. & Gadd, E. M. (1990). Home treatment for acute psychiatric illness. *British Medical Journal*, **301**, 1021–3.

Dedman, P. (1993). Home treatment for acute psychiatric disorder. *British Medical Journal*, **306**, 1359–60.

Dowell, D. A. & Ciarlo, J. A. (1983). Overview of the community mental health centers program from an evaluation perspective. *Community Mental Health Journal*, **19**, 95–125.

Goldberg, D. & Huxley, A. (1992). *Common Mental Disorders: A Biosocial Model.* London, Tavistock/Routledge.

Goldberg, D. & Huxley, P. (1980). *Mental Illness in the Community: The Pathway to Psychiatric Care.* London, Tavistock Publications.

Jarman, B. (1983). Identification of underprivileged areas. *British Medical Journal*, **286**, 1705–9.

Jarman, B. (1984). Validation and distribution of scores. *British Medical Journal*, **289**, 1587–92.

Merson, S., Tyrer, P., Onyett, S., Lack, S., Birkett, P., Lynch, S. & Johnson, T. (1992). Early intervention in psychiatric emergencies: a controlled clinical trial. *The Lancet*, **339**, 1311–14.

Merson, S., Tyrer, P., Carlen, D. & Johnson, A. L. (1995). The cost of treatment of psychiatric emergencies: a comparison of hospital and community services. *Psychological Medicine*. (In press.)

Onyett, S. (1992). *Case Management in Mental Health.* Chapman and Hall, London.

Onyett, S., Tyrer, P., Connolly, J., Malone, S., Rennison, J., Parslow, S., Shia, N., Davey, T., Lynch, S. & Merson, S. (1990). The Early Intervention Service: the first eighteen months of an inner London demonstration project. *Psychiatrric Bulletin*, **14**, 267–9.

Stein, L. I. & Test, M. A. (1980). Alternative to mental hospital treatment. 1. Conceptual model, treatment program and clinical evaluation. *Archives of General Psychiatry*, **36**, 1073–9.

Tyrer, P. (1992). Schizophrenia: early detection, early intervention. In *The Primary Care of Schizophrenia*, ed. R. Jenkins, V. Field & R. Young, London, HMSO.

Tyrer, P. (1993). Who is failing the mentally ill? *The Lancet*, **341**, 1199–201.

Tyrer, P., Ferguson, B. & Wadsworth, J. (1990). Liaison psychiatry in general practice: the comprehensive collaborative model. *Acta Psychiatrica Scandinavica*, **81**, 359–63.

Tyrer, P., Merson, S., Onyett, S. & Johnson, T. (1994). The effect of personality disorder on clinical outcome, social networks and adjustment: a controlled clinical trial of psychiatric emergencies. *Psychological Medicine*, **24**, 731–40.

Tyrer, P., Turner, R. & Johnson, A. L. (1989). Integrated hospital and community psychiatric services and use of inpatient beds. *British Medical Journal*, **299**, 298–300.

11

Psychiatric emergencies in the casualty department

Sonia Johnson and Howard Baderman

Introduction

The accident and emergency (A & E) department of the general hospital differs from other settings for emergency intervention as patients with acute psychiatric problems will present here whether or not a specific service for their management is provided. Whatever their treatment history and familiarity with local health services, most people know where to find their local general hospital A & E department, and know that it is a source of urgent help available day and night. Further, it has been observed that some patients and their carers continue to come to the A & E department even if they are aware of other, sometimes more appropriate, services which they may contact in crisis (Bartolucci & Drayer, 1973).

However, whilst the A & E department figures prominently in the minds of the public as a source of help, it has not always been so central in discussion and research on psychiatric emergencies, or in the development of innovative services. In the 1960s and 1970s, at least in North America, the general hospital emergency room was for a time a major focus for research and service development, as numbers of patients presenting here increased and as psychiatric services began to shift from the large mental hospital to general hospital units. More recently, the assessment and management of self-poisoning has received considerable attention in Britain. Apart from this, there has been little more general discussion of needs for psychiatric care in the casualty department (in the UK referred to as A & E department and in the United States as emergency room), perhaps partly because attention has shifted to development of acute services based in the community. However, while casualty department emergency psychiatry may appear less fashionable, less exciting and less innovative to clinicians and researchers than community interventions, it continues in practice to be an important component in psychiatric emergency care in most areas.

In this chapter, we will begin by briefly describing the main groups of patients who present in the casualty department. We will then discuss current patterns of service provision in this setting. Common management difficulties and resource deficiencies will then be identified. Finally, we will discuss ways in which more effective provision might be developed. This chapter principally refers to the UK and North America, as we have found few reports on the structure and activity of psychiatric services elsewhere, and the discussion of current problems and possible improvements refers largely to Britain.

Psychiatric problems in accident and emergency department practice

On the basis of their principal presenting problems, three main groups of patients may be distinguished in the A & E department. These are discussed below.

Presenting problems with physical and psychiatric components

Whatever emergency psychiatric facilities are provided elsewhere, a group of patients who are likely to continue to need to be seen in the A & E department are those with urgent needs for both physical and psychiatric assessment and intervention. The most prominent are patients who deliberately harm or poison themselves. During the 1970s and 1980s, there was concern about the large increase in the number of people presenting, having taken overdoses. Hawton and Catalan (1987) described a four-fold increase in casualty attendances following overdoses or deliberate self-harm in Oxford between 1963 and 1973. Whilst patients who survive deliberate self-harm have different clinical and social characteristics from completed suicides and will not always have a high level of suicidal intent, parasuicide is a substantial risk factor for suicide. Hawton and Fagg (1988) studied suicide and other causes of death in 1959 patients who had attended a casualty department following deliberate self-harm or self-poisoning, and found that over a mean follow-up of eight years, 2.8% had died through suicide or probable suicide, with around 1% killing themselves during the year after the index attempt, 27 times the rate expected from general population statistics. As described below, this group has therefore been identified as a promising target for interventions aimed at suicide prevention.

Other patients, with mixed needs for urgent physical and psychological intervention, present in A & E from time to time (Ellison *et al.*, 1989). The homeless mentally ill and other patients with mental illness and severe self-neglect may present with concurrent severe physical and severe psychiatric pathology, requiring the collaboration of general and psychiatric services. Distressed victims of rape or violence may require some form of social or psychological assessment and intervention. Particularly where communication and collaboration between services are poor, acrimonious boundary disputes may arise between psychiatric staff and general medical and A & E staff about patients with both organic pathology and behavioural disturbances, as in confusional states, encephalopathies and dementias.

Primarily somatic complaints with a background of psychiatric morbidity

Psychiatric morbidity also seems to be common among those who come to the casualty department with apparently exclusively physical complaints. A range of presentations will be found, from those who present with clear acute physical pathology, but concurrently have significant psychological symptoms, to patients with somatisation disorders who repeatedly present with physical symptoms despite reassurance that they have no organic pathology. As with general hospital in-patients, A & E attenders appear to have higher levels of psychiatric morbidity than the general population. Bell *et al.* (1990) found that psychiatric diagnoses could be made for 24 out of 120 daytime attenders with physical complaints at a central London A & E department, although in most cases the psychopathology was not severe and was categorised as an indication for intervention at a primary care level. Salkovskis *et al.* (1990) have also found high levels of psychiatric symptoms on screening patients attending A & E with medical complaints, and found that these symptoms tended to persist at one month follow-up.

Overtly psychiatric presenting problems

As A & E departments are accessible and well known, some patients will refer themselves or be brought here by carers. In addition, in some areas the A & E department is the officially designated setting for the provision of psychiatric emergency services, so that general practitioners (GPs) and other professionals wishing to make referrals for specialist assessment are directed to send patients here. Thus in most areas, some patients with severe mental illness are likely to present in this setting, and in some places, most psychiatric emergency assessments will take place here.

Whilst there is a substantial body of good research on deliberate self-harm and self-poisoning (Hawton & Catalan, 1987), there seems, at least in the UK, to have been little work on the overall psychiatric case-load of the A & E department: the numbers of patients with primarily psychiatric problems, their clinical and social characteristics, their needs for intervention and their disposition and outcome have not recently been clearly described. Although modern information systems might make this task considerably easier, the bulk of published work in this area is rather old. Bartolucci and Drayer (1973) reviewed North American and UK work on this subject, and suggested that in most centres around 5% of visits to the casualty department or emergency room involved primarily psychiatric complaints. Bassuk *et al.* (1983) studied attenders at the emergency room in a hospital in Boston, USA and in the A & E department in Bristol, UK. They identified 3.9% of Boston attenders (1400 psychiatric visits in one year) as presenting with psychiatric complaints, whilst in Bristol the proportion was 3% (504 visits in a year). Of the psychiatric attenders in Bristol, around two-thirds had harmed or poisoned themselves and one-third presented with other psychiatric complaints. They noted that these figures did not include patients in whom overtly physical complaints masked psychiatric symptoms, and that around 2.5% of visits involved vague physical complaints for which no specific diagnosis or treatment was recorded. A further detailed study was made of 50 patients in each of the centres. In Bristol, 20% had psychoses, 33% depression, 22% personality disorder and 16% generalised anxiety, whilst in Boston, 16% had psychotic illnesses, 29% depression, 14% personality disorders and 6% generalised anxiety. Patients were often not in contact with any other health services, and study of the social characteristics and psychiatric histories of these patients showed more limited social networks than in other treatment settings, particularly in Bristol, where only 19% of patients had at least weekly contact with a relative or friend.

North American studies have identified a number of clinical and social attributes which seem more prevalent in emergency room attenders than in patients in other treatment settings. Both in psychotic and non-psychotic patients, substance abuse has been identified as a frequent complicating factor (Barbee *et al.*, 1989; Wolfe & Sorensen, 1989). A substantial literature has accumulated on the characteristics of frequent attenders in the psychiatric emergency room. Bassuk (1985) suggests that this setting is now a last resort for the most difficult patients, with between 7 and 18% of visits involving 'chronic crisis patients' who have a variety of diagnoses, including psychotic illnesses and personality disorders, but share a tendency to have few social supports, very limited engagement in other treatment systems and poor rapport with clinicians. An important characteristic of A & E attenders is that their clinical and social problems are often complex and long-standing, with attendances sometimes precipitated by relatively minor failures of fragile support systems or coping strategies. The chronic nature of their problems and the relatively minor precipitants to visits can be a potent source of frustration to clinicians, who may feel that these presentations are not 'true emergencies'.

Current service provision in the accident and emergency department

Whilst a fairly similar spectrum of psychiatric problems is likely to present in most general hospital casualty departments, the nature and extent of services provided for their management varies. A single psychiatric trainee may be responsible for assessment of all emergency referrals, combining this with duties on the in-patient wards. On the other hand, particularly in larger urban hospitals in the United

States, the psychiatric emergency room may be a distinct department, with its own 24-hour multidisciplinary team. A range of arrangements exists between these two extremes.

A nationwide survey of psychiatric emergency provision in England and Wales carried out in 1991 (Johnson & Thornicroft, 1991) elicited some basic information about current arrangements for psychiatric cover for the A & E department. Responses were obtained from 87% of district health authorities in England and Wales. Respondents were asked who was the first point of contact for A & E doctors making referrals to the psychiatric services, and the results suggest that junior psychiatric staff remain the main professionals involved, at least initially, in A & E assessments. In office hours, a senior house officer or registrar on the same site was the first contact in 57% of districts, whilst a more senior psychiatrist (senior registrar or consultant) was the contact in 21% and a psychiatric nurse in 4%. In most of the remaining 19%, doctors at various grades were the main contact. At night, junior psychiatric staff were the initial contact in 72%. Particularly at night, there was little evidence of any extensive use of multidisciplinary assessments. Senior house officers and registrars usually have concurrent responsibilities apart from seeing these urgent referrals: only 9% of districts had junior staff dedicated solely to emergency work 24 hours a day. It was also common for psychiatric staff covering the A & E department to be based on a different site, particularly at night, when 46% had to travel to the general hospital from another, sometimes distant, site.

Johnson and Thornicroft's (1991) survey suggests that the A & E department retains an important role not only in the assessment of patients who present initially to A & E doctors, but also in the management of patients referred from the community to psychiatric professionals. Sixty-six per cent of districts reported that they made use of the casualty department for emergency assessment of patients referred by GPs for specialist psychiatric assessment at night and at weekends, whilst 50% used it routinely for this purpose during office hours. It was notable that during the working day, many districts offered some alternative sites for assessment outside the hospital, but at night, these largely ceased to operate. Sixty-three per cent of districts provided some daytime assessments at a community site such as a community mental health centre or day hospital, whilst only 1% provided such services at night or at weekends. Similarly, where specialist psychiatric emergency clinics, multidisciplinary assessments or crisis intervention teams were provided, these were almost exclusively functioning in office hours only. Thus whilst innovative emergency services are beginning to develop during the day, most districts appear to revert outside office hours to the traditional model of a single junior doctor assessing referrals alone in the A & E department, or sometimes on in-patient psychiatric wards.

In the United States, Hopkin (1985), Goldfinger and Lipton (1985) and Wellin *et al.* (1987) have documented an increasing tendency for the general hospital emergency room to be used as the primary site for emergency intervention. This trend may in part be related to the increasing adoption in psychiatry of more biological models, and the accompanying tendency to seek greater integration with general medical services at a time when there seems to have been a decline in faith in the crisis intervention model. As Solomon and Gordon (1986) point out, the move to the general hospital emergency room as the primary site for the delivery of psychiatric services has also been advanced by the tendency of community mental health centres to contract the local general hospital to operate the emergency part of their service, and, in the 1980s, by a general diminution in community mental health care funding. Perhaps partly because the much weaker primary care structure makes the range of alternative sources of help in psychiatric emergencies still narrower, emergency room psychiatric services are often more developed than those in UK A & E departments. At least in large urban centres, psychiatric emergency rooms have often developed as distinct departments within or next to the general emergency room, and they may have a multidisciplinary team dedicated 24 hours a day to emergency work, a triage officer, specific security staff and their own purpose-built interviewing suites.

Resource and management problems in the accident and emergency department

Specialist services for psychiatric emergency intervention, such as psychiatric emergency clinics and crisis intervention services, are designed specifically to meet the needs of those with acute mental illness. In contrast, the A & E department has generally not been planned with this group particularly in mind, but has come to be widely used for emergency psychiatry because it is convenient and already available in every district. It is thus not surprising that the difficulties arising in its use can be considerable. In a national survey of the views of two major voluntary organisations concerned with mental health (MIND and the National Schizophrenia Fellowship), A & E departments were rated as one of the poorest elements in acute psychiatric services, with only 25% of groups rating their local service as adequate or good (Johnson & Thornicroft, 1991). Some of the difficulties which may arise are described in this section.

Local availability of psychiatric resources

The availability of services to which patients can be referred from the A & E department necessarily has a crucial effect on service effectiveness and staff morale. The development of high quality facilities and staffing within the A & E department will achieve very little if in-patient beds are in very short supply and take many hours to find, or if intensive community treatment is unavailable. Weissberg (1991) describes the poorer mentally ill as 'chained in the emergency room', arguing that the emergency room of the general hospital is now almost the only treatment site available for the chronically mentally ill in the United States, so that they often spend many hours under physical restraint there whilst increasingly irritated staff experience great difficulties in finding any appropriate disposal. Similar situations are often encountered in UK A & E departments, and where this is the case, clinicians are likely mainly to concentrate on considering where they can send patients rather than how they can help them.

Continuity of care

As well as needing resources to which patients may be referred, good mechanisms for ensuring that patients engage with these services are needed. The main decision on which psychiatrists often focus in A & E is whether the patient is at immediate risk and requires admission, with little attention given to establishing some continuity of care for those who are not admitted. When junior staff have finished their day or night of emergency duty, they are not generally assigned any continuing responsibility for following up patients they have assessed, and often there are no permanent psychiatric A & E staff to whom this task might be passed on. Psychiatric staff, particularly trainees who rotate frequently between placements, may lack a thorough knowledge of local resources and their referral procedures. Solomon and Gordon (1986) reviewed literature on compliance with onward referrals of patients assessed but not admitted, and found generally poor rates of contact with the services to which referrals were made, sometimes as low as 30%. Assertive attempts to engage patients swiftly with other services may not be given a high priority where patients' main difficulties are longstanding, and their attendance is not seen as a 'true emergency'. However, patients with largely chronic difficulties who use the emergency services will include people with severe and persistent mental illnesses. Particularly in city centre departments, they are often very mobile, socially isolated and not engaged with any more long-term treatment. Thus their sporadic appearances in the A & E department may be the main opportunity for making contact and endeavouring to provide them with continuing care.

Effects of the accident and emergency department environment

Patients with psychiatric problems differ from those with other complaints in that the A & E department environment may make their symptoms worse. Gerson and Bassuk (1980) write that this setting is 'a unique context for psychotherapeutic intervention: unlike other psychiatric settings, in which the environment is structured with the purpose of increasing the possibilities of calm enquiry into the patient's problems, the emergency room environment is the locus of a variety of influences that may have a negative impact on patient care.' The atmosphere of A & E departments tends to be noisy, highly charged and busy. Interruptions are common and privacy difficult to obtain. Accompanying family members and friends may be perceived as, or feel themselves to be, in the way, and may be moved out of the main clinical areas, rather than being actively involved in assessment and treatment planning. Patients with psychiatric problems may be disturbed and alarmed by seeing those who have life-threatening physical conditions, and patients with physical complaints may find the presence of disturbed psychiatric patients distressing. The needs of psychiatric patients for appropriate physical facilities have tended to be overlooked both in central policy and by local planners: whilst well-equipped cubicles for resuscitation, for children and for patients with gynaecological problems are standard, psychiatric patients are very often seen in a standard A & E cubicle, or in an interview room which has been minimally modified, and which may sometimes have been chosen as the psychiatric cubicle largely because it is an area too small, barren and inconvenient to be allocated for other clinical use. The harmful effects of the A & E environment will be exacerbated where patients have very long waits for assessment, admission or other appropriate disposition.

The A & E department setting may also mould the interaction between patient and clinician in ways which are sometimes unhelpful. Patients' and psychiatrists' expectations about consultations in the A & E department may be influenced by the swift assessments and decisive and directive management characterising the assessment of patients with physical complaints in A & E. Stereotypical doctor and patient roles may be adopted, with the clinician tending to assume complete control over the patient and the patient taking an attitude of helplessness and fear. The social context of the emergency and the nature of the patient's support network are less visible and less easily investigated than in an assessment in the community, and assessment is often purely medical rather than multidisciplinary. Both these factors may produce a tendency to view emergencies purely as exacerbations of illness, when it might be useful in some instances to view them as breakdowns in patients' usual social support systems or as failures of their usual coping and problem solving strategies.

Safety in the accident and emergency department

Safety is an aspect of the setting for emergency psychiatric assessment which has special importance for good clinical management and for staff morale. Adequate consideration is not always given to making rooms used for psychiatric assessment safe for patients who are actively trying to harm themselves and safe for the staff who attend them. Careful planning is also needed to ensure patients cannot readily abscond if they are at risk of harming themselves or others. The possibility of violence towards staff may be a considerable source of anxiety in managing psychiatric emergencies in this setting. In fact, violence in the A & E department is frequent, but the perpetrators are much more often intoxicated young men than people with mental illnesses (Cembrowicz & Shepherd, 1992). However, psychiatric patients become violent from time to time, and this possibility will be a perpetual source of anxiety where, as often occurs, staffing levels, physical setting and staff training are not adequate for the safe management of very behaviourally disturbed patients. The problem of safety is particularly acute in A & E departments which are designated 'places of safety' for Section 136 of the 1983 Mental Health Act, so that the police bring to them people whose behaviour in a public place suggests that they are suffering from a mental disorder and are in need of immediate care and control, or require assessment in their own interest or for the protection of others. The facilities and staffing levels of A & E departments are often such that they fall far short of really being the 'places of safety' required by the Act, either for patients or for staff.

Accident and emergency clinicians' difficulties in the management psychiatric problems

Considerable hostility to patients with psychiatric problems is often encountered among the general staff of the A & E department. A number of potential sources of this hostility have already been alluded to: they include difficulty in arranging adequate disposals for these patients, the feeling that many patients have mostly chronic difficulties and are thus not 'true emergencies' and the perceived threat of violence which the department is inadequately equipped to manage. Particularly following deliberate self-harm or substance abuse, patients may be blamed for their difficulties, leading to a punitive attitude. The mental states of many patients presenting in casualty also have aspects which are likely to provoke frustration and irritation: patients tend to be at their most regressed and helpless when they present in crisis in this setting, and in this state they often have a powerful capacity for transmitting to others their feelings of hopelessness, fear and hostility. The difficulties in establishing good rapport and productive therapeutic relationships which characterise repeat attenders (Bassuk & Gerson, 1980) make this sub-group of patients particularly likely to frustrate and annoy clinicians. These negative feelings often give rise to very cursory assessments, irritable interactions with patients and with mental health staff and an eagerness to pass on or remove patients as rapidly as possible.

A & E clinicians are also often handicapped by lack of knowledge and confidence about mental health problems. The psychiatric element in casualty officer induction courses or in A & E nurse specialist training is usually very limited. In higher training for career specialists in A & E medicine, psychiatry is again often neglected. Whilst a secondment to an acute psychiatric facility is often mentioned in training schemes, relatively few senior registrars in A & E medicine actually gain this experience, and these working attachments are not always very easy to arrange. A perception of emergency psychiatry as a low status area which does not require great attention is often reinforced by the fact that A & E work is often relegated almost exclusively to junior psychiatric staff. Appearances in the casualty department by consultant psychiatrists are uncommon, and a lack of interest and involvement among senior A & E staff in planning and providing appropriate services for psychiatric patients again strengthens the perception of psychiatry as a poor relation of emergency medical and surgical specialities.

Psychiatrists' difficulties in working in accident and emergency

The hostility towards psychiatric patients and their doctors found among A & E staff is often accompanied by a distaste for A & E work among junior psychiatrists. Ellison *et al.* (1989) review several studies which suggest that junior psychiatrists in casualty departments are often demoralised and see this placement as a 'rip-off' in which there are large demands on them for service provision, but little contribution is made to their training. Again, several reasons have already been identified which make these feelings very understandable: they include difficulties in disposition, hostile and dismissive attitudes among A & E staff, an inappropriate environment for assessments, frequent interruptions, patients' helpless states and unrealistic expectations that all their difficulties may be resolved through some decisive emergency intervention, and the fact that duties on the wards often compete with the A & E department. A particularly important factor in the development of negative attitudes to A & E duties is the frequent lack of specific training and senior supervision for this work. There is often very little opportunity for junior psychiatrists to discuss and receive guidance on their emergency assessments, particularly when they are carried out on call at night or at the weekend, and teaching on emergency psychiatry may be limited.

Developing effective psychiatric services in the casualty department

Thus, the A & E department continues to occupy a central position in emergency psychiatry, but a variety of major hazards impede good practice in this setting. In this final section, we will consider service models which have been implemented or proposed for the improvement of these services, and will make some suggestions about important considerations in A & E service planning.

In the UK, work on developing more effective services has mainly focused on assessment and management of deliberate self-harm. A number of studies have addressed the question of who should assess patients following self-poisoning. The Hill Report (Central and Scottish Health Services Councils, 1968) advocated the establishment of poisoning treatment centres to which all patients were to be referred, for assessment by a psychiatrist and a social worker. In practice, these official recommendations were widely disregarded, and several studies have subsequently shown that psychiatric nurses (Catalan *et al.*, 1980), social workers (Newson-Smith & Hirsch, 1979) and physicians (Gardner *et al.*, 1978) can assess patients competently following attempted suicide. An essential point about each of these studies, however, was that specific training was provided before these professionals began to assess patients who had taken overdoses. In a number of centres in the UK, specialist psychiatric liaison nurses are now beginning to play an important part in assessment and management of deliberate self-harm.

A number of reports have also appeared in the past 20 years evaluating model services for intervention following parasuicide, for example offering problem solving treatment by nurses, domiciliary visits or a social work service (Gibbons *et al.*, 1978; Hawton *et al.*, 1981). However, the results of these interventions have generally been disappointing, with very few gains reported in improving psychiatric symptoms or preventing repetition of parasuicide (Hawton & Catalan, 1987; Moeller, 1989). Two major factors are likely to be important in explaining the very limited benefits apparent in these model programmes. Firstly, the interventions offered to control groups have often been substantial, so that it may well be the case that some intervention in this group is better than no intervention, but that there are no very great differences in efficacy for the various interventions which have been used. Secondly, for ethical reasons, these studies necessarily do not focus on those who are at highest risk of self-harm or of considerable deterioration. Those who require admission or who have serious mental illnesses cannot generally be included in studies where interventions provided are of quite low intensity, so that much of the recent work on interventions following A & E attendances excludes those who are most at risk and likely to have the highest levels of unmet need. Interventions mainly targeting those who present in the A & E department with physical complaints, but who are found to have substantial anxiety or depressive symptoms, such as the brief cognitive behavioural treatment programme described by Atha *et al.* (1992), may have similar weaknesses; they again may not show very great gains because they do not target those most in need.

A new emphasis thus seems timely on the role and functioning of the A & E department as a place of assessment and intervention for the seriously mentally ill, who may present or be referred here not only following self-harm but also at other times when an acute deterioration in their mental state has occurred or their social support network has broken down. Recent research, public policy and local planning have paid little attention to the general requirements for an effective A & E psychiatric service, or to ways of remedying the deficiencies identified above. A central requirement prior to the planning of better services is for better information about the current psychiatric activity and patient populations of A & E departments, including data concerning patients' unmet needs and engagement with other services prior to and following A & E attendance. Information from a number of centres would be helpful, as demographic characteristics and the extent and organisation of other local services are likely to affect use of the A & E service.

However, even without better information on A & E activity, there are a number of ways in which local initiatives might alleviate some of the problems we have identified. One way of resolving some of the difficulties inherent in working in this setting is to move emergency assessments out of this setting altogether to a specialist emergency clinic or a base in the community. However, whilst referrals from GPs and the police and some self-presentations might be directed elsewhere, there will still be a need for A & E department assessments for patients who harm themselves or who have referred themselves initially to A & E doctors. Also, in many areas, there are currently few obvious alternatives to the A & E department, particularly at night and at weekends. No imminent end to the central position of A & E in out-of-hours emergency cover currently seems probable.

In engaging patients with continuing treatment after casualty department attendances, North American authors have described two strategies which have been found helpful. Firstly, Gillig *et al.* (1989) have described the use of a short stay psychiatric holding area within the emergency room, in which extended evaluation and mobilisation of community supports may take place over a period of up to 24 hours. Secondly, patients not admitted may routinely be followed up through a planned series of repeat appointments with emergency service psychiatric staff, as described by Blane *et al.* (1967). However, strategies which prolong patients' involvement with the casualty department seem likely to be less useful than the promotion of rapid engagement with services which can provide longer term care. Staff working in A & E need to have access to very good information about local psychiatric resources and how to mobilise them, and, particularly for those with severe mental illnesses, community psychiatric services need to have the capacity to engage A & E attenders swiftly and assertively with their services. The availability of a permanent staff member in A & E who can ensure effective follow-up after A & E attendance and develop links with other psychiatric agencies may be very useful in improving continuity of care. At University College Hospital, London, a recently appointed psychiatric liaison nurse has extended her role considerably beyond the assessment of patients who have taken overdoses: she has an important role in arranging admissions and in general acts as a link between A & E and other local services, with whom she has established good communication. She also provides staff working in A & E with information on local resources and on how to admit patients. For example, she has produced a booklet giving information for on call junior psychiatrists, which is helpful when they are not familiar with local services.

Better physical facilities may also go some way towards improving patients' and staff experience of A & E psychiatric services. Interview rooms need to be safe: it should be possible to remove any furniture or fittings with which patients may harm themselves or others, rooms need to be reasonably damage-proof and they should not be located in obscure corners of the department from which it is easy to abscond unnoticed. Comfort and privacy also have to be carefully considered: rooms should be pleasant, without harsh lighting, and conversations should not be overheard. There should be enough space for accompanying family or friends to be comfortably accommodated.

Training and supervision of both A & E psychiatric staff is another crucial area. Acute psychiatry needs to be incorporated into induction courses for A & E staff, and regular input from psychiatric staff be incorporated into continuing education. At University College Hospital, the psychiatric liaison nurse has taken the lead role in providing teaching for A & E and psychiatric staff; monthly early morning tutorials and case conferences with a psychiatric senior registrar or community psychiatric nurse, have proved to be successful. Both formal teaching on important topics such as the management of violence and the assessment of suicide risk and opportunities for discussion of problems which have arisen are helpful. The training needs of paramedical, ancillary and administrative staff need to be considered as well as those of medical and nursing staff. For career A & E medicine specialists, a psychiatric placement needs to become mandatory. Greater knowledge and confidence are likely to diminish negative feelings towards psychiatric patients. However, it should also be acknowledged that the anger, fear and hopelessness sometimes provoked in staff by very distressed patients with difficult and longstanding problems are natural responses: staff should not be blamed for experiencing these feelings, but be helped to understand and manage them. For junior medical and nursing staff, their experience in the A & E department may be the time in their training when they are most exposed to severe psychiatric problems. If they receive enough teaching and supervision to prevent this being an aversive experience, it represents a valuable opportunity to gain confidence and expertise in the assessment and management of psychiatric problems.

Psychiatric staff also need specific training and supervision for their work in the A & E department. The requirements for effective work in this setting differ from other settings, in that ways of helping patients need to be found in the course of only one interview, there is often little time, patients may be particularly distressed and disturbed, and substance abuse, physical illness and homelessness are frequent complicating factors. Again, teaching on important topics in emergency psychiatry, opportunities to discuss patients and a willingness on the part of senior psychiatric staff to become involved with difficult problems will be helpful. It should also be considered whether combining A & E duties with ward duties (sometimes on another site) may create an unreasonable burden for the junior psychiatrist on call and that perhaps a more multidisciplinary approach to A & E assessments might be feasible and fruitful.

Finally, the development of good A & E services is likely to require good communication at senior levels between A & E staff and psychiatrists. The formation of a liaison group involving managers and senior nursing and medical staff has been found to be a way of improving the two groups' understanding of one another's difficulties, developing a joint approach to problems which arise, and planning ways of improving services. Senior involvement may also raise the status of emergency psychiatry and indicate to junior staff that it is an important and valued service. At a national as well as a local level, little attention has been given to developing policy on good practice and on resources needed for A & E psychiatric services, and collaboration between professional bodies such as the Royal College of Psychiatrists and the Faculty of A & E Medicine would be helpful in defining good practice and stimulating the development of central policy.

Conclusions

In summary, the A & E department remains an important site for the provision of emergency services to patients with a wide range of psychiatric problems, including an important group of people with serious mental illnesses who are poorly engaged in services elsewhere. However, little specific planning has generally gone into making it an appropriate setting for this work, and this is reflected in inappropriate facilities, inadequate attention to safety, poor mechanisms for establishing continuity of care following attendance and limited confidence and negative attitudes among A & E and psychiatric staff. Good information is needed about the extent and nature of the current psychiatric workload in the general hospital A & E department.

In the meantime, strategies which may prove helpful in alleviating some of these problems include better training and supervision, improved interviewing facilities, the appointment of permanent staff who can establish good liaison with other agencies and improve continuity of care, and discussion and collaboration, both at local and at national levels, between senior A & E and psychiatric staff.

Acknowledgement

We are grateful to Ms Sara Murphy for very helpful discussion, particularly of her role and experience as Psychiatric Liaison Nurse at University College Hospital, London.

References

Atha, C., Salkovskis, P. M. & Storer, D. (1992). Cognitive-behavioural problem solving in the treatment of patients attending a medical emergency department: a controlled trial. *Journal of Psychosomatic Research*, **36**, 299–307.

Barbee, J. G., Clark, P. D., Crapanzano, M. S., Heintz, G. C. & Kehoe, C. E. (1989). Alcohol and substance abuse among schizophrenic patients presenting to an emergency psychiatric service. *Journal of Nervous and Mental Diseases*, **177**, 400–7.

Bartolucci, G. & Drayer, C. S. (1973). An overview of crisis intervention in the emergency rooms of general hospitals. *American Journal of Psychiatry*, **130**, 953–9.

Bassuk, E. L. (1985). Psychiatric emergency services: can they cope as last resort facilities? *New Directions for Mental Health Services*, **28**, 11–20.

Bassuk, E. L. & Gerson, S. (1980). Chronic crisis patients: a discrete clinical group. *American Journal of Psychiatry*, **137**, 1513–17.

Bassuk, E. L., Winter, R. & Apsler, R. (1983). Cross-cultural comparison of British and American psychiatric emergencies. *American Journal of Psychiatry*, **140**, 180–4.

Bell, G., Hindley, N., Rajiyah, G. & Rosser, R. (1990). Screening for psychiatric morbidity in an accident and emergency department. *Archives of Emergency Medicine*, **7**, 155–62.

Blane, H. T., Muller, J. J. & Chafetz, M. E. (1967). Acute psychiatric services in the General Hospital. II – Current status of emergency psychiatric services. *American Journal of Psychiatry*, **124**, 37–45.

Catalan, J., Marsack, P., Hawton, K. E., Whitwell, D., Fagg, J. & Bancroft, J. H. J. (1980). Comparison of doctors and nurses in the assessment of deliberate self-poisoning patients. *Psychological Medicine*, **10**, 483–91.

Cembrowicz, S. P. & Shepherd, J. P. (1992). Violence in the Accident and Emergency department. *Medicine, Science and the Law*, **32**, 118–22.

Central and Scottish Health Services Councils (1968). *Hospital Treatment of Acute Poisoning*. London, HMSO.

Ellison, J. M., Hughes, D. H. & White, K. A. (1989). An emergency psychiatry update. *Hospital and Community Psychiatry*, **40**, 250–60.

Gardner, R., Hanks, R., Evison, B., Mountford, P. M., O'Brien, V. C. & Roberts, S. J. (1978). Consultation-liaison schemes for self-poisoned patients in a general hospital. *British Medical Journal*, 1978(2), 1392–4.

Gerson, S. & Bassuk, E. (1980). Psychiatric emergencies: an overview. *American Journal of Psychiatry*, **137**, 1–10.

Gibbons, J. S., Butler, J., Urwin, P. & Gibbons, J. L. (1978). Evaluation of a social work service for self poisoning patients. *British Journal of Psychiatry*, **133**, 310–12.

Gillig, P., Hilliard, J. R. & Bell, J. (1989). The psychiatric service holding area: effects on use of resources. *American Journal of Psychiatry*, **146**, 369–72.

Goldfinger, S. M. & Lipton, F. R. (1985). Emergency psychiatry at the crossroads. *New Directions for Mental Health Services*, **28**, 107–10.

Hawton, K., Bancroft, J., Catalan, J., Kingston, B., Stedeford, A. & Welch, N. (1981). Domiciliary and out-patient treatment of self-poisoning patients by medical and non-medical staff. *Psychological Medicine*, **11**, 169–77.

Hawton, K. & Catalan, J. (1987). *Attempted Suicide: A Practical Guide to its Management*. Oxford, Oxford University Press.

Hawton, K. & Fagg, J. (1988). Suicide and other causes of death following attempted suicide. *British Journal of Psychiatry*, **152**, 359–66.

Hopkin, J. T. (1985). Psychiatry and medicine in the emergency room. *New Directions for Mental Health Services*, **28**, 47–53.

Johnson, S. & Thornicroft, G. (1991). *Psychiatric Emergency Services in England and Wales*. Report to the Department of Health. London, PRiSM, Institute of Psychiatry.

Moeller, H. J. (1989). Efficacy of different strategies of aftercare for patients who have attempted suicide. *Journal of the Royal Society of Medicine*, **82**, 643–7.

Newson-Smith, J. G. B. & Hirsch, S. R. (1979). A comparison of social workers and psychiatrists in evaluating parasuicide. *British Journal of Psychiatry*, **134**, 335–42.

Salkovskis, P. M., Storer, D., Atha, C. & Warwick, H. M. (1990). Psychiatric morbidity in an accident and emergency department: characteristics of patients at presentation and one month follow-up. *British Journal of Psychiatry*, **156**, 483–7.

Solomon, P. & Gordon, B. (1986). The psychiatric emergency room and follow-up services in the community. *Psychiatric Quarterly*, **58**, 119–27.

Weissberg, M. (1991). Chained in the emergency department: the new

asylum for the poor. *Hospital and Community Psychiatry*, **42**, 317–19.
Wellin, E., Slesinger, D. P. & Hollister, C. P. (1987). Psychiatric emergency services: evolution, adaptation and proliferation. *Social Sciences and Medicine*, **24**, 475–82.
Wolfe, H. L. & Sorensen, J. L. (1989). Dual diagnosis patients in the urban psychiatric emergency room. *Journal of Psychoactive Drugs*, **21**, 169–75.

12

Acute crisis respite care

William H. Sledge, Jack Tebes and Jaak Rakfeldt

Introduction

Acute crisis respite care involves the provision of mental health services in a short-term residential setting that functions as an alternative to acute voluntary psychiatric hospitalisation. For the past two decades, short-term residential alternatives to psychiatric hospitalisation have grown steadily in both the United States and the UK despite the lack of a coherent definition, purpose, or conceptualisation for their use. As employed here, the term 'acute crisis' respite care does *not* include the use of acute hospital stays to provide respite for family members of a severely mentally ill adult (Geiser *et al.*, 1988) or the brief placement of such patients with carefully selected families in the community in order to provide respite to families or residential service providers (Britton & Mattson-Melcher, 1985). Although 'crisis hostels' (Brook, 1973) may have represented an early form of acute crisis respite care, crisis respite services are distinct from 'hostel' services because the latter usually functions as an alternative to hospital-based institutionalisation for long-stay patients (Gibbons, 1986; Hyde *et al.*, 1987; Simpson *et al.*, 1989).

There is considerable evidence in the literature of the need for acute crisis respite care. Studies of family members of de-institutionalised mental patients consistently indicate a need for respite care among family members (Zirul *et al.*, 1989), including families with members living in board and care homes (Segal & Kotler, 1989). Evidence for this need is also provided by the requests from community providers of severely ill patients (Ghaziuddian, 1988).

Thus far, acute crisis respite care has been found to be appropriate for a wide range of adults with psychiatric difficulties. Although services are most commonly designed for persistently mentally ill adults who experience an acute exacerbation of their illness, acute respite care also has been found to be appropriate for young adults experiencing a first acute episode of major mental illness (Brunton & Howthorne, 1989), long-stay users of day hospitals (MacCarthy *et al.*, 1989), adolescents with psychiatric difficulties (Schwartz, 1989), and individuals in acute psychiatric emergency resulting from a life crisis (Brunton & Harwthorne, 1989). In the only study thus far to report on the 'failures' of acute crisis respite care (i.e. those patients who required more intensive care in a psychiatric hospital), Walsh (1986) found that patients who transferred to in-patient care were more likely to have abused drugs or be non-compliant with their medication while receiving respite services.

A number of authors (Shadoan, 1985; Fields, 1990) have argued that acute crisis respite care should be part of a full range of residential treatment programmes which function to maintain severe mentally ill (SMI) adults in the community. The emphasis in such models is the integration of various levels of residential care within a service system. In such a conceptualisation, residential care should not be regarded as merely 'housing' but rather as 'treatment in a residential setting' in the community, regardless of its focus or length (Fields, 1990). Levels of care are conceptualised in terms of the staff–patient ratio and the degree of structure required: high intensity (crisis housing and lodge programmes), moderate intensity (board and care homes), low intensity (co-operative living arrangements) and psychiatric outreach for patients living independently (Shadoan, 1985). In all instances, treatment services for patients in acute crisis respite care are provided on-site or through an out-patient setting.

Until recently, there has been only limited systematic evaluation of the effectiveness of acute crisis respite and its impact on the service system. In the only known comparative outcome study, Brook (1973) compared patients served in a seven-day crisis respite alternative to a non-equivalent comparison group of patients who received hospital services. Crisis respite patients were found to have a lower readmission rate than the control patients and to have better outcomes on 11 out of 12 measures of functioning. Descriptive accounts of the effectiveness of crisis respite services have also reported their effectiveness, under specific circumstances. Walsh (1986) has suggested that medication compliance and substance use problems do not predict favourable outcomes, and Brunton & Harwthorne (1989) have noted that such residences work best when located in or near a residential neighbourhood and are staffed by a multidisciplinary clinical team.

Thus far, no published reports have examined the effectiveness, impact and costs of acute crisis respite care in a randomised comparative trial with acute psychiatric hospitalisation, and no reports of any kind have described the use of acute crisis respite care in combination with day hospital services. Below we describe such a trial and provide preliminary evidence of its relative efficacy involving clinical outcomes, service utilisation impact and costs. The programme we have implemented is a combined day hospital and crisis respite living situation that is structured to serve as an alternative to conventional in-patient treatment for some patients. The research is a random design comparison between the day hospital/crisis respite (DH/CR) treatment and conventional in-patient treatment on efficacy and costs. Patients are followed up after a standardised diagnostic and research interview at admission with re-interviews at discharge, two months, five months, and nine months follow-up. Before giving preliminary data on the evaluation of these two programmes, we will describe the experimental DH/CR programme. This report is not meant to be a comprehensive description of the study or the results of the research, rather it is a preliminary report of the results to date in order to give an example of a programme designed to be an alternative to psychiatric hospitalisation.

Connecticut Mental Health Center day hospital/crisis respite programme

Our rationale for providing clinical services through an acute day hospital setting was based on recent literature which indicated that acute day hospital services produce equivalent clinical outcome when compared to in-patient services (Dick *et al.*, 1985, 1991; Creed *et al.*, 1989a,b 1991). Our goal was to extend this work to investigate the clinical efficacy and cost effectiveness of a combined DH/CR home model which we believed could be an alternative for most voluntary patients who required acute hospitalisation.

Clinical programme description

The DH/CR programme has two components: the day hospital of the Connecticut Mental Health Center (CMHC) and the Brownell

House of the Continuum of Care. These two elements are administratively separate but are closely integrated for clinical care.

Connecticut Mental Health Center

The CMHC is a collaboration between the State of Connecticut, Department of Mental Health and the Yale University School of Medicine, Department of Psychiatry. Funded and owned by the State the facility is operated by Yale faculty through a contract between Yale and the State of Connecticut. One of the missions of the CMHC is to provide comprehensive mental health services for poor and severely mentally ill on a catchmented basis in south central Connecticut. In order to carry out this mission, there exists within CMHC several clinical programmes, one of which is the CMHC day hospital (DH) programme the primary purpose of which is to serve as an alternative to acute in-patient hospitalisation for appropriate patients. A secondary purpose is to provide transition for persons being discharged from in-patient units. Seventy per cent of admissions are for acute patients having been referred as an alternative to in-patient hospitalisation. The DH has a maximum census of 20 patients with about 220 admissions per year. The programme is geared to a 30-day cycle and the average length of stay in the programme is 30 days. The treatment goals are to stabilise patients and reconnect them to the community and/or other components of the mental health service system. Patients are encouraged to continue to see their out-patient therapists while they are in the DH, and to maintain involvement in volunteer or work placements while enrolled in the DH.

The DH staff is comprised of psychiatry, psychology, nursing, social work, recreational therapy and pastoral services. There are roughly 12 full-time equivalent staff. The disciplines collaborate throughout the process of providing care to patients through careful assessment and individualised treatment plans. The treatment is multimodal including individual, family and various groups. Patient's social supports are emphasised requiring the active participation of family or others who are important to the individual. In addition, the referring clinician or agency participates in the treatment planning process. These supports serve as resources for patients after discharge. Patients are expected to attend regularly and participate actively in the various aspects of the programme. Treatment goals include helping patients reduce symptoms, learn new ways of coping with problems, re-engage in daily tasks and connect with community resources that can assist them after leaving the DH.

Important aspects of the programme at the DH include the Family Programme, which includes individual family therapy, evaluation of family resources and a family issues group. Goals of the family issues group are to evaluate family resources, identify family systems issues, process ways to deal with difficult situations and feelings, and assist patients to identify potential supports in their lives.

In addition, there are therapy groups that have as goals to provide safe environments for patients to discuss interpersonal problems with their peers, to reduce feelings of hopelessness and isolation, and to help patients identify areas of their lives over which they may exercise control.

The DH also runs groups for people who have a dual diagnosis of a major psychiatric disorder as well as a substance abuse problem. The goal in this group is to allow patients to discuss their coexisting and interrelated problems, help identify symptoms and behavioural patterns that contribute to relapse, explore alternative coping mechanisms, stress importance of ongoing self-help groups, and to highlight choice and the importance of decision making related to taking personal responsibility.

Other groups included a community meeting as well as a health issues group focusing on specific information and techniques that promote good health. A very important experience for patients is the medication education group. The goal of the medication group is to encourage adherence to prescribed medications through promoting a greater understanding of the need for them. There is also a sexual issues group that deals with such topics as intimacy and relationships, sexually transmitted diseases and birth control. In terms of skills development groups, there are life skills planning groups, life skills outings in which patients are reintegrated into the community through outings to shops and community resources. A skills building group also deals with meal preparation. And because the effective use of leisure is a problem for many patients, there is a leisure time counselling group. In addition, occupation and recreational therapies provide a variety of treatment groups, activities and outings which focus on independent life skills, pre-job training, leisure time management and exploration of community resources.

Programme hours are from 9.30 a.m. to 2.30 p.m. for four days per week with one day's hours running from 1.30 p.m. to 7.00 p.m., to enable family members to participate in a scheduled treatment meeting.

Patients are expected to attend regularly and participate actively in the various aspects of the programme. A variety of groups are offered to assist patients in discussing their problems, learning new skills and making discharge plans.

In times of crisis, patients may call a 24-hour emergency number and talk with one of the staff who is on call. When necessary, patients may be admitted to a back-up bed on the in-patient unit of CMHC. In such circumstances the patient who is unable to safely remain in his or her usual residence without significant clinical or personal risk is allowed to board on the in-patient unit without being formally admitted to the hospital. In such circumstances the DH staff continue to manage the patient and to be responsible for the treatment planning. If the patient is unable to leave the back-up bed within two days, they are formally transferred to the in-patient unit.

The DH also provides formal education and training to full-time staff, and to clinicians from various academic institutions. It is the clinical site for training of psychology interns, psychiatric residents and graduate nursing and social work students. The staff consists of two faculty psychiatrists who are available for three and a half days per week. In addition, there is a psychiatry resident who is assigned to the DH for three days each week. The DH has two social work full-time equivalents who are masters level clinicians. There is also one clinical nurse specialist who is available for three days each week. In addition, there are two staff nurses. There are three mental health worker positions, one full-time occupational therapist and one full-time recreation therapist.

Brownell House

Brownell House is owned and operated by Continuum of Care Inc., a non-profit service organisation that provides residential services to clients of the Department of Mental Health through contracts. Brownell House is an environment similar to that of a private home. Brownell staff establish a warm and attractive setting that is inviting, yet with minimal stimulation, in an appartment within a three-family dwelling in a middle class neighbourhood. The apartment comprises three sleeping rooms, an office/interview room, a kitchen, one bathroom, a living room and a large dining room.

The individual daily routine of the patients is maintained as nearly as possible. If patients can function well enough to return to their established daytime activity after an initial evaluation at the CMHC DH, transportation is provided by Brownell staff. However, it is expected that all the Brownell patients who are not able to continue in work or school will be enrolled full-time in the CMHC DH Programme during most of the day (9.00 a.m. to 2.30 p.m.). While in the DH, the patient receives a complete psychiatric evaluation including a needs assessment for community living.

Patients take care of their own personal needs to whatever degree they are able, given their clinical conditions. Intensive staff assistance is always available. Patients are expected to participate in activities of daily living such as meal preparation, upkeep for the facility and shopping to the extent that is appropriate.

Brownell staff also work with patients' families by providing appropriate linkages and counselling whenever needed or requested. Linkages with CMHC DH, ongoing case management, or out-patient services are facilitated by close linkages and daily contact between the Brownell and DH staff. Indeed, Brownell staff help cover some DH functions during a daily wrap-up meeting. While clinical responsibility rests with the CMHC DH personnel, Brownell staff work closely with DH personnel in both formulating and implementing individualised treatment plans and monitoring the administration of treatments such as medication. Furthermore, Brownell staff monitor patient symptoms as closely as is appropriate while the patient is in residence at the Brownell House.

The programme is in operation seven days per week 24 hours per day with a maximum capacity of four patients.

Methods

The in-patient service that is the comparison treatment comprised two separate units (36 beds total) providing acute in-patient services to public sector patients from three geographically defined contiguous catchment areas in south central Connecticut covering a population of about 200,000 citizens. One unit is oriented towards clinical problems of patients who have co-morbid conditions of psychiatric and substance abuse. The other unit is oriented towards patients with acute psychotic conditions. Both units have an active milieu programme that emphasises adaptation and activities of daily living. The in-patient units are well staffed (roughly 41.5 full-time equivalent staff – FTES – during the week and 25.5 FTES on the weekend) and serve as a training site for Yale residents in psychiatry as well as other mental health professional trainees and is a setting for a variety of research programmes.

Planning for discharge begins soon after admission. On the in-patient service there are staff who specifically deal with developing housing dispositions for patients who do not have an appropriate place to stay. The in-patient services are oriented towards acute treatment. The combined average length of stay for 1992 for the two units was 26 days. Some patients are not able to recover within three to four months; some of these patients are referred to the regional large state hospital, Connecticut Valley Hospital (CVH) in Middletown (about 20 miles away) for longer duration inpatient treatment. Approximately 4% of CMHC in-patient admissions were transferred to CVH during 1992. Other patients are referred to out-patient or partial hospital programmes, either at CMHC or other local institutions, as a transition from in-patient to out-patient treatment.

The possible relationships between the DH/CR and the in-patient services as far as patient care are concerned are outlined in Fig. 12.1.

Research methods

Recruitment, selection and randomisation of subjects

Admission to the DH/CR is through the Entry Crisis Service (ECS) of CMHC. All patients who are requesting admission to a public sector psychiatric hospital are screened by the ECS of the CMHC. ECS staff serve as the single point of entry for in-patient beds as well as the DH/CR. The CMHC provides medical back-up to the Brownell House during DH off hours for emergencies through the ECS, the Yale–New Haven Emergency Room (YNHH-ER) and consultation with DH senior staff who are continuously available on a rotating on call system.

Subjects

Research subjects are drawn from the Department of Mental Health target population, namely those adults who have a prolonged mental

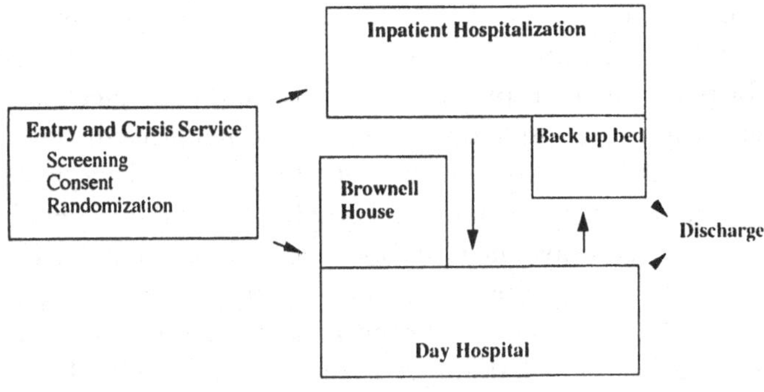

Fig. 12.1. Patient flow for day hospital/crisis respite study

illness and who are poor (family income no more than 150% of the poverty level established by the federal government) and/or those who are at risk for psychiatric hospitalisation.

- **Inclusion criteria:** Patients must be at least 18 years of age, give informed consent and reside in the New Haven or two adjoining catchment areas. Potential subjects are those who are evaluated by clinical staff as needing psychiatric hospitalisation. The criteria for psychiatric hospitalisation are: (1) presence of a psychiatric disorder with active signs or symptoms of psychiatric illness, (2) symptoms that are severe enough to cause moderate disturbance of role performance in more than one area, and/or to jeopardise a person's residential or financial status, and/or (3) are dangerous to the patient or others, (4) the available non-hospital clinical treatments have not been effective in preventing a progressive deterioration and (5) there are no other clinical services available to the patient except those of DMH.
- **Exclusion criteria:** Clinically, patients are excluded who have any one of the following: (1) have been committed to involuntary hospitalisation on a physician's Emergency Certification and who continue to refuse to become voluntary, (2) a condition that requires, or is likely to require, physical restraints or demand one-to-one attention; (3) acute intoxication or (4) a significant and active medical illness that requires active, hospital-based medical treatment.

  A non-clinical exclusion criterion is that patients who are able to afford private psychiatric services will not be invited to participate.
- **Recruitment:** All patients referred to the ECS during daytime

hours and the Yale–New Haven Emergency Room (after hours and at weekends) who are evaluated to be clinically appropriate for psychiatric hospitalisation and who do not meet the exclusion criteria are considered for the study. When the clinical evaluation to determine whether or not the patient is appropriate for psychiatric hospitalisation is completed and the patient is found to meet the inclusion and exclusion criteria for the research programme, the patient is invited to participate in the research programme. Since the design entails a random assignment either to DH/CR or to traditional in-patient care, the patient is offered the option to participate in the research. Consent is obtained before he or she knows the treatment assignment. Patients who agree to participate in the project are paid $10.00 per interview for the duration of the project.

For those who refuse to participate or who are not eligible, we record demographic data and clinical facts such as presumed diagnosis, presenting complaints and psychiatric history.

Recruitment and retention experience

Of the 146 participants recruited, 21 (14%) dropped out of the study prior to completing either in-patient or DH/CR treatment. This resulted in a total of 125 participants who constitute the study panel for this report. The attrition rate remained relatively stable at approximately 20% at each measurement time, despite the passage of time.

After the patient has consented to participate in the study, the randomisation is accomplished by the evaluator calling the CMHC switchboard operator who opens a numbered envelope and reads the assignment to the evaluator. The envelopes are numbered sequentially and are prepared by research staff using a random numbers table to generate the contents of the envelope. Only the research staff member who prepared the envelopes is aware of their contents.

The randomisation takes place independently of any consideration of bed availability in either of the two sites. If a patient is randomised into a site for which there are no beds available, the patient will wait in the Emergency Room of Yale New Haven Hospital if the site is likely to have a free bed within the next 12 hours. If there is no bed and there are no plans to have a bed within the next 12 hours, the patient is assigned to the other setting (if there is a bed). We believe this procedure maintains the randomisation in as much as the condition of the site being without beds is in itself a random event as far as patients who are in the Emergency Room seeking admission are concerned. Close inspection of our demographic and diagnostic data reveals that the randomisation seems to be working (see below). However, it should be noted that this differential availability to admit to a programme is the source of our higher numbers of subjects in the in-patient condition. Once a patient has been assigned to one condition or another, if the patient returns in need of an acute intervention, he or she will be assigned to the originally assigned treatment unless the patient requires (in the case of DH/CR) a more intensive level of care because of a worsening of clinical condition.

Measures

Patient measures

Patient level outcome is assessed as follows:

- Symptom measures – Brief Psychiatric Rating Scale (BPRS; Overall & Gorham, 1962); Symptom Checklist-90 (SCL-90; Derogatis *et al.*, 1973); Global Assessment of Functioning (GAF; Endicott, *et al.*, 1976); Structural Clinical Interview for DMS-III (SCID; Spitzer & Williams, 1988); Mini Mental State Examination (Folstein *et al.*, 1975); the Substance Abuse Screening Form.
- Social-psychological measures – Social Adjustment Scale (SAS-SR; Weisman *et al.*, 1981); Quality of Life Interview (modified from The Client Survey, Mental Health Policy Studies Program, University of Maryland, 1988 and the work of Susan Essock, Ph.D.); Rosenberg Self-Esteem Scale (Rosenberg, 1965); Self-Efficacy Scale (SES; Sherer *et al.*, 1982); and Cognitive Adaptation Survey (Tebes, 1991, unpub. data).

Cost measures

Cost measures for this report include costs of health care of the index episode, with attention to the costs of readmissions and transfers to prolonged hospitalisation or more intensive care. Cost measures depend on an accurate account of the costs of units of service and an accurate account of the units of service consumed by the participants. At this point our cost account is preliminary and not yet comprehensive since this portion of the study is not yet complete.

Data collection

Within 48 hours of admission the patient is interviewed by a research assistant, at which time the symptomatic and self-esteem measures are completed and demographic data is gathered. The admission interviews include the SCID, Mini Mental State Examination, BPRS and GAF. Patients are interviewed just prior to discharge from the programme at which time the symptomatic measures (BPRS, GAF and SCL-90), the social adjustment measures (Quality of Life Interview and the SAS), and the self-esteem measures are completed. The measures conducted at the discharge interview are repeated at two, five and nine month follow-up times.

Utilisation of service data are obtained from clinicians on a monthly basis and cross-checked in follow-up interviews with patients. The family burden questionnaire is completed at discharge and at 2 and 9 month follow-up.

Cost data addressing CMHC actual expenses are collected bi-annually from the fiscal controllers office at CMHC; cost data from other hospitals is obtained through telephone contact with their business offices concerning costs to the DMH and/or the State of Connecticut; cost data concerning the Brownell House are obtained from the Continuum of Care Inc.

Results

This report uses the data on the 125 patients who were enrolled in the programme between April, 1991, and the end of August, 1992, with admission, discharge and follow-up data collected and available for analysis. Again, these data should be considered preliminary and are not a comprehensive report of the results of the study.

Sample characteristics

During the period under consideration (17 months), 672 patients presented to the ECS and were admitted to the CMHC in-patient services or the DH/CR; 168 (25%) were eligible for admission to the study and 146 were enrolled (87% of those eligible and 22% of those admitted). The major reasons why patients were not eligible for this project were: 50% were not voluntary admissions, 20% required

Table 12.1. *Demographic features of the study groups*

Feature	Overall sample (n=125)	DH/CR program (n=58)	In-patient units (n=67)
Females (%)	51	55	48
Males (%)	49	45	52
Race			
African-American (%)	34	27	39
Asian-American (%)	2	2	2
Caucasian (%)	56	59	53
Native American (%)	9	12	6
Hispanic origin (%)	8	10	6
Age (mean years)	33.8	34.6	33.1

restraints, 5% were intoxicated, 10% required one-to-one management, and 2% required 24-hour medical surveillance/treatment. Patients met the inclusion criteria with an active psychiatric disorder (98%) and/or a severe disorder (90%); a substantial number were considered dangerous to self (66%) or others (22%) and out-patient treatments had been tried and found to be ineffective (82%).

Demographic data by treatment condition are indicated in Table 12.1. There are no differences between the treatment conditions.

We characterised patients diagnostically with the SCID. In the DH/CR programme there were 39% with psychotic disorder, 52% with a mood disorder, and 2% with an anxiety disorder; assigned to the inpatient condition, there were 49% with psychotic disorder, 47% with mood disorders and 3% with anxiety disorders. There were no statistically significant difference by DSM-IIIR diagnoses by treatment condition. Carrying a diagnosis of substance abuse were 45% of the DH/CR patients and 68% of the in-patients.

Treatment results

We will present the studies that address patient outcomes and utilisation and costs of the treatment conditions overall.

Symptoms and functions by treatment condition overall

Three types of analyses were conducted to examine the differential of the intervention and the relationship of mediators to selected patient characteristics at discharge, and at the 2, 5, and 9 month follow-ups. Analyses of covariance were employed to assess the impact of condition and selected characteristics on participant outcome, with the relevant outcome variable assessed at admission entered as a covariant (e.g. admission BPRS, admission GAF). A second set of analyses examined outcome effects focused on determining the **change** in participant status over time in relation to condition and selected patient characteristics. To examine this factor, a repeated measures analyses of variance was conducted with the same set of variables used in the first analyses.

There were no differences between DH/CR and in-patient at admission, discharge, 2, 5, and 9 month follow-up for the BPRS (Fig. 12.2), the SCL-90, and the GAF (Fig. 12.3) indicating that, at least in terms of symptoms and function measured by these instruments, there is no difference in efficacy of these two programmes. In all instances patients improve overtime with an initial rapid improvement at the beginning of treatment.

Utilisation of services by treatment condition overall

The length of stay averaged 17.2 (10.4) days in the DH/CR programme with an average length of stay for patients who were admitted to the in-patient service of 24.4 (14.2) days; the difference is significant (t test $= 3.28$, $p < .002$).

The readmission rate for the two treatments is 43% and 31%, respectively for DH/CR and in-patient treatment (chi square $= 2.28$, df $= 1$, p $=$ ns). The overall readmission rate is 34.4%. The details of the utilisation record for the two conditions are summarised in Table 12.2.

Social adjustment, self-esteem, self-efficacy and quality of life outcome by treatment condition-overall

Other measures of outcome available for analysis at this stage include social adjustment, the happiness scale from the Quality of Life Interview, the Rosenberg Self-Esteem Scale, and the SES. There is no difference between the treatment conditions on any of these measures.

Costs outcome

We have estimated the cost of care per episode and have limited the definition of cost as the cost to the Department of Mental Health for

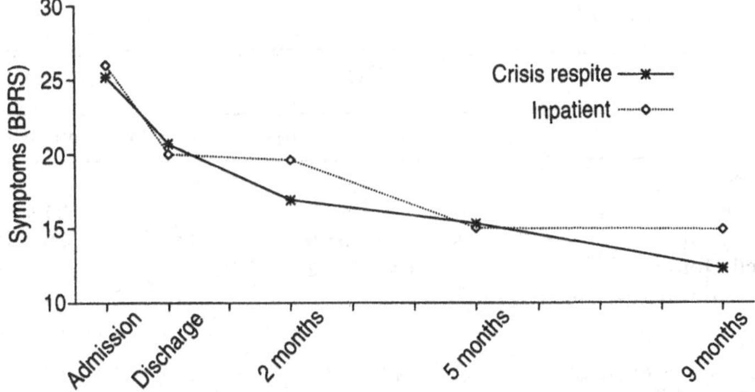

Fig. 12.2. Symptoms over time as measured by the Brief Psychiatric Rating Scale (BPRS) for day hospital/crisis respite and in-patient care

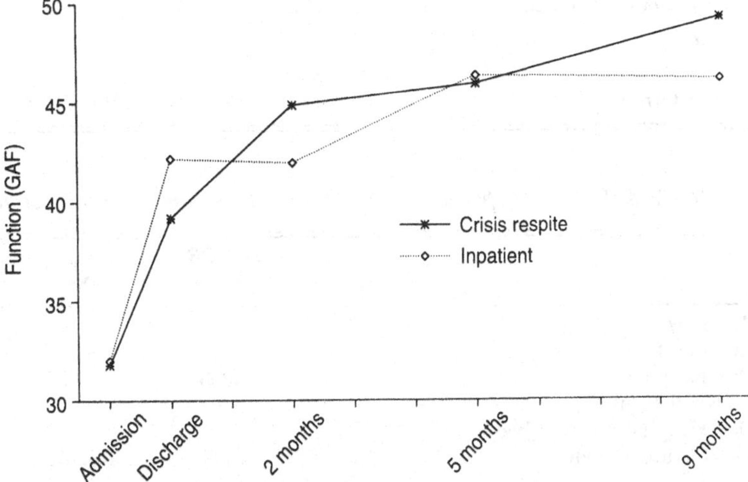

Fig. 12.3. Function over time as measured by the Global Assessment Form (GAF) for day hospital/crisis respite and in-patient care

mental health services. To date we have only analysed the use of acute services such as hospitalisation and DH use (or alternatives) since we believe these costs are the most likely to demonstrate differences. Eventually, we will be able to determine total mental health costs. Costs per patient by treatment condition are presented in Table 12.3.

The unit cost of the different treatment conditions expressed as per patient per day costs are as follows: in-patient at CMHC, \$514; DH at CMHC, \$157; Brownell House, \$192; CVH, \$479; other acute psychiatric hospitals, \$699. These data are preliminary estimates

Table 12.2. *Utilisation experience*

	DH/CR			Inpatient		
	n	%	mean/part	n	%	mean/part
Index admission						
In-patient				67	100	24.4
Day Hospital	58	100	31.9	11	16	26.5
Brownell House	58	100	17.2			
Day Hospital back-up bed	17	29	2.7	1	1	4
Readmission						
Number of readmissions	25	43	2.1	21	31	2
to the DH/CRP	10	17	13.4	0	0	
to the day hospital alone	12	21	38.5	15	22	36.1
to day hospital back-up bed	3	5	1.3	6	9	4.7
to the in-patients units	14	24	36.4	16	24	40.7
to other acute in-patient	10	17	22.2	11	16	33.5
Transfers						
to acute in-patient	4	7	34.5			
to long-term in-patient	3	5	144	6	9	121.5

Table 12.3. *Costs ($) per patient by treatment condition of acute services*

	DH/CR ($)	In-patient ($)
Admission		
In-patient		13,200
Day Hospital	5008	586
Brownell House	3302	
Day Hospital back-up bed	407	
Total acute episode	8717	13,786
Readmissions		
to the DH/CRP	444	
to Day Hospital	1088	1170
to the Day Hospital back-up	36	
to the In-patient Units	4208	4481
to other acute in-patient care	2675	3845
Total readmissions	8451	9496
Transfers		
Transfers to acute in-patient care	1706	
Transfers to long term in-patient care	3568	5372
Total costs	22,442	28,654

based on the best data available to us. The CMHC data were based on CMHC financial data but are incomplete since some of the personnel indirect costs are paid out of another State account. The CVH and other hospital expenses are based on records made available to us by the financial officers at these institutions and have not been verified by a close audit. We expect these estimates to be revised as we have access to the actual costs of the CMHC programmes. The costs per episode are calculated by multiplying the unit cost by the amount of service utilised.

Inspection of the total costs reveals there is a substantial difference (the DH/CR total cost per episode is 78% of the in-patient costs) between the programmes. If one examines the cost per episode without including the transfer and readmission costs, one sees a greater difference (the DH/CR cost per episode is 63% of the cost for the in-patient treatment) between the costs of the two programmes.

Discussion of results

Our data indicate that the DH/CR alternative is effective for at least 25% of all those who would normally be hospitalised in an urban, inner city treatment system in terms of standard measurements of symptoms and function. Furthermore, the patient population treated effectively by the DH/CR programme are severely mentally ill and carry a high incidence of dual diagnosis. The DH/CR, however, is 22% more cost effective than the conventional in-patient setting. Most of the difference in cost can be found in the treatment of the initial episode as opposed to differences in readmission or transfer use of services. The DH/CR does not simply delay hospitalisation for those who need it but functions as a true alternative to hospitalisation.

Implementation considerations

The creation of an acute crisis alternative to psychiatric hospitalisation begins with careful specification of the goals of such a programme, the target population of patients to be served and the clinical service context in which the programme is to exist. Once these considerations are resolved, subsequent decisions concerning funding, location, staffing, programme features, policies and procedures, and other matters will follow logically. While the push for alternative programmes may be fuelled largely by possible financial savings such programmes offer, we want to note that the claim frequently has been made that for many patients community-based, alternative programmes are superior to acute psychiatric hospitalisation in terms of symptom relief as well as rehabilitative re-integration into the community. If the purpose of the crisis respite programme is to serve as a true alternative to psychiatric hospitalisation, it is important for there to be a clear, gatekeeping function at the admission process that evaluates and triages patients according to predetermined characteristics.

Individuals are hospitalised because they are perceived to require in-patient-level care or because there are no suitable alternative, community-based services available (Oldham *et al.*, 1990). Patients may be diverted from hospitalisation by intervening at the earliest signs of an exacerbation of the disorder or assigning them to a viable alternative to hospitalisation. Since many mental health professionals are unfamiliar with the growing literature indicating that alternatives are cost effective and safe, they are inclined to seek to hospitalise patients who are very ill. Thus, for an acute crisis respite programme to be utilised effectively, it is essential for there to be a strong admissions function that will be able to screen and triage patients appropriately. Furthermore, if the acute crisis programme is to serve as a true alternative to hospitalisation, it is critical that the admissions function should not be allowed to drift into admitting patients, who would normally not be hospitalised (unless such a patient group is part of the target population, see below), into the respite programme. The triage function and hospitalisation decision is best accomplished by a single point of entry, managed by staff who are not part of the treatment staff of the unit referring to the patient or receiving the patient. Such a triage unit could be crisis personnel, hired by the mental health authority but not connected directly to the hospital or alternative programme.

Another function an acute crisis programme can serve is as a crisis setting for people in distress before they need to be hospitalised. In this instance the indications for admission into the programme will be considerbly less stringent in terms of intensity of need in comparison to the programme that functions as an alternative to psychiatric hospitalisation. While such a crisis programme may indeed serve to divert hospitalisation, it may be more costly than other less intensive community-based services that do not include a residential component.

To our knowledge, such a programme has not been systematically investigated.

Another goal that could be served by an acute CR alternative programme is to function as a referral site for patients who are admitted for very brief stays to the hospital. Such patients may be admitted to the hospital for one to five days and then 'transitioned' into a CR-like programme. Again, this seems to be a reasonable way of structuring care which would be appropriate for a substantial number of patients who are otherwise hospitalised. However, as far as we know, such a configuration of services has not been systematically evaluated.

In designing an alternative it is important to consider that in some instances the alternative may simply function as a delay for needed hospitalisation. In such instances the alternative is not cost effective and should be avoided. A close consideration of the factors below will ensure that a minimal number of people will fall into this category of delayed, inevitable admissions.

Target population

A clear definition of the people that a programme is intended to serve is necessary. Firstly, any programme should be culturally and ethnically sensitive, which can be achieved in a variety of ways including staffing, decorating and the provision of multilingual materials and staff. If the majority or a substantial number of patients are poor, then the programme will need to have a case management function that will ensure that patients are being enrolled in suitable entitlements in order to provide food and shelter. Another population consideration is the age range (i.e. whether adolescents or elderly patients are included). Obviously, special programming needs must be instituted if these populations are a part of the primary patient mix. Other considerations are the functional level of the patients in terms of disability. The more functionally impaired the higher the staff–patient ratio necessary in order to ensure safety and an adequate clinical and rehabilitative approach. The level of psychopathology of the patients is another major consideration. From our study it is clear that people who are depressed are most cost effectively treated in the CR alternative. Perhaps this is because they are relatively easy to manage and they respond well to the structure and the home-like quality of the setting. Patients with dual diagnosis are also efficiently managed in the CR programme. Patients with psychosis can also be well managed in the DH/CR alternative but the difference in cost between crisis respite and in-patient is only about 10%. Acute manic excitement is the most difficult to manage in an alternative programme. Indeed, patient acuity more than psychopathology or functional impairment seems to be the most important feature in determining the management difficulty. Manic patients require substantial levels of structure.

Other considerations in terms of psychopathology are whether or not substance abusers are admitted. Including primary substance abusers in the target population would require a programme that would be able to work effectively with this patient group. Combining primary substance abusers and patients with major psychiatric disorder is very challenging and generally believed to be ineffective.

Staffing

The qualifications of staff are an important consideration. Highly trained professional staff bring the advantage of their professionalism and their understanding of mental illness from a formal perspective. However, many of the concrete and everyday tasks of assisting people with major mental illness and in helping them care for themselves may be less attractive to people with advanced or higher professional degrees. Consequently, mental health workers or staff who have no professional training in the mental health disciplines may be better suited for some of the tasks necessary in any kind of residential setting. It is important for there to be highly trained mental health professionals who are responsible for the evaluation, diagnosis and treatment planning functions. However, the residential site itself can be staffed by personnel without a formal mental health professional degree.

Wherever possible, it is important to have the gender and racial characteristics of the patient population reflected in the staff. It is extremely helpful for patients to be cared for by those who understand their cultural and ethnic background. Such a racial and cultural diversity makes it easier for patients to feel welcomed and to be emphatically engaged in a collaborative treatment process.

The ratio of staff to patients in our alternative programme has been roughly two patients to one staff so that there are two staff on duty at all times in a programme for four patients. To some extent the staff ratio should be a function of the acuity of the patients and the capacities and qualifications of the staff. There should always be at least two staff on duty in order to cope with the unexpected and untoward. However, it is possible that two staff can easily manage six patients if these patients are not psychotic and/or the acuity level is not high.

Programme design features

The alternative to a hospitalisation programme must have a strong working connection to other services within the mental health system. These other services include case management, residential resources, rehabilitative services as well as ongoing clinical care. Essential design features are an admission screening/gate-keeping function that ensures that only people for whom the programme is designed are admitted. Furthermore, there has to be an exit function which includes discharge planning making certain that the appropriate housing and clinical services are available when the patient is ready to leave the programme (see below). Another exit function that must be a part of the design, is a provision of a ready and easy access to a higher level of care for those patients for whom the CR programme is not structured enough or otherwise inappropriate. We found that approximately 12% of our DH/CR patients required transfer to one or another form of in-patient care.

Treatment functions include medical evaluation and treatment addressing conditions and medication requirements as well as habilitative and rehabilitative functions addressing psychosocial rehabilitation and vocational rehabilitation. The rehabilitation functions in the hospital alternative must emphasise aspects of self-care, autonomy and/or bulwarks against the compelling pull towards regression which is a feature of many psychopathological states. The rehabilitative functions that can be usefully addressed can center on activities of, for example, daily living, including self-care, meal and food preparation, budgeting, shopping and grooming.

Medical and psychiatric evaluation is essential in order to make a proper diagnosis and to guide a proper medical treatment approach. Such an approach depends on a careful psychopathological diagnosis as well as a functional assessment of social and rehabilitative needs. Diagnosis and evaluation should be an ongoing activity but these functions also need to be organised to occur rapidly during the admission and early treatment phase. A psychiatrist must be a part of this programme approach who can adequately evaluate, judge medication need and prescribe accordingly.

It is important for the staff to have immediate and quick access to security and a higher level of intensity of care should either of these be necessary. We have found the availability of the local municipal police to be adequate to provide the security back-up for our programme.

Security and clinical back-up, however, are usually achieved in a substantially more complex way. When it becomes clear that patients are not able to tolerate being in the crisis respite programme without some danger either physically to themselves or others or clinically in terms of a progressive deterioration, they are transferred to the in-patient setting. There they are boarded on the in-patient setting but their management continues from the staff of the DH. If after two days the patient is not able to return to the crisis respite programme, they are formally transferred to the in-patient setting.

House rules and policies concerning the programme and acceptable patient behaviours should be carefully considered and written up for both patients and staff. Such rules in a concrete form are important aides in guiding the treatment and setting the tone of the milieu. These rules should be simple, clear and should also address the consequences of breaking the rules. Obviously, violence and the presence of illicit drugs cannot be tolerated. Other rules should be formulated to be consistent for the clinical mission and appropriate for the target population.

The length of stay for such a programme is frequently an administrative issue and should be consistent with the goals of the programme. Length of stay in general should be kept to a minimum utilising as much as possible the natural strengths of the patient and his or her resources.

Discharge planning

This should begin with admission to the programme and should include a careful assessment of the patient's current living arrangements. It is essential that a decision be made early as to whether or not the patient can return to these arrangements. If such return is not possible or in the patient's best interests, then alternative arrangements must be secured. One major consideration, of course, is whether or not the patient lives with his or her family of origin. This question should be addressed in the evaluation function early in the stay. Family treatment and family management should be a part of the treatment programme as well.

Location

Alternatives to hospitalisation should be placed in a setting that allows as much normalisation as feasible. A safe residential setting near the DH is advisable. Such a setting should be rendered to be as home-like as possible, with separate sleeping rooms for each patient if possible; a common room, a living room for group meetings and recreation, a dining room for meals and a kitchen appropriately supplied to carry out basic meal preparations and function but with an eye towards safety concerning the securing of sharps and other instruments that can be used in self-injurious behaviour. The challenge for the staff is to maintain a home-like atmosphere in the face of the security and safety issues necessitated by some forms of mental illness, mainly depression and suicide.

Another aspect of location usually involves the opinion of the neighbours about the location of a treatment programme for the mentally ill in their neighbourhood. It is generally quite desirable to locate such a programme in a residential area which then means that the programme must be consistent with local zoning laws. In addition, it is a good idea for there to be open and frank discussion with the neighbours and local politician before a programme is located in a setting. It is essential to have good neighbours and one way is to treat them with respect concerning their fears about mental illness.

A programme needs to be located conveniently to public transportation and to other institutions that are a part of the normalisation process such as easy shopping for basic items of living, programmes for ongoing rehabilitation and recreational activities.

Conclusion

Crisis respite programmes can be an effective and safe alternative to psychiatric hospitalisation for many patients who find themselves admitted to a psychiatric hospital. The DH/CR we developed has worked well with an urban, poor and severely disturbed patient group in a manner comparable to in-patient care for about 25% of those who are presently admitted. We believe this is a modest estimate of the percentage of the population that can be effectively served by a crisis respite programme. In our study there were strict requirements for the ability to give consent and patients had to be voluntary in order to participate in the research. Furthermore, the programme is not designed to take patients who are not voluntary. Under non-research conditions we believe the proportion of voluntary patients who can be effectively and safely served by this programme could be 70 to 80%.

Acknowledgement

This project was supported by SAMSHA Grant R18-MH47638 to William Sledge, MD, principal investigator.

References

Britton, J. G. & Mattson-Melcher, D. M. (1985). The crisis home: sheltering patients in emotional crisis. *Journal of Psychosocial Nursing and Mental Health Services*, **23**, 18–23.

Brook, B. D. (1973). Crisis hostel: an alternative to psychiatric hospitalization. *Hospital and Community Psychiatry*, **24**, 621–4.

Brunton, J. & Harwthorne, H. (1989). The acute non-hospital: a California model. *Psychiatric Hospital*, **20**, 95–9.

Creed, F., Anthony, P., Godbert, K. & Huxley, P. (1989a). Treatment of severe psychiatric illness in a day hospital. *British Journal of Psychiatry*, **154**, 341–7.

Creed, F., Black, D. & Anthony, P. (1989b). Day Hospital and community treatment for acute psychiatric illness: A critical appraisal. *British Journal of Psychiatry*, **154**, 300–10.

Creed, F., Black, D., Anthony, P., Osborn, M., Thomas, P., Franks, D., Polley, R., Lancashire, S., Saleem, P. & Tomanson, B. (1991). Randomised controlled trial of day and in-patient psychiatric treatment. II. Comparison of two hospitals. *British Journal of Psychiatry*, **158**, 183–9.

Derogatis, L. R., Lipman, R. S. & Covi, L. (1973). The SCL-90: an outpatient psychiatric rating scale. *Psychopharmacology Bulletin*, **9**, 13–28.

Dick, P. H. *et al.* (1985). Day and full-time psychiatric treatment: a controlled comparison. *British Journal of Psychiatry*, **147**, 246–9.

Dick, P. H., Sweeney, M. L. & Crombie, I. K. (1991). Controlled comparison of day-patient and out-patient treatment for persistent anxiety and depression. *British Journal of Psychiatry*, **158**, 24–7.

Endicott, J., Spitzer, R. L., Fleiss, J. & Cohen, J. (1976). The Global Assessment Scale: a procedure for measuring overall severity of psychiatric disturbance. *Archives of General Psychiatry*, **33**, 766–71.

Fields, S. (1990). The relationship between residential treatment and supported housing in a community system of services. Special issue: Supported housing: new approaches to residential services. *Psychosocial Rehabilitation Journal*, **13**, 105–13.

Folstein, M., Folstein, S. & McHugh, P. (1975). Mini-mental state: a practical method for grading the cognitive state of patients for the clinical. *Psychiatric Research*, **12**, 189–98.

Geiser, R., Hoche, L. & King, J. (1988). Respite care for mentally ill patients and their families. *Hospital and Community Psychiatry*, **39**, 291–5.

Ghaziuddin, M. (1988). Referral of mentally handicapped patients to the psychiatrist: a community study. *Journal of Mental Deficiency Research*, **32**, 491–5.

Gibbons, J. S. (1986) Care of 'new' long-stay patients in a district general hospital psychiatric unit: the first two years of a hospital-hostel. *Acta Psychiatrica Scandinavica*, **73**, 582–8.

Hyde, C., Bridges, K., Goldberg, D. *et al.* (1987). The evaluation of a hostel ward: a controlled study using modified cost-benefit analysis. *British Journal of Psychiatry*, **151**, 805–12.

MacCarthy, B., Lesage, E., Brewin, C. R., Brugha, T. S., Mangen, S. & Wing, J. K. (1989). Needs for care among the relatives of long-term users of day care: A report from the Camberwell High Contact Survey. *Psychological Medicine*, **19**, 725–36.

Oldham, J. M., Lin, A. & Breslin, A. (1990). Comprehensive psychiatric emergency services. Special Issue: Redesigning a public mental health system. *Psychiatric Quarterly*, **61**, 57–67.

Overall, J. & Gorham, D. (1962). The brief psychiatric rating scale. *Psychological Reports*, **10**, 799–812.

Rosenberg, M. (1965). *Society and the Adolescent Self-Image*. Princeton, NJ, Princeton University Press.

Schwartz, I. M. (1989). Hospitalization of adolescents for psychiatric and substance abuse treatment: Legal and ethical issues. *Journal of Adolescent Health Care*, **10**, 473–8.

Segal, S. P. & Kotler, P. L. (1989). Do we need board and care homes? *Adult Research in Care Journal*, **3**, 24–32.

Shadoan, R. A. (1985). Levels of care for residential treatment in an urban setting. *Psychiatric Annals*, **15**, 639–41.

Sherer, M., Maddox, J. E., Mercandte, B., Prentice-Dunn, S., Jacobs, B. & Rogers, R. W. (1982). The Self-Efficacy Scale: construction and validation. *Psychological Reports*, **51**, 663–71.

Simpson, C. J., Hyde, C. E. & Faragher, E. B. (1989). The chronically mentally ill in community facilities: A study of quality of life. *British Journal of Psychiatry*, **154**, 77–82.

Spitzer, R. & Williams, J. (1988). *Structured Clinical Interview for DSMIII-R*. New York, Biometrics Research Department, New York State Psychiatric Institute.

Walsh, S. F. (1986). Characteristics of failures in an emergency residential alternative to psychiatric hospitalization. *Social Work in Health Care*, **11**, 53–64.

Weisman, M. M., Sholomskas, D. & John, K. (1981). The assessment of social adjustment: an update. *Archives of General Psychiatry*, **31**, 1250–8.

Zirul, D. W., Lieberman, A. A. & Rapp, C. A. (1989). Respite care for the chronically mentally ill: focus for the 1990s. *Community Mental Health Journal*, **25**, 171–84.

13

Family placement schemes as an alternative to short-term hospitalisation

Russell Bennett

> I really liked the Crisis Home. Staying with a regular family kept me from feeling abnormal, and helped me feel like a regular person.
>
> *'Mary'*

Introduction

For thousands of years people in crisis have found support by staying with concerned and caring neighbours. This was achieved without staff, formal programmes, quarterly fiscal reviews or programme criteria; help was needed, help was offered. It is therefore logical that community families are a component of contemporary community mental health care, yet this type of service is rarely found in mental health systems.

This chapter will explore the role of community families in providing emergency support to people with mental illness. After some background and a review of the literature, the Crisis Home Program of the Mental Health Center of the Dane County will be described in detail, with an emphasis on practical considerations. The chapter will conclude with observations about why this option is not more prevalent despite its tremendous potential.

Historical overview and review of literature

The 'innovative' ideas of the current age are often the direct descendants (and bear a striking resemblance) to notions of previous generations. This is certainly the case with the idea of using family homes to help those with a mental illness. The most famous example is that of the village of Gheel, Belgium, where for perhaps 1300 years families have opened their homes to people with mental illness (Aring, 1974). This was most commonly done on a long-term basis. More recent examples include the use of adult foster care for the mentally ill in Scotland during the 1860s (McCoin, 1983). Dorothea Dix brought the concept to the United States, where it was first used in Massachusetts in the early 1880s, and then by the Veterans Administration in Tennessee in the 1930s and 1940s (Searight & Searight, 1988). By 1959, one-quarter of the chronically mentally ill population of Norway was living in community family homes (McCoin, 1983). The advent of effective neuroleptic medications in the late 1950s combined with changing societal perspectives on civil rights to create an impetus for more of the mentally ill to live in the community, but it was unclear where, or who would treat them.

The 1963 Community Mental Health Act in the United States provided for one treatment modality (Rubin, 1990) and paved the way for supportive living options such as the halfway house, an idea which originated in London in 1959 (Weisman, 1985). The concept of the halfway house was grounded in the idea that this was far more than mere housing, it was considered a preferred treatment modality, superior to the hospital in many regards (Plotinsky, 1985). This early example of non-institutional housing was the foundation for more recent efforts to provide emergency residential treatment options, as an alternative to even short-term hospitalisation.

In addition, one study (Shadoan, 1985) estimated that one-half to three-quarters of psychiatric readmissions could have been avoided if comprehensive services, including Crisis Homes, had been in place. Keisler (1982) reviewed 10 studies of psychiatric patients randomly assigned to in-patient or out-patient. None of the studies found that in-patient treatment was more effective than out-patient treatment.

There are two broad models for emergency residential mental health treatment. The group approach, where anywhere from 6 to 50 clients are accommodated, is more prevalent. They are usually owned and run by community mental health centres, and try to provide a non-institutional atmosphere. Such an approach is described in detail by William Sledge (chapter 12). In this chapter the use of family homes as the supportive setting is reviewed; throughout the chapter this option will be referred to as a crisis home.

The Crisis Home Program of the Southwest Denver Mental Health Center began in 1972 in Colorado, and appears to be the first of its kind in recent times. It began as an outgrowth of the historical forces mentioned above, and established the parameters for many of the family based systems to follow, including some of the key features of how such a family home interfaces with the mental health system. The success of the programme and published research helped spread the concept around the world (Polak & Kirby, 1976; Brook *et al.*, 1976; Brook, 1980). Another early model programme is the Crisis Home Program of Hennepin County, established in 1980 in Minneapolis, Minnesota (Leaman, 1987). There is also increased interest in the use of family homes as an alternative to in-patient care, for children with mental illness.

An extensive overview of the topic is to be found in *Crisis Residential Services in a Community Support System* by Beth Stroul (1987), available through the US National Institute of Mental Health. Information on crisis response systems in general is described by Stroul (1991) in a later volume.

Outcome studies

There is little published research about this type of programme, reflecting both the scarcity of such programmes and the difficulties endemic in the evaluation of any mental health care. Polak and Kirby (1976) studied outcome measures completed by clients, staff and family members of crisis home clients, both at the time of discharge and four months later. Results indicated that crisis homes were more effective than in-patient care, across a range of outcome measurements. Brook *et al.* (1976) described the results of independent researchers looking at the same programme in Denver. During the first two years, 100 clients in crisis were randomly assigned to either a crisis home or an in-patient setting. The staff ratings of discharge outcomes revealed no differences between the groups. In contrast, the ratings by the clients and by others in the community were that the crisis home was more beneficial than in-patient care.

Leaman (1987) writes that clients in the Hennepin County Crisis Home Program reported significant improvement on five different self-rating scales: general neurotic feelings, somatisation, cognitive performance, depression, fear and anxiety. Programme staff noted on the brief psychiatric rating scale improvement in four areas: anxiety, depression, withdrawal and hostility. A patient satisfaction survey of clients found 94% satisfied with the programme; 77% thought it helped them avoid an in-patient stay.

When looking at a variety of community residential alternatives, Walsh (1986) found the rehospitalisation rate was 15–25%, with drug abuse and medication non-compliance as the strongest predictors of failure. Writing on the more general area of adult foster care, Rubin (1990) cautions against evaluating these programmes negatively just because of subsequent hospital admissions; qualitative experiences from the point of view of the client are difficult to measure, but ultimately more important in overall evaluation. This is in keeping with a broad new paradigm emerging in community mental health, where the preferences and self-assessments of the client are being given more weight (Livingston & Srebnick, 1991; Carling, 1993; Diamond, 1993; Tanzman, 1993). Finally, positive relationship building is essential for successful involvement in the lives of those with long-term mental illness (Brown & Wheeler, 1990; Terpstra & McFadden, 1993); it is a key component of crisis homes, but difficult to measure.

Community mental health in Dane County, Wisconsin

Dane County is located in southern Wisconsin in the upper mid-west of the United States. The population of 367,000 is roughly split between those living in rural areas and those living in Madison, the urban capital of the state. The mental health system has a strong out-patient focus, with approximately 80% of its budget being spent on such services (Table 13.1). Many developed countries spend that proportion, or more, on their in-patient system. The 'Madison Model' has been extensively researched, and reviews are generally very positive (Thompson *et al.*, 1990). The overall approach of this system is to offer a wide variety of services, a continuum on which people can move as need and circumstance dictate. These services include community support programmes, supportive living arrangements, crisis intervention, vocational services, psychotherapy and various levels of case management. These services are provided by 40

Table 13.1. *The mental health services of Dane County, Wisconsin*

- Population 93% Caucasian, 7% other.
- Long-term psychiatric in-patients 10 per 100,000 (50–75 in United States).
- Total mental health budget $9,833,048, ($24 per taxpayer in Dane County).
- 3,867 (5.27%) of population served by mental health service.
- 85% of budget spent on 1500 clients with serious long-term mental illness (average annual cost in this group $6133, 22% under involuntary commitment).

different programmes in 18 organisations (LeCount, 1992). The intent is for people to have services available to meet their changing individual needs and preferences.

One essential service is the Emergency Services Unit (ESU), a team of suicide prevention phone staff, social workers, support staff, nurses, psychologists and psychiatrists. The Crisis Home Program is 'nested' within this unit, which provides the 24-hour support for the Crises Home families and their guests. This team is available to respond to emergencies at any time. ESU staff are in a unique position to consider whether a Crisis Home is an option, as they also function as gatekeeper to the inpatient system for many clients. In addition, local police consult with ESU staff prior to any involuntary hospitalisations. Of the 1500 or so people with serious mental illness in treatment in the county, 22% are receiving compulsory treatment under civil commitment. The majority are treated in the community rather than institutions.

Crisis Home Program of Dane County

The fundamental goal of the Crisis Home Program is to provide a safe, supportive, family-based alternative to clients who might otherwise be hospitalised. It began in 1987, when we recognised that our mental health system needed such a component. Crisis homes are normal homes in Madison, owned by individuals and families who have been certified and trained to offer this service. These families are willing to have mental health clients as guests in their homes, usually for less than a week at a time. Only one clients is in the home at any given time. These home providers are paid $55 per day of occupancy. They provide a bedroom, meals, a tremendous amount of empathy and a wide array of other support, such as monitoring medication, teaching basic living skills and transportation. The support they offer is often far beyond the programme expectations: helping with physical health needs, teaching parenting skills, help in applying for jobs or other social services. They are in close contact with the ESU clinicians, and help staff understand clients by providing additional information.

The crisis homes have three major roles:

- As an alternative to an in-patient stay.
- To facilitate an early release from an in-patient stay.
- As pre-crisis intervention to de-escalate a situation.

Some specific examples:

- Paula, a young woman with schizoaffective disorder, decided 'I don't need to take all these pills anymore', and is now hearing voices and feeling agitated in her small apartment. The landlord, who is unsympathetic to Paula's illness, is threatening to evict her 'the next time she causes any trouble'. She has numerous past hospitalisations that were preceded by a similar scenario, and has a history of suicide attempts, some potentially lethal.
- Mary has had numerous hospital admissions in the past, and has been given a variety of diagnosis. Recently, she is most often described as having a borderline personality disorder. When feeling terrible, she sees cutting herself and overdosing as a means to ensuring that she is admitted to hospital. After discharge, staff usually feel that the admission has resulted in little or no improvement. At times, Mary will agree that the hospital 'brought out the worst' in her.
- Steve, an 18-year-old man, was seen following an overdose. He said he took the overdose because his girlfriend had just left him. He appeared to have some healthy coping skills, but also some impulsive and dependent personality traits. He does not want to be admitted to the psychiatric ward, but the medical staff are reluctant to 'just let him go'.

None of these people were admitted to the hospital. This is not to say that hospitals are never needed, but even if someone is admitted for a short stay, discharge to a crisis home is helpful in allowing clients to return safely to the community sooner.

The families and their guests

The families

Most of the providers came to our programme through an advertisement in the local paper, although other programmes have noted 'word of mouth' as a primary point of entry (Miller, 1987). The text of the advertisement can be very general:

> The Crisis Home Program offers support and very short-term housing to people in crisis. The program is currently looking for families willing to open their homes to such people, most of whom have some kind of mental illness. Reimbursement is $55/day, tax exempt. For more information call Russ Bennett at 251-2341.

The financial incentives are a legitimate motivation for recruitment and retention, and do not necessarily imply that the provider is 'only in it for the money' (Carling, 1984).

After initial telephone screening of the family, details of the programme are sent, and if the family are still interested, a home visit is arranged. After more discussions (which are part of the training), they are asked to complete an application to be certified as an adult foster home. If all the information and references are acceptable, the potential home provider receives further information and subsequent training dates are arranged.

Training

Experienced home providers are an important part of such training, they often share insights and practical advice not considered by professionals. Often current or former clients of the programme participate in the training of new families. Much of the training is 'on the job', with an emphasis on the fact that they are not expected to become mental health professionals, and that they are expected to call if they have any questions or concerns.

Retention rates

Less than 10% of the people who respond to the initial advertisement go on to become certified as crisis homes, and many others only stay in the programme for a short time. Over the past six years there has been a total of 20 different crisis home providers, and six were in the programme for less than three months. There are currently ten individuals and families providing crisis homes in the programme;

eight for at least a year. Two of the families have been with the programme for seven years. In the past, we have been able to maintain an effective programme with as few as two families. Three of the current homes have children; it has been noted that this feature is a significant predictor of a successful milieu for the guest with mental illness (Rubin, 1990).

The clients

Demographic data about the clients who use the Crisis Home Program are listed in Table 13.2. Such figures, while relevant, do not give the whole story about what is important to, and about, the clients who use the homes; such numbers say little about the particular personalities, likes and dislikes of the crisis home guests. Such unique characteristics are as important for the mentally ill as they are to the rest of us, and underscore the benefits of the crisis home system, which can offer an individualised match between a client and provider family.

Approximately 40% of the crisis home admissions are an alternative to a hospital admission, 40% facilitate earlier transition out of the hospital and 20% are primarily a housing issue or 'pre-crisis' intervention. In 1992, there were 140 separate crisis home admissions, with a total of 443 days of Crisis Home usage. The average length of stay is three to five days, with two weeks the maximum. Roughly 70% of the clients are on disability income, and have a diagnosis of a major mental illness such as schizophrenia, bipolar disorder, or depression. Of special interest is the finding that people who have a diagnosis of borderline personality disorder have not been particularly difficult guests for the crisis home families. The normalising home environment, combined with the high degree of individual attention seems to enhance the person's coping skills, and this contrasts sharply with their behaviour when admitted to hospital.

Crisis home admission of 'Mary'

Mary has presented at a hospital emergency room with some superficial cuts on her wrists and some thoughts of suicide. She also reports hearing voices, but has been unwilling to take therapeutic doses of neuroleptic medications. Past hospitalisations have resulted in some dependency and learned helplessness. We would never force

Table 13.2. *Characteristics of crisis home clients*

Characteristic	Percentage
Diagnosis:	
Schizophrenia/schizoaffective disorder	43
Affective disorders	13
Personality disorders/adjustment disorders	40
Other	5
Age (years):	
18–25	20
26–35	54
36–50	22
50+	4
Living situation	
Apartment	48
None	36
Family	13
Group Home	3
Length of stay (days)	
1–3	37
4–7	44
7–10	11
11+	8

Mary to use a crisis home, but we do not want her to have yet another in-patient stay. She is initially sceptical, but willing to 'give it a try'. Giving her precise details about the home appears to be very helpful for her – 'They have a green house on a quiet street, two children, a dog named Freud, . . .'.

Before arranging admission to a crisis home we complete the necessary paper work. This includes an assessment of risk factors, a brief treatment plan, a signed release, and a copy of the crisis home guidelines for Mary. We then call a home provider who seems to best match her specific requests and needs. Families always have the option of not accepting guests for any period of time or any specific client situation. Admission to crisis homes generally occurs between 8.00 a.m. and 10.00 p.m. (If the crisis happens at 3.00 a.m., a safe but temporary alternative plan is needed.)

After hearing about Mary and her situation, Tom and Sandy say they are willing to have her in their home, so we arrange a time to bring Mary over. At the home, staff introduce everyone and go over the plan for the stay before leaving Mary. We make it very clear that the stay must feel safe for both Mary and the family; if either has questions or concerns, they call our 24-hour crisis line.

Our original idea was that we needed home providers who could provide 24-hour support in their homes. This quickly proved to be unnecessary and even inappropriately paternalistic in many situations. Once Mary felt safe and supported in a crisis home, she was able to spend some time either alone in the home or in one of the other supportive programmes in the community.

There is daily telephone 'check-in' contact between the ESU and the crisis home, with both home provider and Mary. It is an opportunity for ESU to monitor how things are going, and make changes in the care plan as needed. It also helps to remind the home provider and guest that they are not 'alone out there', and helps to confirm our support and concern. During the following days ESU staff meet with Mary to try and sort out her numerous and overlapping problems of finances, housing and psychiatric symptoms. Because of the recent crisis, Mary's medication has been changed, and we assess how it is working, and make changes as needed.

For clients like Mary who have become overly dependent on being admitted to hospital, we can arrange for her to stay at a crisis home two or three days a month; Mary has got to know several crisis home families, and she will often request to be with a specific household, and if this is reasonable we will try to arrange it. Mary mainly decides herself when to use these days, and this helps to avoid a power struggle and the situation where she has to 'prove' to the clinician that she really needs help. This type of regular use of the homes brings the average length of stay down to only three days; if such admissions are excluded, the average stay is around 5 days.

Why does it work?

There are several positive psychological factors that may have varying degrees of significance in any given crisis home admission:

- **The name itself.** The word 'crisis' acknowledges the feelings of uncertainty and hurt. 'Home' implies a sense of belonging and safe haven from that confusion. When the client goes through the front door, they become a 'guest', a word that is rich in its implication of

being welcome, as well as introducing implicit behavioural expectations.
- **Using private homes.** The client often feels very honoured to be a guest in a private house. In many cases, it will have been years (if ever) since the client has been in a pleasant living situation, and it is appreciated. In such a setting the principles of normalisation are better able to take hold. Even a severely dysfunctional client will rise to the occasion and try hard to be a safe and welcome guest. Environmental factors have been found to be more important than client characteristics in predicting level of social functioning (Levin & Brekke, 1993). For some of the clients the home environment seems to plant a seed of hope for some degree of 'recovery'; hope that may be undermined by some aspects of the traditional mental health system.
- The fact that **only one client is in the home at a time** offers a truly individualised approach. Surveys have shown that clients prefer not to live with other mental health consumers, and desire flexible and individually tailored support (Tanzman, 1993). Graduated expectations with positive low-key interactions are essential (Ranz *et al.*, 1991), and are part of the crisis home philosophy.
- **Non-professional home providers.** Just as the client becomes a 'guest' once in the home, the home providers are just 'nice people'. They are often immediately seen as an ally, and tend not to get into the power struggles that occur with the professionals (Polak *et al.*, 1977). At times, non-professionals may have a greater potential to look beyond the various diagnoses, and see the real human being (Mosher & Reifman, 1973).

Over the years we have been impressed how each home has a unique approach to providing their service. The formality and depersonalising aspects of professional mental health care dissolve in the context of how a family relates to someone in their own home. Effective crisis home support needs the following from the families:

- To be able to accept and welcome someone into their home without being tense or 'fake' (Segal *et al.*, 1991).
- To be able to acknowledge the problems of the client without feeling obligated to try to solve the problems.
- To know when they need to call us for advice or intervention.

- To recognise and hopefully draw out the strengths of even the most severely disabled clients.

Potential problems

Given the difficulties of assessing the mental health needs of people in crisis, problems are to be expected.

- **Violence.** We have never had a home provider attacked in his or her home, but staff have had one physical confrontation with an intoxicated client, and we have removed clients from homes because of fears over the safety of the family.
- **Neighbourhood opposition.** The home provider can help reduce the anxieties of neighbours by talking to each of them, and explaining that the guests are carefully screened. Unlike other residential models, there is usually no legal requirement for any sort of public hearing prior to a family agreeing to share its home in this fashion (Stroul, 1987).
- **Liability.** Establishing a family placement raises a range of liability issues (McCoin, 1987). In our service, home providers are now covered under the insurance of the mental health centre, but for many years each provider dealt with this individually through their own insurance agencies. The risks of offering a crisis home are fairly clear, but need to be considered in light of the fact that psychiatric wards are not devoid of risk. It is critical that everyone involved in the programme acknowledge the importance of responsible risk-taking, and values it as a necessary part of anyone's quality of life (and any quality mental health system).
- **Psychological dependency on crisis homes.** In our experience this has not been as much of a problem as we had expected. People seem to appreciate that these homes are only for short stays.
- **Tragedy.** Several suicidal clients who have used crisis homes have killed themselves in the days or weeks following their stay. Other tragedies have also occurred. This has been very difficult for our home providers, but as far as we know none have left the programme for this reason. The home providers have joined professionals and client family members in processing the impact of such a loss.

Summary

Despite a wide interest in minimising unnecessary use of in-patient services, admissions to such psychiatric programmes continue to rise (Slagg, 1993). Our experience over the years is that family crisis homes can help people through many different mental health emergencies. A review of the literature also supports this contention. Why are there not more such programmes?

Some of the reasons have already been discussed: concerns over liability, difficulty in recruiting families and the numerous problems associated with helping people with mental illness. But there are other reasons, which tell us more about society in general (and mental health professionals in particular) than they do about the problems of having a mental illness. Community mental health systems must examine these more systemic issues. It has been noted that it is sometimes difficult to find psychiatrists willing to admit someone to such a programme (Cutler, 1986). Part of the problem seems to be 'professional insecurity'. Historically, psychiatry has fought hard to be seen as on equal ground with other medical disciplines (Mosher, 1983); to lend too much credence to a more psychosocial model of treatment can be threatening to professionals who see their power as emanating from hospitals and a strict medical model of mental illness (Piers, personal correspondence).

A related problem is the increasing tendency for society to only reward professional assistance to people with a mental illness (Rubin, 1990). The United States government programmes will not reimburse agencies for non-professional support such as crisis homes; they will pay for in-patient care, despite the much higher cost (Randolph *et al.*, 1986). Also, while agencies often speak about offering a 'continuum of services', they rarely have the funding to actually implement such a system (Randolph *et al.*, 1991). Family crisis homes may wrongly be viewed as an unnecessary part of the out-patient system, whereas in fact they offer a unique contribution.

Others have noted that the broad concept of using community families for the treatment of the mentally ill will never become popular without a strong endorsement from the government (Belcher, 1987) and a 'moral crusader' to strongly advocate for this option (Rubin, 1990). As the United States moves towards a national health care system it would appear sensible to consider this cost-effective alternative to unnecessary in-patient treatment. Countries with a well-developed national health system should reflect on whether they should include such an option in their out-patient mental health system.

Our Crisis Home program can never be the perfect option for every mental health crisis; we will continue to use the hospital for those who need it. Nonetheless, it can be the option of choice for many people in different situations, and can offer advantages over the hospital. To be truly welcomed into a home is something we all deserve to experience.

It is what we see and hear from the people directly involved that prove to us that what we offer is successful. In an exit survey, 90% of the clients report being pleased to have the option of going to a crisis home. 'Having a time out from a stressful situation' was most often identified as what was helpful, as was 'being treated like a normal person'. In the words of one guest:

> Being in an environment where support and safety could be obtained outside the sterile walls of the hospital is always the better alternative. The crisis home family did more for me than any hospital could have ever offered me.

The provider families also give the programmes high marks, feeling personally enriched from the experience (Leaman, 1987). What follows are some of the thoughts of our first crisis home provider, who is still in the programme six years later.

> When my family and I took the plunge to become a crisis home, I wondered if we (not our guests) could be 'normal' enough for the job. How would it be to have a stranger showering in my bathroom who would also partake in the chaos that sometimes passes for domesticity in the kitchen? And, more importantly, would we be 'good for' the people who would come to our home as guests?
>
> Now that we have weathered six years together, I have tentative answers.
>
> Concerns about appearances long ago gave way to the inescapable yet comfortable truth that we can't stay dressed-up for long at our house. If mom and kids are skirmishing over dirty socks in the corner, or engaged in lively discussion as to the merits of practising this week's least favourite piano tune – well, welcome to our world.
>
> Somehow our guests have not stayed strangers for long. With the kaleidoscope of personalities who have come to stay with us, I'm struck by the fact that overwhelmingly we have enjoyed their presence. Yes, there is fragility, awkwardness at times and wrenching pain that also touches our family in surprising ways. But our guests have been so accepting of us and our fragility, that, far from feeling invaded by

people with 'problems' it's more as though our family enlarges a little at intervals.

Finally, it turns out that, in spite of ourselves, we often are 'good for' the person staying with us. As it is for everyone, there are days when a lot happens in our family; we have a lot of chores to tackle, a lot of turmoil to handle in our own lives. There's not always time to consciously channel energy into the role of helper for someone else. Though we acknowledge the emotional challenge facing our guest, it's almost as if circumstances conspire to leave the 'disorder' behind for periods in the day; taking such a break seems to fortify the person. It is clear to me that often I have ended up on the receiving end of the helping that happens here; this has been the lesson most useful to me about living in a Crisis Home.

Krista Roys

And how does the family Crisis Home programmes of community mental health centres apply to the concept of the broader 'community' and its 'mental health'? The undue professionalisation of human caring and support can rob a community of both the responsibility and the opportunity to grow, through helping others, and through being touched by those who are in some way different. Ending this chapter where it began, in the town of Gheel, here are the words of Dr. Charles Aring (1974), reflecting on his visit there many years ago:

> Were it possible to disseminate the spirit of Gheel, there would be little problem in gracefully phasing out the population of mental hospitals ... Thomas Szasz has long maintained that there is no aspect of life more precious than the freedom and opportunity to steer one's own bark, however erratic the direction. A contribution to be made by these patients is to render us more tolerant and accordingly, more civilised. In this case, mental patients might be considered to be among the expanders of civilisation.

Our hope is that crisis home programmes can contribute to this process, by helping to civilise our support that we offer to those with mental illness, as well as ourselves.

References

Aring, C. D. (1974). The Gheel experience: eternal spirit of the chainless mind. *Journal of the American Medical Association*, **230**, 998–1001.

Belcher, J. R. (1987). Adult foster care: an alternative to homelessness from some chronically mentally ill persons. *Adult Foster Care Journal*, **1**, 212–25.

Brook, B. (1980). Community families: a seven year program perspective. *Journal of Community Psychology*, **8**, 147–51.

Brook, B., Cortes, M., March, R. & Sundberg-Stirling, M. (1976). Community families: an alternative to psychiatric hospital intensive care. *Hospital and Community Psychiatry*, **27**, 195–7.

Brown, M. A. & Wheeler, T. (1990). Supported housing for the most disabled: suggestions for providers. *Psychosocial Rehabilitation Journal*, **13**, 61–7.

Carling, P. J. (1984). *Developing Foster Care Programs in Mental Health: A Resource Guide.* Rockville, Maryland, University of Vermont.

Carling, P. J. (1993). Housing and supports for persons with mental illness: emerging approaches to research and practice. *Hospital and Community Psychiatry*, **44**, 439–49.

Cutler, D. (1986). Community residential options for the chronically mentally ill. *Community Mental Health Journal*, **22**, 61–73.

Diamond, R. J. (1993). The psychiatrist's role in supported housing. *Hospital and Community Psychiatry*, **44**, 461–4.

Keisler, C. A. (1982). Mental hospitals and alternative care. *American Psychologist*, April, 349–60.

Leaman, K. (1987). A hospital alternative for patients in crisis. *Hospital and Community Psychiatry*, **38**, 1221–3.

LeCount, D. (1992). *The Dane County Model Adult Mental Health System Overview.* Madison, Wisconsin, Dane County Department of Human Services.

Levin, S. & Brekke, J. S. (1993). Factors related to integrating persons with chronic mental illness into a peer social milieu. *Community Mental Health Journal*, **29**, 25–33.

Livingston, J. A. & Srebnick, D. (1991). States' strategies for promoting supported housing for persons with psychiatric disabilities. *Hospital and Community Psychiatry*, **42**, 1116–19.

McCoin, J. M. (1983). *Adult Foster Homes: Their Managers and Residents.* New York, Human Services Press.

McCoin, J. M. (1987). Adult foster care: old wine in a new glass. *Adult Foster Care Journal*, **1**, 21–39.

Miller, M. (1987). Small towns and country lanes. *Adult Foster Care Journal*, **1**, 56–65.

Mosher, L. & Reifman, A. (1973). Characteristics of nonprofessionals serving as primary therapists for acute schizophrenics. *Hospital and Community Psychiatry*, **24**, 391–6.

Mosher, L. (1983). Alternatives to psychiatric hospitalization: why has research failed to be translated into practice? *New England Journal of Medicine*, **309**, 1579–80.

Plotinsky, I. (1985). Conard House: the halfway house as transitional residential facility. *Psychiatric Annals*, **15**, 648–52.

Polak, P. & Kirby, M. (1976). A model to replace psychiatric hospitals. *Journal of Nervous and Mental Disease*, **163**, 13–22.

Polak, P., Deever, S. & Kirby, M. (1977). On treating the insane in sane places. *Journal of Community Psychiatry*, **5**, 380–7.

Randolph, F. L., Lindenberg, R. E. & Menn, A. Z. (1986). Residential facilities for the mentally ill: needs assessment and community planning. *Community Mental Health Journal*, **22**, 77–89.

Randolph, F. L., Ridgeway, P. & Carling, P. J. (1991). Residential programs for persons with severe mental illness: a nationwide survey of state-affiliated agencies. *Hospital and Community Psychiatry*, **42**, 1111–15.

Ranz, J. M., Horen, B. T., McFarlane, W. R. & Zito, J. M. (1991). Creating a supportive environment using staff psychoeducation in a supervised residence. *Hospital and Community Psychiatry*, **42**, 1154–9.

Rubin, J. S. (1990). Adult foster care for people with chronic mental illness. *Adult Residential Care Journal*, **4**, 5–19.

Searight, H. R. & Searight, P. R. (1988). The homeless mentally ill: overview, policy implications, and adult foster care as a neglected resource. *Adult Foster Care Journal*, **2**, 235–57.

Segal, S. P., Kotler, P. L. & Holschuh, J. (1991). Attitudes of sheltered care residents toward others with mental illness. *Hospital and Community Psychiatry*, **42**, 1138–43.

Shadoan, R. A. (1985). Levels of care for residential treatment in an urban setting. *Psychiatric Annals*, **15**, 639–41.

Slagg, N. B. (1993). Patients that predict hospitalization or disposition to alternative treatments. *Hospital and Community Psychiatry*, **44**, 252–6.

Stroul, B. A. (1987). *Crisis Residential Services in a Community Support System.* Rockville, Maryland, National Institute of Mental Health.

Stroul, B. A. (1991). *Profiles of Psychiatric Crisis Response Systems.* Rockville, Maryland, National Institute of Mental Health.

Tanzman, B. (1993). An overview of surveys of mental health consumers' preference for housing and support services. *Hospital and Community Psychiatry*, **44**, 450–5.

Terpstra, J. & McFadden, E. J. (1993). Looking backward: looking forward/new directions in foster care. *Community Alternatives*, **5**, 115–33.

Thompson, K. S., Griffith, E. E. H. & Leaf, P. J. (1990). A historical review of the Madison model of community care. *Hospital and Community Psychiatry*, **41**, 625–33.

Walsh, S. F. (1986). Characteristics of failures in an emergency residential alternative to psychiatric hospitalization. *Social Work in Health Care*, **11**, 53–63.

Weisman, G. K. (1985). Crisis-oriented residential treatment as an alternative to hospitalization. *Hospital and Community Psychiatry*, **36**, 1302–5.

14

Acute home-based care and community psychiatry

LORENZO BURTI AND MICHELE TANSELLA

Introduction

Before it was believed to foster dependency and promote chronicity, hospitalisation was the main strategy for helping the mentally ill in any situation, including a crisis. Until the mid-1950s, hospitalisation was mainly in remote mental hospitals. Custodial mental health care had expanded during the previous century, even though pre-eminent psychiatrists such as Griesinger (1845) in Germany had warned of disastrous consequences (see in Häfner & an der Heiden, 1989). Unhappy with traditional mental hospital care, professionals began to look at alternative community-based strategies, and to compare the effectiveness with standard hospitalisation (Tyrer, 1985; Hoult, 1986; Kiesler & Sibulkin, 1987; Tansella & Zimmermann-Tansella, 1988; Mosher & Burti, 1989; Thornicroft & Bebbington, 1989).

In emergency situations, community care must offer a rapid response to urgent requests for help, with a minimum use of the hospital. To achieve this, a gatekeeper to the hospital is needed, and care must be offered to the client in his or her own environment. Acute home-based care typically meets both of these requirements. An early example is the 'psychiatric first aid service', established by Querido in Amsterdam, during the early 1930s (Querido, 1968). Other early examples of community home visiting and treatment services are reported to have existed since 1949 in Nottingham, UK (MacMillan, 1958), and in Worthing (Carse *et al.*, 1958) and in Boston, USA, since 1957 (Meyer *et al.*, 1967).

The need to care for patients discharged from mental hospitals expanded the practice of home visits both for crisis intervention and follow-up. Home visiting became an **everyday routine** for community psychiatric nurses (CPNs), since the 1950s in England (Woof *et al.*, 1988), and from the 1960s in France (Fournaise, 1988; Maurin, 1990), in Russia (Singer *et al.*, 1969) and in Italy (Jervis, 1975). Home visits were also provided by other professionals, but 'house calls' by psychiatrists are reported as being generally rare (Talbott & Manevitz, 1988), although there are exceptions (Brown, 1962; Mickle, 1963; Levy, 1985; Strathdee, 1990).

A team approach to home visiting resulted in mobile crisis units. These services have been refined, extensively studied and publicised by a number of authors (Stein & Test, 1978; Ratna, 1982; Reynolds & Hoult, 1984; Hoult, 1986; Muijen *et al.*, 1992) and have become the reference approach to emergency home care. Psychiatric home care is now considered a crucial programme of a comprehensive mental health service (Falloon & Pederson, 1985; Leff *et al.*, 1985; Pelletier, 1988).

The aim of this chapter is two-fold: firstly, to review the published programmes of home-based care and to outline the main characteristics of this component of community psychiatry and secondly, to describe briefly the 10-year experience of home care offered in South Verona by a new community-based psychiatric service.

The need for integrating emergency and continuous community care

A psychiatric emergency will often either be an aggravation of a pre-existing condition, or else the beginning of a path towards psychiatric chronicity (Reynolds *et al.*, 1990). The treatment of acute episodes must, therefore, include urgent intervention as well as careful follow-up treatment. In acute situations admission to hospital provides treatment and refuge to patients and respite to families, but will usually be of short duration. Traditional aftercare, i.e. without an intense (**assertive**) outreach orientation, will rarely result in an effective follow-up: new emergencies will ensue, often resulting in further admissions. In contrast, a community treatment team provides ongoing care, and is available at all times for emergencies. The team's readiness to respond to early worries of patient and/or family may even **prevent** emergencies: in Madison, USA, a **pre-crisis intervention service** is provided by the crisis intervention/emergency team (Mosher & Burti, 1989). Community care must be provided without time limits, otherwise patients are likely to return to former levels of functioning and relapse. In other words, there is no 'forever' treatment for this population. Stein and Test (1980) conclude that 'we should change our treatment strategy from preparing patients **for** community life to maintaining patients **in** community life.'

The ideal crisis service would provide high quality and specialised skills close to the population, 24 hours a day. This is clearly utopian: specialisation has to be traded for accessibility and prompt availability, and vice versa. It should be noted that chronic patients, who originate the highest number of psychiatric emergencies, require ongoing aftercare as well. It is extremely unlikely that specialised services can offer such aftercare.

Comprehensive community services, instead, may provide emergency care and crisis intervention as one of their manifold responsibilities. Community staff become effective in following up their patients, by getting to know them well and by fully exploiting local resources. However, there are legitimate doubts about the ability of these comprehensive general-purpose local services to provide optimum care for patients with acute psychiatric episodes of organic origin, or the most severe acute psychosocial crises. A possible answer is to supplement the system with a hospital backup and specialised crisis programmes (e.g. telephone lines for the suicidal, adolescent clinics) which cover a wider area.

Acute home-based care and the mobile crisis team

Chiu and Primeau (1991) stated that, essentially, a mobile crisis team is 'a van staffed by health professionals, typically a psychiatrist, a social worker and a registered nurse who provide at-home crisis intervention for patients suffering psychiatric trauma'. A more formal definition was given by Sullivan *et al.* (1984) 'a front line outreach multiprofessional crisis intervention team based in a neighbourhood health care centre'. In the service described by Reynolds and Hoult (1984), 'The community treatment team consisted of three psychiatric nurses, two social workers, one occupational therapist, one psychologist and one part-time psychiatrist, none of whom had previous experience with this kind of treatment program. The staff were rostered on duty for two shifts every day.

One staff member remained on call from 11.00 p.m. until 8.00 a.m.'

We view home care as a general purpose treatment option, but others have described its use with specific groups of patients, such as those who cannot, or do not want to, leave their home (Chiu & Primeau, 1991), including the elderly (the 'homebound aged' of Grauer *et al.*, 1991). Discussing his 24-hour home crisis service for geriatric patients in the London Borough of Barnet, Ratna (1982) stresses the low mortality rate he found among his patients followed up at home (29% mortality at one year), compared with the mortality and occurrence of complications reported in other published studies on old people admitted to psychiatric hospitals: 35 to 60% at one year follow-up (Baker & Byrne, 1977; Turner & Sternberg, 1978). Ratna's results are even more impressive, considering he used a mainly non-medical, problem-oriented social approach. Other suggested appropriate clients of home crisis intervention are non-responders to hospitalisation, patients with both medical and psychiatric disorders, isolated rural families (Heiman, 1983); families who prefer the sick relative to stay at home; patients in serious crisis, cases where collaborative family therapy (Bloch, 1973) or the treatment of family members, other than the identified patient are indicated (Soreff, 1983, 1985); children abused and neglected (Amundson, 1989); people living in urban ghettos (Chappel & Daniels, 1970, 1972) and patients who are known to easily develop dependence on the hospital when they are admitted.

In developing countries, where hospital facilities and trained psychiatrists are scarce or non-existent, home treatment by semi-professionals or non-professionals may be the only available alternative (Pai & Kapur, 1983). The homeless present particular challenges for a mobile crisis team. Project HELP based at Gouverneur Hospital in New York since 1982, was established to provide medical and psychiatric services to the impaired homeless, but found them to be difficult to treat because of their distrust and unwillingness to provide information about themselves (Cohen *et al.*, 1984).

Home visits have also been found useful to engage reluctant patients, conduct more comprehensive assessments, strengthen support networks and maintain patients in the community when their condition deteriorates (Kates *et al.*, 1991), and to train medical students (Wells *et al.*, 1987).

When acute home care is viewed as a general-purpose alternative to traditional hospitalisation and aftercare, only very general selection criteria are described. For instance, in Hoult's (1986) programme and follow-up study, access was open to all patients who presented voluntarily, or were taken involuntarily for admission to the local psychiatric hospital, and who met the following criteria: (1) resident in the catchment area; (2) aged between 15 and 65 years; and (3) not having a primary diagnosis of drug or alcohol dependence, organic brain disorder or mental retardation.

Techniques for home-based care

The 'foreign' territory of a patient's home may be taxing in terms of techniques that should be mastered by an ideal home-care professional (Lesseig, 1987; Bowers, 1992); however, personal characteristics, open-mindedness and enthusiasm remain the basic ingredients of all new alternative services even in the absence of previous specific experience (Reynolds & Hoult, 1984; Mosher & Burti, 1989).

Techniques reported as relevant span from those typical of general psychiatry and case management to those typical of a psychodynamic training: interfacing with other agencies and staff; attention to fine details of the home environment, assessment and reassessment through reframing, reviewing and updating observations (Sullivan *et al.*, 1984), resolving resistances by joining feelings, assuming personal responsibility and encouraging communication (Hazel, 1987, quoted by Chiu & Primeau, 1991). Experience, discernment and determination may uncover and endure the efforts of those close to the patient to transfer all the responsibility for the patient, and even their own problems, to the psychiatric services (Katschnig *et al.*, 1993). Skilfully interpreting, and fully understanding the reasons behind a request for help, and uncovering any hidden agendas, is both a technique and an art. Careful questioning during the initial phone call will save time by providing vital information to guide any following action. Useful formats to collect and organise information on referrals and during an interview with a natural group, usually a family, have been developed in the field of family therapy (Selvini-Palazzoli *et al.*, 1978, 1980).

Training on the delivery of psychosocial intervention to families can change the role and function of the community psychiatric nurse (Brooker, 1990; Brooker & Butterworth, 1991; Brooker *et al.*, 1992). Families can also help in 'case management' tasks such as assessments, linkage, monitoring, assistance with daily problems, crisis intervention and advocacy. But their efforts must be acknowledged, valued and supported by the professionals (Chiu & Primeau, 1991). Emergency service providers must include families in the assessment, decision making and treatment (Morgan, 1990).

Examples of community-based psychiatric services providing acute home-based care

In the programme described by Chiu and Primeau (1991) the team is usually alerted on the telephone by the family, the neighbours, an emergency medical service or the police. Depending on urgency, either an appointment is given or the team visits immediately. The average home visit takes about an hour, and treatment involves simply talking, or else medication. Hospital admission is a last resort, when all attempts of domiciliary treatment have failed. Even when in hospital the team remains in contact with the patient and the hospital staff throughout the admission. Once initial contact has been established, the mobile team will be responsible for him or her, until the situation has settled and the family is prepared to care for, and monitor the patient competently, or the case is taken over by another agency for regular follow-up. The authors describe three stages of stabilisation: building trust and confidence, establishing a therapeutic alliance, and fostering acceptance and compliance.

Training in Community Living, the model of home care developed by Stein and Test (1978, 1980), has been extensively investigated in controlled studies and widely replicated (Hoult & Reynolds, 1984; Reynolds & Hoult, 1984; Hoult, 1986; Muijen *et al.*, 1992). It is characterised by a strong commitment to prevent hospitalisation, a strong emphasis on the psychosocial dimensions of emergency, a long-term outlook, and an **assertive** support system and follow-up style. As Reynolds and Hoult (1984) report,

> The initial interview sometimes lasted several hours. An assessment was made not only of the patient's clinical symptoms leading to a diagnosis, but also of the events precipitating the admission request, the patient's behaviour, interpersonal relationships, social circumstances, and support and willingness to co-operate with treatment.

The team administered medication, including rapid tranquillisation if necessary, but also paid attention to significant interpersonal problems and to immediate practical problems,

> Patient and relatives were given information about the illness, explanation about the Community Treatment Team's methods of working and, for the relatives, guidance about how to deal with the patient's symptoms and behaviour. Threats of violence and suicide usually subsided with support, firmness and medication. If the psychiatrist considered it feasible, the team then returned with the patient to the community setting and immediately continued treatment. However, if the situation in the home appeared untenable, the team took the patient to alternative accommodations such as a boarding house and was responsible for his or her care there. Initially they may have stayed with the patient for many hours, monitoring his or her behaviour and the side-effects of medication given and reassuring patient and relatives. Once the patient became more settled, the staff withdrew, but still visited frequently for the first few days, and even took the patient out for some hours to give relief to families. Relatives and the patient were encouraged to contact staff readily if they were in any way worried, and staff visited willingly. This willingness to be contacted and 24-hour availability for home visiting greatly reassured the relatives. Necessary clinical investigations were carried out at this stage. In most cases, over several days quite a strong and enduring treatment alliance was formed; patient and relatives learned to regard the illness in quite a different light and learned new ways of managing it. As quickly as possible the patient was expected and encouraged to be responsible for himself and resume normal duties. Where necessary, staff accompanied the patient on tasks of community living, in order to assess, supervise, and train him in these tasks in the natural setting. For most patients these activities by the staff soon decreased as the patient became less psychotic, but for those patients with chronic, severe handicaps, they continued on an ongoing basis. Staff assertively trained patients in adequate hygiene and grooming, and use of community facilities such as transportation, supermarkets, day centres and sheltered workshops. The Team remained responsible for all experimental patients. In some cases patients had a recurrence of their symptoms during the study year but the Team was usually contacted early and was able to intervene quickly and deal with both the symptoms and the associated problems without needing to hospitalise the patient.
>
> Some acutely psychotic patients did need admission... Patients who were admitted remained in the experimental group; they were supervised in hospital by the Community Treatment Team psychiatrist and upon discharge [usually after two or three days] were offered the same treatment as those who were not admitted.

Outcome studies

Pasamanick *et al.*, (1967) and Langsley *et al.* (1969), conducted controlled studies demonstrating that crisis intervention and home support are as effective as hospital care and follow-up for the patient. Experimental studies contrasting community alternatives with mental hospital care for the acutely mentally ill were reviewed by Braun *et al.* (1981). In all the studies critically reviewed 'experimental alternatives to hospital care of patients have led to psychiatric outcomes not different from and occasionally superior to those of patients in control groups' but positive results required community-based, comprehensive care without time limits.

The Training in Community Living Program (Stein & Test, 1980) showed striking results: patients in the experimental group were less symptomatic, spent little time in psychiatric institutions (only 12 out of 62 experimental patients were admitted to hospital, compared with 58 out of 65 control patients) and less time unemployed, and were significantly more satisfied compared with the control group treated with hospitalisation and standard aftercare. Similar findings have been described in Australia (Reynolds & Hoult, 1984) and in the UK (Tufnell *et al.*, 1985; Muijen *et al.*, 1992; Dean *et al.*, 1993). (See chapter 2 for details.)

In the report of Kuznetsov and Voskresensky (1982), the implementation of psychiatric teams for emergency interventions brought about a global improvement of psychiatric care in the area covered by the service. In India, Pai and Kapur (1983) compared home treatment by a visiting nurse, monitored by a psychiatrist, with initial standard hospitalisation and subsequent aftercare, for first episode schizophrenic patients. Follow-up at six months revealed that home treatment gave better clinical outcome, better social functioning of the patient, reduced the burden on the patients' families and was also more economical.

Finally, Burns *et al.* (1993a,b) randomly allocated 94 patients to experimental home-based treatment and 78 to control treatments and followed them up for a year. No differences in clinical or social functioning outcome were found, both groups showed substantial improvement. There were three suicides in the control group and one in the experimental group. In the experimental group access to care was better and there was a substantial reduction in in-patient care, both in terms of proportion admitted and duration of admissions, despite similar out-patient and general practice care. The authors concluded that 'improved use of the resources that already exist within the community mental health team can substantially improve care'.

The South Verona Community Psychiatric Service: an integrated service for community-based treatment of mental illness

The Italian reform of 1978 introduced the phasing out of state hospitals and the establishment of catchment area community services. The Institute of Psychiatry of the University of Verona agreed with the spirit of the Reform Act and took responsibility for one of the districts of Verona with a resident population of 75,000 inhabitants. The South Verona Community Psychiatric Service (CPS) was established and has been operational ever since. It provides a full range of psychiatric interventions for the adult population (14 years and above), including involuntary commitments, long-term care and rehabilitation (Tansella, 1991).

The Service includes the following programmes:

- **Community Mental Health Centre**, open on working days, from 8 a.m. to 8 p.m. (8 a.m. to 4 p.m. on Saturdays) which is considered the hub of the service. Day care, rehabilitation and out-patient care is provided in the Centre.
- **Psychiatric ward** (15 beds), located in the university general hospital (about 1000 beds total).
- **Out-patient department**, providing consultations, individual and family therapy.
- **Mobile community teams**, home visits and other community interventions are made by all staff members, grouped in small mobile teams, in reply to emergency calls (provided by staff on call on a rotation basis) and for follow-up and long-term care (provided by the same staff members who are in charge of that particular patient).
- **Psychiatric emergency room**, which is part of the casualty department of the medical centre, for emergency interventions after workings hours.

- **Psychiatric liaison service**, providing consultations for patients and doctors of other departments of the medical centre.
- **Residential facilities**, three apartments and one 24-hour staffed hostel are available for up to 13 patients needing various types of supervision.

Staff are divided into three multidisciplinary teams, each responsible for a subsector of the catchment area. They work both in the hospital ward and in the community – i.e. staff follow their patients wherever they are treated. This approach encourages close personal relationships between staff and patients and ensures continuity of care through different phases of treatment and the various components of the service. Two or three staff members are assigned to long-term patients, so that at least one will usually be available. Patients are encouraged to come or call whenever they need help. If a patient shows up or is visited at home in an emergency, he is likely to encounter somebody he already knows and trusts – a real advantage in the case of a crisis when personal relationships are a key resource to deal with behavioural disorganisation and environmental confusion.

The principal responsibility of the service is to the more disturbed and disturbing individuals for whom it attempts to provide care in the least restrictive environment – i.e. with a minimum use of the hospital. House calls are considered especially suitable for crisis intervention. The principles are those described above – i.e. crisis resolution rather than crisis intervention alone, and the team assuming full responsibility for as long as needed. This is facilitated by the same team remaining responsible for a given patient indefinitely, and wherever the patient is, including the hospital, there is no need to refer to another team. Lasting personal relationships between staff and patients are regarded as valuable components of treatment; along with carefully designed and reviewed treatment plans. Planning always involves the whole team. There are resocialisation activities available at the Mental Health Centre, however, *in vivo* rehabilitation (training in community living) is more extensively used. As 83% of the patients live with their families, the service works hard to support families and offer family therapy.

In summary, the South Verona CPS, while not yet offering a 24-hour a day mobile crisis team (although one is planned), is an example of community programme integration. The same staff members of mobile teams continue to see the same patient even when he or she is admitted to the hospital. In turn, mobile teams can rely on the specialised backup of a conveniently located psychiatric ward and a University Medical Centre.

The South Verona psychiatric case register

This psychiatric case register was established on 31 December 1978 as a cumulative register of adult psychiatric morbidity defined by specialist service utilisation. The sociodemographic information, past psychiatric and medical history, and clinical data for each resident of South Verona aged 14 years and over, plus the contacting psychiatric services data are collected routinely (Tansella *et al.*, 1991). Diagnoses are assigned according to the International Classification of Diseases (ICD-9) and the World Health Organization (WHO) glossary and guide to the classification of mental disorders (WHO, 1978) and then coded into 11 standard diagnostic groups. From January 1992 diagnoses were assigned according to ICD-10 and coded into 13 diagnostic groups.

All services within the province of Verona report to the register, including the in-patient ward, the community mental health centre, the day hospital, out-patient services, state and private psychiatric hospitals, neurology wards of general hospitals (only for patients with a psychiatric diagnosis), the service for drug addicts and the out-patient service providing psychological and psychiatric care for adolescents older than 14 years. Contacts with all specialist psychiatric staff (nurses, psychiatrists, psychologists, social workers, etc.) are included. Each extramural contact, including home visits, is recorded as 'booked' or 'urgent', according to whether or not an appointment was previously arranged.

Quantitative data on home visits provided in 1982–91

We have analysed data on home visiting during a 10-year period (1982–91) which followed the preliminary phase of our experience with the new service. Although this type of care was provided from the beginning of the service during the three and half years (1978–81) the services underwent many changes, and we have excluded it from our analysis. All patients were considered except those with a diagnosis of drug dependence, who are treated by a specialised service, which is not part of the South Verona CPS.

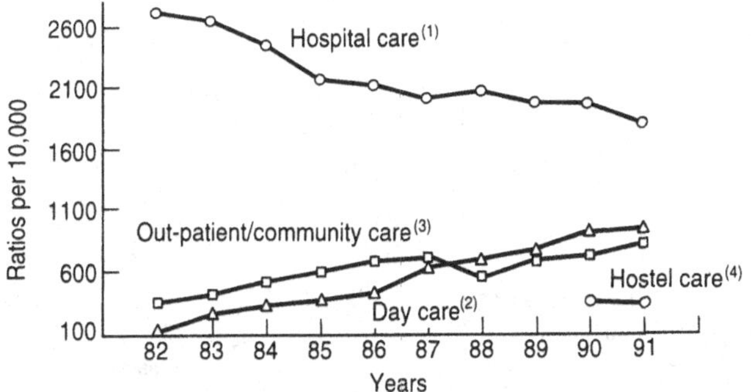

(1) Days in hospital. Long -stay patients in state mental hospitals and patients admitted to neurological wards (with psychiatric diagnosis) are included.
(2) Days in the day hospital and in the day centre and sessions of rehabilitation groups at the community mental health centre.
(3) All out-patient attendances and home visits. Contacts with the Service for drug dependence are excluded.
(4) Days in the 24-hour staffed hostel.

Fig. 14.1. Patterns of extramural and intramural care in South Verona, 1982–91. Ratios per 10,000 adult population

Figure 14.1 shows that, while an increase in out-patient/community care (data on out-patient attendances and home visits pooled together) and day care was taking place there was a parallel fall in the use of public and private hospital beds. The mean number of occupied beds per day (ratio per 10,000) was 4.8 in 1991, i.e. 28.6% lower than the 1982 ratio (6.7 per 10,000) and 48.8% lower than the 1979 ratio (9.3 per 10,000). On the other hand the number of home visits provided in 1991 (n=1824) was 786% higher than in 1982 (n=232) and in 1979 (n=233).

However, Fig. 14.2 (all visits, A), demonstrates that the increase over the years in the provision of home-based care was not consistent across age and sex groups. In 1991 the number of home visits was much higher in females aged 45–64 years, than in younger female patients or in males. Also the patterns of home visits provided on an urgent basis (without appointment) were not consistent over the years in the various age and sex groups and again in 1991 most interventions of this kind were provided to females aged 45–64 years (Fig. 14.2, urgent visits, B).

Also when considering the patients who received home-based care over the study period the increase of the rates was consistent and substantial for the females aged 45–64 but not so in younger females and in males (Fig. 14.3, A). This trend is also confirmed when the

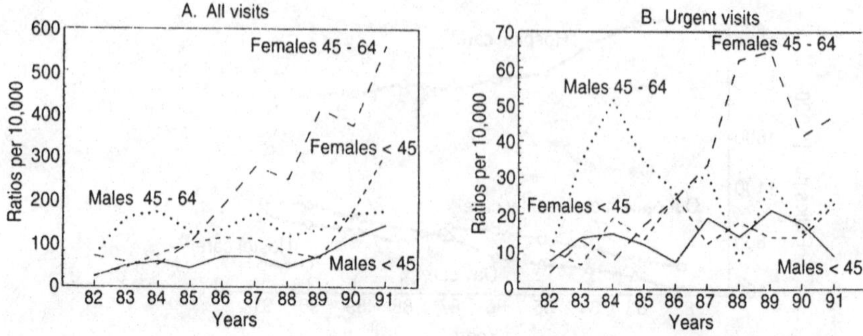

Fig. 14.2. All home visits (A) and urgent home visits (B) provided to adult South Verona residents in 1982–91. Age and sex specific ratios per 10,000 adult population

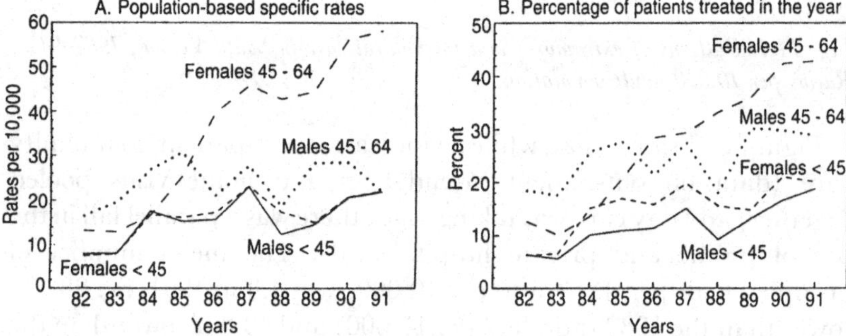

Fig. 14.3. South Verona patients who received home visits in 1982–91. Population-based age and sex specific rates per 10,000 adult population (A). Percentage of patients treated each year, by sex and age (B)

patients treated at home were calculated as a percentage of all patients in the same age and sex groups who were in contact with psychiatric services in the year (Fig. 14.3, B).

Data were therefore analysed by diagnosis. Three diagnostic groups were considered. Schizophrenia and related disorders (ICD-9 codes 295,0-1-2-3-4-5-6-7-8-9; 297,0-1-2-3-8-9; 298,2-3-4-8-9 and 299,0-1-8-9); affective disorders (ICD-9 codes 296,0-1-2-3-4-5-6-8-9; 298,0-1; 300,4; 309,0–1) and all other diagnoses. Fig. 14.4 (A) concerns patients with schizophrenic disorder and shows that again an increasing number of visits were provided to females aged 45–64 and (from 1989 only) to younger females, while the increase in home visits provided to male patients with schizophrenia was smaller. The

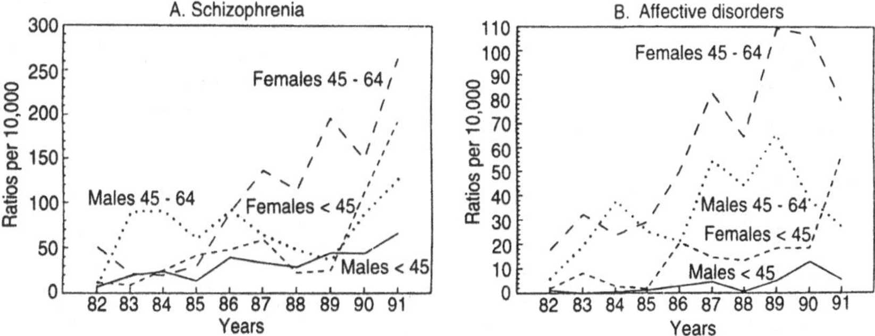

Fig. 14.4. Home visits provided in 1982–91 to South Verona patients with diagnosis of schizophrenia and related disorders (A) or of affective disorders (B). Age and sex specific ratios per 10,000 adult population

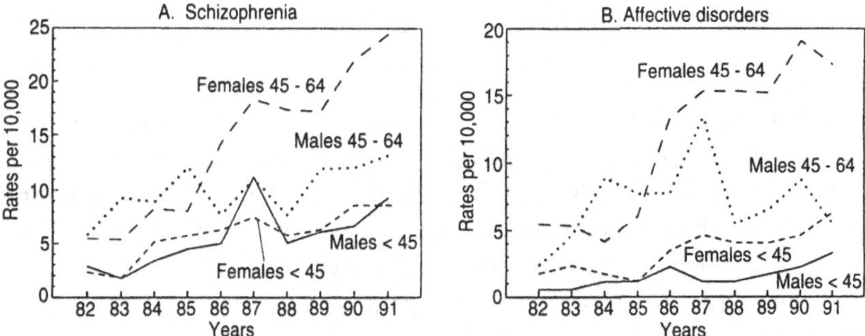

Fig. 14.5. South Verona patients with a diagnosis of schizophrenia and related disorders (A) or of depressive disorders (B) who received home visits in 1982–91. Age and sex specific rates per 10,000 adult population

patterns of home visits to patients with affective disorders (Fig. 14.4, B) are similar. Finally Fig. 14.5 shows data concerning rates of patients with schizophrenia (A) or affective disorders (B) treated at home. The most consistent change over the years is again the increase of home care provided to females aged 45–64.

It is not clear why home care has been concentrated on older women. One hypothesis is that in our society these patients, along with most other women in the same generation, tend to be passive-dependant, and prefer this type of care to traditional visits to the out-patient department. Another hypothesis is that it is more difficult for them to leave their houses and reach the services, either because they live alone (although, only 10% of all South Verona

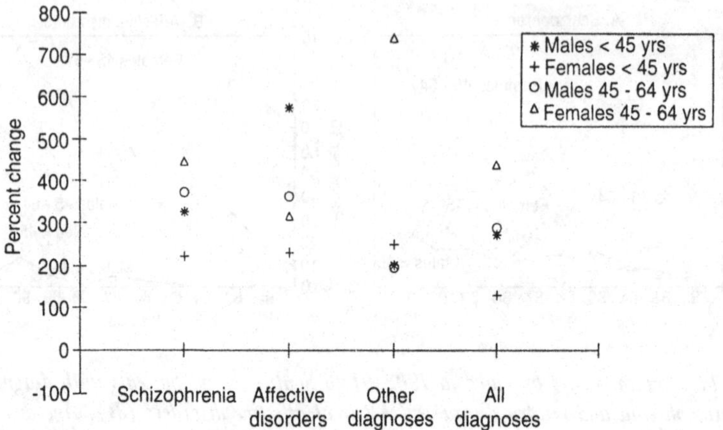

Fig. 14.6. Percentage change in 1991 versus *1982 in the rates of patients who received home visits per 10,000 adult population, by diagnosis, sex and age.*

patients aged 45–64 years who received home care in 1991 lived alone) or, more likely, they still have a large role in looking after their families and households, and therefore have to be supported in their home more than women of other age groups, or men. Further studies are necessary to confirm or reject these hypotheses.

Figure 14.6 shows the percentage changes (1991 *versus* 1982) in the age and sex specific rates (per 10,000 adult population) of patients who received home visits. The biggest increase (more than 700%) concerned the older female group with 'other diagnoses', followed by young males with a diagnosis of affective disorders and by females older than 45 years with a diagnosis of schizophrenia. The smallest increase (still more than 100%) concerned young females with all diagnoses.

As reported above in South Verona during the 10-year study period, while the amount of care provided in the community increased, a parallel decrease in the use of hospital beds occurred. An important component of community care was home-based care. In order to evaluate the relation between the increasing provision of home care and the decreasing utilisation of in-patient care (the availability of beds in public and private hospitals remained constant over the years), the correlation coefficients between number of home visits (separately for all visits and for urgent visits) and number of days in hospital provided in each trimester were calculated ($n=40$).

Table 14.1. *Correlations between number of days in hospital and number of home visits provided each trimester in 1982–91 (n=40).*

	r	Significance
All diagnoses		
Males 14–64 yrs	−0.55	**
Females 14–64 yrs	−0.51	**
Males <44 yrs	−0.50	**
Females <44 yrs	−0.43	*
Females 45–64 yrs	−0.61	**
Affective disorders		
Females 14–64 yrs	−0.45	*
Females 45–64 yrs	−0.46	*
Other diagnoses, excluding schizophrenia and related disorders		
Females 14–64 yrs	−0.44	*
Females 45–64 yrs	−0.56	**

* $p<0.05$; ** $p<0.01$.

Separate calculations were performed by sex, age and diagnosis. Only significant correlations found for all home visits are reported in Table 14.1.

In female patients many significant correlations emerged. All were negative and concerned, for all diagnoses, all patients (14–64 age groups) and both age groups (<44 yr and 45–64 yr), and for affective disorders, as well as other diagnoses (excluding schizophrenia), all patients (14–64 yr) and the older age group (45–64 yr). In males the only significant correlations were two negative correlations found for all diagnoses when all patients (14–64 yr) and the younger group (<44 yr) were considered. No significant correlations were found in patients of either sex with schizophrenic disorders.

For urgent home visits only the correlations concerning females with all diagnoses (all and both those belonging to the younger and to the older groups) were significant ($r=-0.52$; -0.40 and -0.44, respectively). In 1991, 280 home visits per 10,000 adult inhabitants were provided and 31 patients per 10,000 received this type of care (28% of those in contact with psychiatric services in the year). However, the ratio of urgent home visits in the same year was 22 per 10,000 inhabitants and 13 patients per 10,000 received this care on an urgent basis (12% of all patients treated in 1991).

The above results show that home-based care, increasingly

provided in the 1982–91 period to all South Verona patients (particularly to older females) was associated with a decreasing use of hospital beds in female patients (all diagnoses) and in female patients with affective disorders and with other diagnoses, but not in those with schizophrenia and related disorders. In males the negative correlation between home care and in-patient care emerged only when all diagnoses were considered. In discussing these findings the possibility that the statistically significant relation which was found was not a causal one cannot be ruled out without further studies. Moreover, it should be considered that, over the study period, while home-based care was increasing, there was also an increase in other types of non-hospital care, such as day care, out-patient care and rehabilitation programmes. Therefore, before concluding that the decrease in hospital care was 'specifically' related to the increasing provision of psychiatric and psychological help in the patients' homes we are conducting further studies and analysis of case-register data.

Conclusions

The main finding of our case-register data analysis is the substantial increase, over the years, of home visits and the number of psychiatric patients treated at home. As well as the apparent affect of this community-based type of care on the use of hospital beds which decreased over the same period, there was a distinct improvement in our psychiatric service as a result of more home-based care. As Cooper (1993) pointed out, a more frequent use by psychiatrists and their co-workers of provisions for domiciliary visiting within the terms of the mental health service, i.e. the possibility that they have to explore the situation where patients live and work, and where pathogens may be active, 'offer a potential framework for clinical epidemiology. The fundamental concept of disease as a result of population exposure to environmental pathogens has served for generations as the lodestar of preventive medicine. Latter-day trends away from segregation of the mentally ill in institutions, in favour of their treatment and care in the community, could serve to foster similar approaches to the problems of mental disorder, and one may hope that they will find greater application in psychiatry in the future'.

Acknowledgements

We are grateful to Mr. Giuliano Meneghelli (South Verona Psychiatric Case Register) for data collection; to Dr. Giulia Bisoffi (statistician) for data analysis and to Dr. Renato Fianco and Mrs. Paola Bonizzato for their help in the preparation of the manuscript.

This study was partially supported by the Consiglio Nazionale delle Ricerche (CNR, Roma), Progetto Finalizzato Fattori di Malattia (FATMA), Sottoprogetto 'Stress', Contracts No. 93.00743.PF41 and No. 94.00659.PF41 to Professor M. Tansella.

References

Amundson, M.J. (1989). Family crisis care: a home-based intervention program for child abuse. *Issues in Mental Health Nursing*, **10**, 285–96.

Baker, A. A. & Byrne, R.J. F. (1977). Another style of psychogeriatric service. *British Journal of Psychiatry*, **130**, 123–6.

Bloch, D. A. (1973). The clinical home visit. *Seminars in Psychiatry*, **5**, 159–65.

Bowers, L. (1992). Ethnomethodology II: a study of the community psychiatric nurse in the patient's home. *International Journal of Nursing Studies*, **29**, 69–79.

Braun, P., Kochansky, G. Shapiro, R., Greenberg, S., Gudeman, J. E., Johnson, S. & Shore, M. F. (1981). Overview: deinstitutionalization of psychiatric patients, a critical review of outcome studies. *American Journal of Psychiatry*, **138**, 736–49.

Brooker, C. (1990). A new role for the community psychiatric nurse in working with families caring for a relative with schizophrenia. *International Journal of Social Psychiatry*, **36**, 216–24.

Brooker, C. & Butterworth, C. (1991). Working with families caring for a relative with schizophrenia: the evolving role of the community psychiatric nurse. *International Journal of Nursing Studies*, **28**, 189–200.

Brooker, C., Tarrier, N., Barrowclough, C., Butterworth, A. & Goldberg, D. (1992). Training community psychiatric nurses for psychosocial intervention: report of a pilot study. *British Journal of Psychiatry*, **160**, 836–44.

Brown, B. S. (1962). Home visiting by psychiatrists. *Archives of General Psychiatry*, **7**, 46–55.

Burns, T., Beadsmoore, A., Bhat, A. V., Oliver, A. & Mathers, C. (1993a). A controlled trial of home-based acute psychiatric services. I: Clinical and social outcome. *British Journal of Psychiatry*, **163**, 49–54.

Burns, T., Raftery, J., Beadsmoore, A., McGuigorn, S. & Dickson, M. (1993b). A controlled trial of home-based acute psychiatric services. II:

Treatment patterns and costs. *British Journal of Psychiatry*, **163**, 55–61.
Carse, J., Panton, N. E. & Watt, A. (1958). A district mental health service: the Worthing experiment. *Lancet*, **1**, 39–41.
Chappel, J. N. & Daniels, R. S. (1970). Home visiting in a black urban ghetto. *American Journal of Psychiatry*, **126**, 1455–60.
Chappel, J. N. & Daniels, R. S. (1972). Home visiting: an aid to psychiatric treatment in black urban ghettos. *Current Psychiatric Therapies*, **12**, 194–201.
Chiu, T. L. & Primeau, C. (1991). A psychiatric mobile crisis unit in New York City: description and assessment, with implications for mental health care in the 1990s. *International Journal of Social Psychiatry*, **37**, 251–8.
Cohen, N., Putnam, J. & Sullivan, A. (1984). The mentally ill homeless: isolation and adaptation. *Hospital and Community Psychiatry*, **35**, 922–4.
Cooper, B. (1993). Single spies and battalions: the clinical epidemiology of mental disorders. *Psychological Medicine*, **23**, 891–907.
Dean, C., Phillips, J., Gadd, E. M., Joseph, M. & England, S. (1993). Comparison of community based service with hospital based service for people with acute, severe psychiatric illness. *British Medical Journal*, **307**, 473–6.
Falloon, I. R. H. & Pederson, J. (1985). Family management in the prevention of morbidity of schizophrenia: the adjustment of the family unit. *British Journal of Psychiatry*, **147**, 156–63.
Fournaise, V. (1988). La psychiatrie de secteur: La visite à domicile en milieu rurale. *Soins Psychiatrie*, No. 96 (Octobre), pp. 16–18.
Grauer, H., Kravitz, H., Davis, E. & Rodrigue, C. (1991). Homebound aged: the dilemma of psychiatric intervention. *Canadian Journal of Psychiatry*, **36**, 497–501.
Griesinger, W. (1845). *Die Pathologie und Therapie der Psychischen Krankheiten.* Stuttgart, Krabbe.
Häfner, H. & an der Heiden, W. (1989). The evaluation of mental health care systems. *British Journal of Psychiatry*, **155**, 12–17.
Hazel, E. (1987). *A Modern Psychoanalytic Approach to Program Development*, Doctoral Dissertation. The Union for Experimenting Colleges and Universities.
Heiman, E. M. (1983). The psychiatrist in a rural CMHC. *Hospital and Community Psychiatry*, **34**, 227–9.
Hoult, J. (1986). Community care of the acutely mentally ill. *British Journal of Psychiatry*, **149**, 137–44.
Hoult, J. & Reynolds, I. (1984). Schizophrenia: a comparative trial of community orientated and hospital orientated psychiatric care. *Acta Psychiatrica Scandinavica*, **69**, 359–72.
Jervis, G. (1975). *Manuale Critico di Psichiatrica.* Milano, Feltrinelli.
Kates, N., Webb, S. & LePage, P. (1991). Therapy begins at home: the psychiatric house call. *Guardian Journal of Psychiatry*, **36**, 673–6.
Katschnig, H., Konieczna, T. & Cooper, J. E. (1993). *Emergency Psychiatric and Crisis Intervention Services in Europe: A Report Based on Visits to Services in Seventeen Countries.* WHO Document EUR/ICP/PSF 030 04025.

Copenhagen, WHO Regional Office for Europe.

Kiesler, C. A. & Sibulkin, A. E. (1987). *Mental Hospitalization. Myths and Facts About a National Crisis*. Newbury Park, CA, Sage Publication.

Kuznetsov, M. & Voskresensky, V. (1982). Emergency aid as part of a system for the delivery of psychiatric aid to the population. *Zhurnal Nevropatologii Psichiatrii*, **82**, 1202–5.

Langsley, D. G., Flomenhaft, K. & Machotka, P. (1969). Follow-up evaluation of family crisis therapy. *American Journal of Orthopsychiatry*, **39**, 753–9.

Leff, J., Kuipers, L., Berkowitz, R. & Sturgeon, D. (1985). A controlled trial of social intervention in the families of schizophrenic patients: two year follow-up. *British Journal of Psychiatry*, **146**, 594–600.

Lesseig, D. Z. (1987). Home care for psychiatric problems. *American Journal of Nursing*, **87**, 1317–20.

Levy, M. T. (1985). Psychiatric assessment of elderly patients in the home: a survey of 176 cases. *Journal of the American Geriatrics Society*, **33**, 9–12.

MacMillan, D. (1958). Mental health services of Nottingham. *International Journal of Social Psychiatry*, **4**, 5–9.

Maurin, F. (1990). Pratique d'infirmier 'aux visites à domicile' du secteur 12. *Soins Psichiatrie*, Nos. 110/111, Décembre 1989–Janvier 1990, pp. 45–8.

Meyer, R. E., Schiff, L. F. & Becker, A. (1967). The home treatment of psychotic patients: an analysis of 154 cases. *American Journal of Psychiatry*, **123**, 1430–8.

Mickle, J. C. (1963). Psychiatric home visit. *Archives of General Psychiatry*, **9**, 379–87.

Morgan, S. L. (1990). Determinants of family treatment choice and satisfaction in psychiatric emergencies. *American Journal of Orthopsychiatry*, **60**, 96–107.

Mosher, L. R. & Burti, L. (1989). *Community Mental Health: Principles and Practice*. New York, Norton.

Muijen, M., Marks, M., Connolly, J., Audini, B. & McNamee, G. (1992). The daily living programme: preliminary comparison of community versus hospital-based treatment for the seriously mentally ill facing emergency admission. *British Journal of Psychiatry*, **160**, 379–84.

Pai, S. & Kapur, R. L. (1983). Evaluation of home care treatment for schizophrenic patients. *Acta Psychiatrica Scandinavica*, **67**, 80–8.

Pasamanick, B., Scarpitti, F. R. & Dinitz, S. (1967). *Schizophrenics in the Community: An Experimental Study in the Prevention of Hospitalization*. New York, Appleton-Century-Crofts.

Pelletier, L. R. (1988). Psychiatric home care. *Journal of Psychosocial Nursing and Mental Health Services*, **26**(3), 22–7.

Querido, A. (1968). The shaping of community mental health care. *British Journal of Psychiatry*, **114**, 293–302.

Ratna, L. (1982). Crisis intervention in psychogeriatrics: a two-year follow-up study. *British Journal of Psychiatry*, **141**, 296–301.

Reynolds, I. & Hoult, J. E. (1984). The relatives of the mentally ill: a comparative trial of community-oriented and hospital-oriented psychiatric care. *Journal of Nervous and Mental Disease*, **172**, 480–9.

Reynolds, I., Jones, J. E., Berry, D. W. & Hoult, J. E. (1990). A crisis team for the mentally ill: the effect on patients, relatives and admissions. *Medical Journal of Australia*, **152**, 646–52.

Selvini-Palazzoli, M., Boscolo, L., Cecchin, G. & Prata, G. (1978). *Paradox and Counterparadox*. New York, Aronson.

Selvini-Palazzoli, M., Boscolo, L., Cecchin, G. & Prata, G. (1980). Hypothesizing-circularity-neutrality: three guidelines for the conductor of the session. *Family Process*, **19**, 3–12.

Singer, P., Holloway, B. & Kolb, L. C. (1969). The psychiatrist-nurse team and home care in the Soviet Union and Amsterdam. *American Journal of Psychiatry*, **125**, 1198–202.

Soreff, M. S. (1983). New directions and added dimensions in home psychiatric treatment. *American Journal of Psychiatry*, **140**, 1213–16.

Soreff, M. S. (1985). Indications for home treatment. *Psychiatric Clinics of North America*, **8**, 563–75.

Stein, L. I. & Test, M. A. (1978). An alternative to mental hospital treatment. In *Alternatives to Mental Hospital Treatment*, ed. L. I. Stein & M. A. Test. New York, Plenum.

Stein, L. I. & Test, M. A. (1980). Alternative to mental hospital treatment: I. Conceptual model, treatment program, and clinical evaluation. *Archives of General Psychiatry*, **37**, 392–7.

Strathdee, G. (1990). Delivery of psychiatric care. *Journal of the Royal Society of Medicine*, **83**, 222–5.

Sullivan, A., Hetrick, E., Blokar, M. & Klot, A. (1984). Psychiatric crisis in the elderly: a systems view. Gouverneur Hospital, Dept. of Psychiatry, New York, NY. *International Journal of Family Psychiatry*, **5**, 233–47.

Talbott, J. A. & Manevitz, A. Z. A. (Eds.) (1988). *Psychiatric House Calls*. Washington, DC, American Psychiatric Press.

Tansella, M. (1991). *Community-based Psychiatry. Long-term Patterns of Care in South Verona*. Psychological Medicine Monograph Supplement No. 19. Cambridge, Cambridge University Press.

Tansella, M., Balestrieri, M., Meneghelli, G. & Micciolo, R. (1991). Trends in the provision of psychiatric care 1979–1988. In *Community-based Psychiatry. Long-term Patterns of Care in South-Verona*. Psychological Medicine Monograph Supplement No. 19. Cambridge, Cambridge University Press.

Tansella, M. & Zimmermann-Tansella, Ch. (1988). From mental hospital to alternative community services. In *Modern Perspectives in Clinical Psychiatry*, ed. J. G. Howells. New York, Brunner/Mazel.

Thornicroft, G. & Bebbington, P. (1989). Deinstitutionalisation. From hospital closure to service development. *British Journal of Psychiatry*, **155**, 739–53.

Tufnell, G., Bouras, N., Watson, J. P. & Brough, D. I. (1985). Home assessment and treatment in a community psychiatric service. *Acta Psychiatrica Scandinavica*, **72**, 20–8.

Turner, R. J. & Sternberg, M. P. (1978). Psychosocial factors in elderly patients admitted to a psychiatric hospital. *Age and Ageing*, **7**, 171–7.

Tyrer, P. (1985). The hive system. A model for a psychiatric service. *British Journal of Psychiatry*, **146**, 571–5.

Wells, K. B., Benson, M. C., Hoff, P. & Stuber, M. (1987). A home-visit program for first-year medical students as perceived by participating families. *Family Medicine*, **19**, 364–7.

Woof, K., Goldberg, D. P. & Fryers, T. (1988). The practice of community psychiatric nursing and mental health social work in Salford: some implications for community care. *British Journal of Psychiatry*, **152**, 783–92.

World Health Organization (1978). *Mental Disorders: A Glossary and Guide to Their Classification in Accordance With the Ninth Revision of the International Classification of Diseases*. Geneva, WHO.

15
Acute day hospital care

FRANCIS CREED

Introduction

This chapter will examine the use of the day hospital for acute psychiatric illness. There are several questions to be addressed. Is it really feasible to treat acutely ill patients in a day hospital? What is the outcome of treatment? Can the findings of the few experimental studies be generalised? If so, can others develop acute day hospital treatment? Finally, is day hospital treatment for acute illness really cheaper than in-patient care? This chapter will examine these questions; there is increasing consensus in the literature about the answers, except, possibly, that concerning cost.

The major problem in trying to tackle these questions is the fact that day hospitals have been used predominantly for support and rehabilitation of patients with chronic disorders rather than as a primary treatment strategy for acute illness (Pryce 1982; McGrath & Tantam 1987); this means that evaluation of their use for acute illness is difficult. The reasons why day hospitals have not changed their role to the care of acute illness are discussed below, they include lack of alternative provision (e.g. day centres) for the chronically ill but also include staff attitudes – acutely ill patients may be perceived as 'demanding and disruptive' in a traditional rehabilitation day hospital (Creed *et al.*, 1989b; Anthony *et al.*, 1991). This resistance to change encourages the attitude that only selected patients are suitable for day hospital treatment.

Some would view day hospitals as having a very limited contribution to make towards the care of acute illness. Evidence quoted in favour of this view includes the repeated finding that only approximately a fifth of patients presenting for admission can be successfully treated in the day hospital as an alternative to in-patient care. The argument is circular, however, as one of the main reasons for this finding is the fact that many clinicians, patients and carers assume that the day hospital is not suitable for acute illness, particularly if it has no means of answering emergency calls for care outside of working hours. For this reason the full potential of the day hospital as an effective treatment facility for acute illnesses may require **access to respite care** (Chapter 12) or be used in conjunction with **short in-patient stay** (Hirsch *et al.*, 1979).

An alternative view, held by the author, is that day hospitals have considerable scope for developing acute care in the community. If day hospital treatment can be used as an alternative to in-patient care (see below), medical, nursing and other staff can begin to offer community-based acute treatments without the potential threats of risk-taking and burnout associated with some more ambitious community treatment approaches (Tyrer & Creed, 1995). For this reason, day hospital treatment may provide a pattern of acute community care that can be replicated throughout the NHS in the UK, and which is more likely to be adopted by many district psychiatric teams than the emergency teams used in the daily living programme (Muijen *et al.*, 1992).

Advantages of day hospital treatment

Over in-patient care

The treatment of patients with acute illness in a day hospital rather than an in-patient unit has several advantages. Firstly, patients are not removed from their homes for any length of time so disruption to their normal routine is minimal. Secondly, it is much cheaper for the hospital service if patients do not stay overnight. Thirdly, day hospital treatment may reduce the stigma, which tends to be associated with in-patient treatment. It may also prevent the development of institutionalised behaviour which can result from prolonged in-patient stay.

Over independent community treatment

The day hospital can also provide important aspects of hospital care (e.g. investigations and treatment facilities, such as electroconvulsive therapy – ECT) **without the patient having to be admitted** for these. Staff used to working in a hospital-based service can continue to do so but gradually extend their treatment to community settings.

Disadvantages of day hospital treatment

The principal disadvantage is the fact that it is not applicable to the great majority of patients presenting with disturbed behaviour, which apparently requires in-patient admission. The call for admission may come from carers in the community who state that they cannot cope any longer. Such a crisis can only be prevented if a community team is already working with the patient; if such a team exists and the need for admission is avoided it might be argued that the day hospital is not needed.

Development of day hospitals in the UK

Although it is nearly 15 years since the Department of Health and Social Security (DHSS) recommended that acutely ill psychiatric patients be treated in day hospitals rather than in-patient units (Department of Health and Social Security, 1975) the development of day hospital treatment in the UK has been described as being 'disordered' (Vaughan, 1983) and determined 'more by fashion than by experimental evidence' (Lancet, 1985). The Lancet review (1985) divided the role of the psychiatric day hospital into three main categories:

- As an alternative to in-patient admission, treating acutely ill patients, admitted directly from the community, though this is not suitable for psychotic patients.
- For treatment of patients with chronic illnesses, mainly schizophrenia. The attendance at the day hospital being mainly for support rather than acute treatment.
- For treatment of patients with personality disorders and neurotic illnesses not considered ill enough for inpatient care.

The first is the subject of this review; the term 'acute' is used to indicate those illnesses that present to psychiatrists for a fresh episode of treatment and not transfers from a long-stay bed. The term 'day hospital' is used in the sense of Rosie (1987), to indicate a facility that provides diagnostic and treatment services for acutely ill patients who would otherwise be treated on traditional psychiatric in-patient units. This distinguishes them from 'day-treatment programmes' for specialised groups of patients, or those with partially remitted illness, and 'day centres' that have the maintenance of chronic psychiatric patients as their primary tasks. The day hospital **can only be used for acute illness** if there is adequate alternative provision for the other groups of patients.

Evaluative research

Previous research in this area has been criticised because it used small numbers of patients, with a selection bias, only partial or no randomisation, and little control of important variables such as diagnosis, medication and treatment between discharge and follow-up (Wilkinson 1984). Day care and in-patient care have not been clearly defined, outcome measures have not been standardised or rated blindly, and too many patients have been lost to follow-up. Therefore evaluation of day hospital treatment requires development of a day hospital with staff and facilities that can cope with acute illness and rigorous research methodology. Part of this chapter is devoted to a description of our work in Manchester but research in other centres will be reviewed first.

Feasibility of day care for acutely ill patients

The results of various studies are summarised in Table 15.1. Most researchers have accepted at the outset that a proportion of patients show disturbed behaviour that was uncontainable in the community and/or would disrupt day-hospital treatment programmes (Vaughan 1985). For example, Dick *et al.* (1985a,b) limited their study to patients with diagnoses of neurosis, personality disorder and adjustment reaction, presumably considering that psychotic patients could not be treated in the day hospital. However, they also excluded many neurotic patients on the grounds that they were 'too ill', but no definition of this term was given. These selection criteria meant that only a small percentage of all admissions would have been included in this study.

Table 15.1. *Proportion of patients excluded from random allocation in studies comparing day hospital and in-patient treatment*

First author of study		Reason for exclusion		
	All admissions included (%)	Too ill	Too well	Refused/social/ other
Wilder (1966)	40	33%	—	—
Herz (1971)	22	38	20	20
Fenton (1979)	19	35		46
Washburn (1976)	15	58		27
Dick (1985a,b)	22	30	12	36
Platt (1980)	12	56	22	10
Kluiter (1992)	40	60	—	—
Schene (1993)	33	63	—	4
Creed (1990)	40	39	—	21
Gudeman (1983)	21	79	—	—

One of the most satisfactory attempts to randomly allocate **all patients presenting for admission** is the oldest. Zwerling and Wilder (1964) attempted to allocate to a day hospital or in-patient unit all patients between 18 and 65 years of age, except those with a primary diagnosis of drug or alcohol dependence, organic brain disorder or mental retardation. Two-thirds of 378 patients were randomly allocated and two-thirds of those referred to day care were accepted for treatment in that facility. The remainder were too ill and had to be transferred to the in-patient unit. This successful study was only briefly described but the high proportion of patients successfully treated in the day hospital may reflect the good morale and large numbers of staff (Wilder *et al.*, 1966). Subsequent attempts to replicate this study have generally not been so successful.

Platt *et al.* (1980) found it impossible to perform a randomised controlled trial because clinicians were conservative and insisted that certain groups of patients were 'mandatory' in-patients (e.g. those with psychotic disorders) and certain groups were 'mandatory' day patients (i.e. too well to be considered for in-patient treatment). This research group therefore switched to a design of brief in-patient care followed by day hospital treatment (Hirsch *et al.*, 1979).

Several American studies have satisfactorily compared day hospital treatment with in-patient care but each excluded the majority of patients presenting to the service for admission. Herz *et al.* (1971)

were only able to randomly allocate 22% of all admissions; the remainder were excluded on the grounds that they were too ill for day patient care, refused to enter the study or were regarded as not ill enough to merit consideration for in-patient treatment (Table 15.1). Fenton *et al.* (1979) had a very similar pattern of exclusions and only included 19% of all potential admissions – this, in spite of the fact that their service had an accompanying community programme, with a 24-hour on-call system. Penk *et al.*'s (1978) study was not a random-allocation one, but individually matched day patients with in-patients in terms of age, type and severity of illness and personal resources; they also included 22% of the total patient population. Washburn *et al.* (1976) randomised patients after several weeks of in-patient care – only 15% were successfully randomised as the remainder were mostly considered to be too ill.

It should be noted that although these studies are described as studies of day hospital treatment, some patients did spend a few nights in the in-patient unit. Wilder *et al.* (1966) found it necessary to 'board' 40% of day patients in the in-patient unit for short periods because of risk to that patient or others; this usually occurred during the first two weeks of treatment. Thus 44% of all patients were treated solely in the day hospital, 34% had one night in hospital and a further 22% were treated in the day hospital but with two or more nights in the in-patient unit. Herz *et al.* (1975) similarly boarded 22% of their day patients because of suicidal or violent behaviour. Such boarding lasted between 1 and 27 (mean 13.7) days. By contrast, Dick *et al.* (1985a,b) did not find it necessary to transfer any of their patients to the in-patient unit following allocation to day hospital – presumably they had excluded all patients with any possibility of severe disturbance or suicidal threat. One other study in the United States (Gudeman *et al.* 1983) represented a prospective attempt to treat all patients primarily as day patients; 79% of all patients were admitted for a mean of 10 days to the intensive care unit at the start of treatment, indicating that only 21% were considered suitable for immediate day treatment. In the Manchester, UK, study described below, approximately half the patients spent up to two nights in the in-patient unit prior to randomisation.

Two recent Dutch studies have used the day hospital as the main focus of treatment, although, once again, some patients spent a few nights in the in-patient unit. Kluiter *et al.* (1992) randomly allocated

152 patients at the point of admission to one of three conditions: (1) immediate transfer to the day hospital, (2) transfer after a short time or (3) continued in-patient care. Their measure of feasibility was the average number of nights spent away from the hospital during the whole treatment episode. Twenty per cent of patients in groups (1) and (2) were treated solely in the day hospital (no nights in the in-patient unit). A further 20% spent an average of three or fewer nights in the in-patient unit and were also counted as satisfactory day hospital treatment (i.e. a total of 40% of all admissions were regarded as primarily treated in this way). All of the patients randomised to group (3) spent an average of four or more nights in the in-patient unit. These authors indicated the similarity of their results with those of Zwerling and Wilder (1964).

The study of Schene *et al.* (1993) used an hierarchical selection scheme. Patients were excluded if they required admission to a locked ward or had a diagnosis of organic mental disorder, substance misuse or mental handicap. Patients were also excluded if day hospital treatment was 'contraindicated' (e.g. home too far to travel; required short-term observation in the in-patient unit). Of 534 patients, 63% were admitted to the locked ward because of serious psychosis, suicidal tendencies, mania, aggression. The remaining 37% were admitted directly to the day hospital; a quarter of these patients made use of a visitor's bed for an average of eight nights and 7% had to be transferred at a later date to the locked ward.

The two Dutch studies and the recent Manchester studies concluded, like Wilder and Zwerling, that 33–40% of all potential admissions could be treated primarily in the day hospital.

Manchester studies

Our own research began with an initial descriptive study (Creed *et al.*, 1989a) and, once we had shown that day hospital treatment was feasible for acute illness, we proceeded to a random allocation study, which was aimed at two questions:

- What proportion of all patients admitted to a psychiatric hospital could in fact be treated in a well-staffed day hospital?
- Are the effects of treatment in a day hospital different from that of an in-patient unit?

Study One

The first study was descriptive, comparing admissions of patients to the day hospital with those admitted to the in-patient unit. The new psychiatric service had been started in 1983 with a 50 place new psychiatric day hospital on the main hospital site at the centre of the district, and a small number of beds 7 miles away. This meant that acutely ill patients were admitted directly from the community to the day hospital because of the small number of beds.

During a nine-month period in 1984–85, each new patient admitted to the day hospital and the in-patient unit was assessed both from the point of view of psychiatric symptoms and social rôle performance. The former was assessed using a standardised interview – the 'present state examination' (PSE) – administered by a research psychiatrist. The individual symptoms recorded at this interview are analysed by a computer programme which groups the resulting syndromes under four headings: behaviour, speech and other syndromes (BSO), delusions and hallucinations (DAH), specific neurotic reactions (SNR) and non-specific neurotic syndromes (NSN).

The social assessment was based on interviews between a social research worker and an informant about the patient's performance in such rôles as household management, employment and spouse/parent. In addition, the burden on the relatives was assessed and the informant asked about any unusual or disturbing behaviour displayed by the patient.

The results of the first study indicated that the patients admitted to the day hospital were nearly as ill as those admitted to the in-patient unit, especially when patients admitted compulsorily under a Section of the 1983 Mental Health Act because of their violent or suicidal behaviours were excluded from the in-patient group (Table 15.2). Table 15.2 also indicates that the patients admitted to the day hospital in Manchester were at least as severely ill as those admitted to the in-patient unit in the London study (Knights *et al.*, 1980).

From these results we concluded that the day hospital at the Manchester Royal Infirmary **was** able to admit seriously ill patients, and it was therefore possible to plan a prospective study in which patients could be randomly allocated either to in-patient or day hospital treatment and we could monitor the proportion of all admissions who could be treated in this way.

Table 15.2. *Mean total and subscore PSE scores and SBAS scores for in-patients and day patients of Manchester study (Creed et al., 1989a) with those of London study (Knights et al., 1980) for comparison.*

	London study all patients	Manchester study	
		in-patients	day patients
	(n=77)	(n=69)	(n=41)
Total PSE Score	24.43	30.64	32.10
DAH	2.68	3.66	4.09
BSO	3.23	3.91	3.02
SNR	4.97	8.00	9.22
NSN	13.65	15.07	15.70
SBAS Scores (*Manchester scores adjusted for comparison*)			
Mean Behaviour	8.7	14.50	12.03
Social Performance	11.9	14.41	13.99

PSE: present state examination; SBAS: social behaviour assessment schedule; DAH: delusions and hallucinations; BSO: behaviour, speech and other symptoms; SNR: specific neurotic reaction; NSN: non-specific neurotic.

Study Two

This study was more ambitious than the first as we had to vary routine clinical practice. As a first step, all admissions were screened; patients who were considered too ill, whose admission was a compulsory one, or where the patient or the relatives refused, were not allocated. All the rest were randomly allocated to in-patient or day hospital. Of 173 admissions during the study period, 102 (55%) patients were allocated; 71 were not allocated on the grounds that they were admitted under a Section of the 1983 Mental Health Act (24%), were considered too ill by the responsible consultant (39%) or were not allocated through social, refusal or other reasons (e.g. no accommodation, carer refused to contemplate day care – 37%).

Of the 51 patients allocated to day care, 10 did not attend regularly so could not become established in day hospital treatment, and a further six had to be transferred to the in-patient unit because their illness was severe and did not settle down rapidly in the day hospital (four of the six had mania). Thus 35 of the 51 patients allocated to day care were successfully treated there. If there were 35 patients in each limb of the trial who could be successfully treated in the day hospital this represents 70 (40%) of all patients (173) presenting for admission who could be treated in the day hospital.

The non-allocated patients who were too ill, were more disturbed than the randomly allocated sample; a greater proportion had schizophrenia or mania and they had significantly more psychotic symptoms (speech/behavioural abnormalities, delusions and hallucinations) and more disturbed behaviour at the time of admission. The one-third of patients who were not allocated because of social reasons were similar to the allocated patients in terms of illness severity, indicating that a total of 55% of all admissions could have been treated in the day hospital if there had been the additional means of support to overcome the difficulties with this group of patients (accommodation, community support, etc).

Herz *et al.* (1971) also provided data on those patients who were excluded from their study because they were too ill; they had more previous admissions to hospital, their illnesses were more severe, particularly in terms of disorganisation and they included more patients with organic brain syndromes.

The outcome of day hospital treatment

The difficulties in performing a randomised trial mentioned above (Wilkinson 1984) mean that only a few recent studies have provided reliable results in terms of outcome. The overall picture from the methodically sound studies is that reduction of symptoms and improved social functioning as a result of day treatment is similar to that of in-patient treatment (Schene *et al.* 1993). In the second Manchester study, patients were assessed exactly as they had been in the first study, with the psychiatric symptoms, social rôle, burden and behaviour measured at the time of admission, after three months and after one year.

Reduction of symptoms and improvement in social functioning

Figure 15.1 indicates the reduction of total psychiatric symptom score for patients allocated to the in-patient unit and the day hospital. It shows that at three months and at one year both groups had improved considerably, and there was no significant difference between these two treatments.

Figure 15.2 indicates the change in social role performance. At

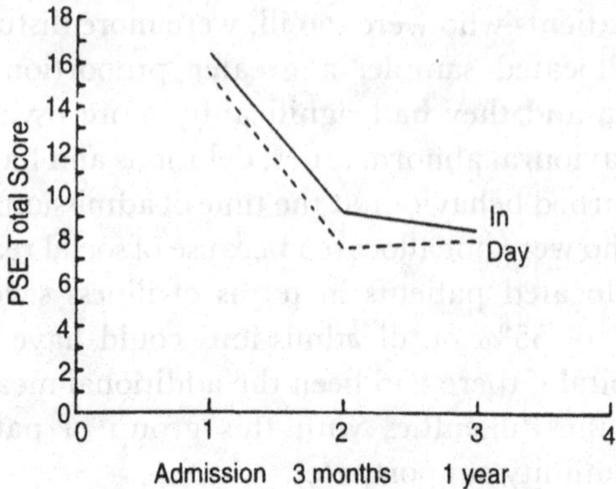

Fig. 15.1. Present state examination (PSE) total score

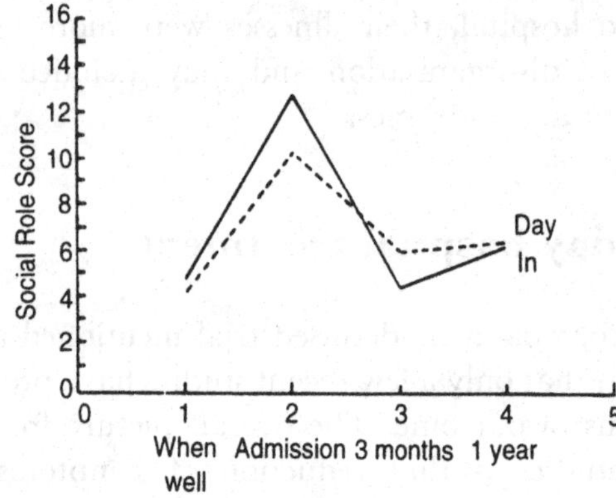

Fig. 15.2. Social role performance

admission, the degree of impairment was not significantly different between day hospital patients and in-patients. During the next three months, both groups improved, but the in-patients showed a greater improvement of social role performance during the first three months of treatment. At the end of one year, however, there was no significant difference between the two groups. Results for burden on relatives and abnormal behaviour observed at home indicated that there was no real difference between in-patient and day hospital treatment at any stage.

Rehospitalisation rate and costs

In line with others studies (Wilder *et al.*, 1966; Fink *et al.*, 1978; Dick *et al.* 1985a,b) the length of stay for the initial admission was significantly longer for the Manchester day hospital patients than for in-patients. However, readmissions during the follow-up year were greater for the in-patients and the total number of days spent in treatment (day or in) was similar (see Creed *et al.*, 1990, for details). Since a day spent in the day hospital is approximately half the cost of an in-patient day (Netten & Smart, 1993; Knapp & Beecham, 1993), this suggests that day treatment is cheaper. However, it is important to note that it is only possible to treat acutely ill patients in a psychiatric day hospital **if there are adequate staff**. This increases the cost and many day hospitals staffed at a minimal level will not be able to treat acute illness (see below). There are other considerations, such as the potential extra burden that acutely ill patients might put on their general practitioner (GP), community psychiatric nurses (CPN) relatives and other carers. These are all included in our current cost-benefit study (Creed *et al.*, 1995). Initial results have indicated that GP visits and burden on carers are not greater for day hospital patients than for in-patients.

Can the findings be generalised?

The Manchester random allocation study was also performed at Blackburn where the day hospital is less well-staffed than at Manchester; it had traditionally been used for rehabilitation purposes and not primarily for direct admissions from the community of acutely ill patients.

The results indicated that (1) the proportion of all admissions who could be randomly allocated was somewhat less (42% as opposed to 55%), and (2) the day hospital only managed to engage those patients who had milder illness – only 16% of all admissions successfully completed a course of day hospital treatment (Creed *et al.*, 1991). Table 15.3 and Fig. 15.3 show the nurses' ratings of disturbed behaviour. For Blackburn, but not Manchester, the day hospital sample shows significantly less disturbance than the in-patients. The conclusion from this study must be that in a less well-staffed day hospital it is not possible to treat acutely disturbed patients. Kluiter et al. (1992) also noted that 'there are no absolute contraindications against day hospital treatment'; they suggested that 'the selection criteria applied in nearly all other controlled studies were unwarranted'. This overstates that case but does indicate that the threshold for

Table 15.3. *Scores on Social Behaviour Rating scale (Wykes & Sturt, 1986) for patients not allocated (primarily because they were regarded as too ill), and for patients successfully allocated to day and in-patient groups. Table shows difference between Manchester and Blackburn with regard to day patients.*

	Score	(median and range)
Manchester		
Non-allocated patients	12	(0–41)
Allocated in-patients	6	(0–25)
Allocated day-patients	7	(0–22)
Blackburn		
Non-allocated patients	11	(0–41)
Allocated in-patients	8	(0–27)
Allocated day patients	2.5	(0–12)*

* significant difference <0.05, for comparison between day patients at Manchester and Blackburn
(From Creed *et al.*, 1991.)

admission to day hospital treatment is not fixed but depends on the nature of the day hospital, and the number and, principally, the attitudes of the staff.

Conclusions from the Manchester studies

The overall conclusions from these studies are (1) that the proportion of all admissions varies between day hospitals and the findings from one cannot be extrapolated to another, (2) that the outcome of treatment in a day hospital is similar to in-patient treatment and (3) there is a suggestion that day hospital treatment will turn out to be cheaper than in-patient care. No studies have yet clearly indicated which patients are best suited to day treatment (Schene *et al.* 1993).

Use of day hospitals for acute psychiatric illness – staff attitudes

Two recent surveys of day hospitals (Schene *et al.*, 1988; Mbaya *et al.*, 1995) have shown that only a minority of patients are admitted as an alternative to in-patient admission – the proportion was as low as 9%

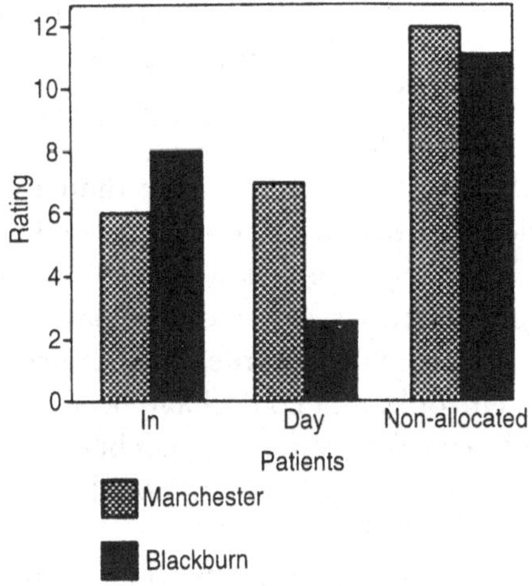

Fig. 15.3. Nurses' ratings of disturbed behaviour

in the Dutch study. Staff attitudes towards suitability are probably particularly important in determining the proportion (Washburn *et al.*, 1976; Platt *et al.*, 1980; Rosie, 1987; Anthony *et al.*, 1991).

Several authors have commented on the attitudes of staff involved in the development of day care for acute illness. Herz *et al.* (1971) noted that the staff were initially antagonistic, later accepting but still preferring in-patient care for seriously ill patients. These authors stated that administrative pressure is necessary to overcome staff resistance. Washburn *et al.* (1976) noted that staff resistance actually prevented random allocation of a proportion of patients. Junior medical staff were especially prone to warn their patients of the problems involved in day care, thereby decreasing the chances that the patient could agree. Platt *et al.* (1980) also recorded this difference between senior and junior medical staff.

Fink *et al.* (1978) specifically identified the bias of the clinicians. Most thought that in-patient care was preferable because it was safer and provided more intensive treatment, and some thought the separation from family was desirable. These authors noted that of 10 clinicians receiving admissions, the three attached to the day hospital admitted 86% of the day hospital patients, so the other seven clinicians must have treated their patients almost exclusively as in-patients.

Both Fink *et al.* (1978) and Hogarty *et al.* (1968) reported that the families of many patients were initially resistant to day care, but later reported more satisfaction from it. Bowman *et al.* (1983) found that family request and patient refusal of day care were important reasons for admitting patients to the in-patient unit rather than the day hospital. Lipius (1973) studied the attitudes of staff and patients; both agreed that two-thirds of in-patient admissions could have been avoided! There was good agreement between staff and patients that most admissions of patients with personality disorders were unnecessary, and that half of those with schizophrenia could have been avoided, but there was disagreement regarding affective psychosis – many more patients than staff felt that these admissions could have been avoided.

Zwerling & Wilder (1964) commented that staff morale must be good to retain psychotic patients through a course of treatment in the day hospital. More importantly is whether staff morale can be maintained over a longer period of time. Our own studies have now been running for nearly 10 years, which suggests that staff can maintain enthusiasm for this type of work.

In our experience, the following are required if acutely ill patients are to be treated in the day hospital.

Staffing level

There must be adequate numbers of staff. The skill mix in our day hospital includes nurses, occupational therapists, psychiatrists and occupational therapists. There must be an adequate total number of staff for a disturbed patient to receive individual attention from one member of staff while groups for the remaining patients continue without disruption. There must be adequate medical staff to provide regular assessments of mental state, side-effects of drugs and perform the necessary intensive treatments, which include, in our own day hospital, ECT. With adequate staff, the day hospital should be able to offer a full range of assessments, including social reports and psychological assessments and treatments.

Treatments

In addition to the above, the day hospital must be on a district general hospital site so that investigations for organic disease are readily available. Consultant opinion or RMO (responsible medical officer) opinion are available. ECT can be administered.

Community support

Acutely ill patients may require additional support at home, overnight accommodation in a hostel and/or help to travel to the day hospital. We have found that a CPN specially attached to the day hospital increased the severity of illness which could be treated there. The CPN can facilitate attendance at the day hospital. A mini bus or taxi can provide transport but if the patient says he or she feels unable to leave their home on a particular day the attendance at the day hospital may cease. In such circumstances, a psychiatric nurse can provide support and encouragement while a patient overcomes his or her fears or difficulties of leaving the home to attend the day hospital. Such fears usually rapidly recede over the first couple of weeks of attendance. In this way, we have found that a CPN can increase the severity of illness treated in this setting.

Staff on call

In addition to the use of a CPN as described above, our CPNs performed an on-call rota so that one was available on the telephone each evening and home visits were possible during daylight hours at the weekend, provided that they were pre-arranged. This meant that a suicidal patient on a Friday evening need not necessarily be admitted to the in-patient unit. He or she could be visited at home on Saturday and Sunday which avoided an in-patient admission and provided the patient with continuity of treatment and support.

Community Day Centres or other continuing care facilities

If the day hospital is used as acute treatment facility, turnover of patients must be rapid. Discharge (usually after two to three months) is facilitated if there are facilities in the community (e.g. day centres, Asian women's centre, art centred rehabilitation facilities, voluntary work organisers). Without such facilities and an energetic policy of discharge, patients can extend their stay in a day hospital for months instead of concentrating on community-based activities that would gradually increase their confidence and which can be continued following discharge. Discharge from the day hospital means the opportunity for another patient to be admitted. Turnover tends to be faster in the in-patient unit, which is where beds may be made available for acutely ill patients. A brisk turnover in the day hospital can lead to specific goals of treatment energetically chased after and the availability of places as needed.

Staff organisation

Each member of staff in the day hospital would normally be a key worker for a number of patients. In addition, two places are kept in reserve for urgent admissions. This policy means that there is always a key worker available for an urgent admission. It is recognised that such patients take additional staff time, which must be catered for.

Role of the day hospital in a community psychiatric service

Only one recent study has examined in any depth the different uses of day hospitals; the study was performed in the Netherlands but the findings can probably be generalised to other countries (Schene *et al.*, 1988). The authors surveyed 85 day hospitals and found that 56% fulfilled the predetermined criteria for one of the four categories (Table 15.4). The categories are: (1) alternative to in-patient units (only 9% of all patients in day hospitals in the Netherlands were admitted for this reason), (2) as a transition from in-patient to out-patient care, (3) as an extension to out-patient care, either for specialised treatment and/or because the condition was becoming chronic and (4) as rehabilitation day care. The most common use was (2), which, if transfer could take place early (Hirsch *et al.*, 1979) is one use of the day hospital as an acute treatment facility. Direct admission to the day hospitals as an alternative to in-patient care was infrequent, as already stated.

Within the range of services offered by a community-orientated district service, the day hospital may reduce length of stay of in-patients. However, this should be seen as making the most use of the potential of day hospital treatment (re-integration into the community, working with family/carers and tackling housing, occupational and relationship problems) not simply as a way of reducing cost of in-patient care. For patients with psychotic disorders in the community, direct admission to the day hospital may be

Table 15.4. *Four different categories of day hospital in the Netherlands (Schene et al., 1988) and their characteristics*

	Alternative to IP	Transition In→day	Expansion of OPD	Rehabilitation
Criterion for classification	20% patients alternative to IP	50% from IP unit	80% from OPD	40% chronic illness/rehab.
Location	In/near IP unit	In/near IP unit	Away from IP unit	In/near IP unit
Orientation	'medical'	'medical'	psycho-therapy	medical/rehab.
Overnight accommodation available	80%	75%	50%	66%
Strict admission criteria?	No	No	Yes	Yes
Treatment period (weeks)	29	28	46	36

IP: in-patient; OPD: out-patient department.

arranged for the early stages of first onset or relapse (before the illness leads to severely disturbed behaviours), for change of medication to Clozapine or for a specific period of rehabilitation. Severe and chronic depressive disorders are well suited to the day hospital, which allows psychotherapeutic, family and other social treatments to be administered (*in vivo*) alongside medication and, if necessary, ECT. Many admissions to the in-patient unit result from short-term crises (e.g. deliberate self-harm); some patients with marked and chronic eating disorders refuse in-patient treatment; other chronic neurotic disorders may lead to dependence if admitted to in-patient units; all are well-suited to day hospital treatment. It must be stressed, however, that there are no definitive admission criteria for the day hospital – the threshold for admission will be determined by other services locally available and the attitude and number of staff in the day hospital. More often there is evidence of underuse of the day hospital. The study of schizophrenic patients one year after discharge (Meltzer *et al.*, 1991) indicated that only 12% attended any form of day care; 55% were psychotic – this raises the possibility that day care for rehabilitation and day hospital treatment for psychotic episodes would both be required. This balance between day hospital and day centre availability on the one hand and day hospital and in-patient treatment on the other will characterise a properly designed comprehensive service.

Conclusion

This review has indicated that day hospital treatment is feasible for acute illness in certain circumstances. One of the primary factors is the number and attitude of staff. There is a large difference between those studies which have only been able to randomly allocate a quarter of all patients to the day hospital compared to those which have successfully allocated one half to three-quarters of patients.

When day hospital treatment is used for acute illness, the social and clinical outcome appears similar. The differences may emerge in cost and patient satisfaction. We are currently researching these. Further intensive studies are needed to understand the different forms of treatments which are actually offered in the day hospital and in-patient unit. We still do not know the effect of the following factors which differentiate day hospital treatment from acute in-patient treatment: remaining in the community and/or remaining in contact with the family; specific programmes aimed at good social adjustment; more involvement of nursing staff in the community; and better compliance with medication after discharge. If these are defined, it will be possible to decide whether the apparently beneficial effects of day care can be included in in-patient programmes, or whether the act of admission itself prevents these. The specific value of 24-hour nursing care needs to be evaluated; it may help because in-patient admission is avoided, or it may allow quite a different form of staff–patient relationship that is helpful in improving social adjustment.

References

Anthony, P., Lancashire, S. & Creed, F. (1991). Side effects of psychiatric treatment: a qualitative study of issues associated with a random allocation research study. *Sociology of Health and Illness*, **13**, 530–44.

Bowman, E. P., Shelley, R. K., Sheehy-Skeffington, A., *et al.* (1983). Day patient versus in-patient: factors determining selection of acutely ill patients for hospital treatment. *British Journal of Psychiatry*, **142**, 584–7.

Creed, F. H., Anthony, P., Godbert, K., Huxley, P. (1989a). Treatment of severe psychiatric illness in a day hospital. *British Journal of Psychiatry*, **154**, 341–7.

Creed, F. H., Black, D. & Anthony, P. (1989b). Day hospital and community treatment for acute psychiatric illness: a critical appraisal. *British Journal of Psychiatry*, **154**, 300–10.

Creed, F. H., Black, D., Anthony, P., *et al.* (1990). Randomised controlled trial comparing day and in-patient psychiatric treatment. *British Medical Journal*, **300**, 1033–7.

Creed, F. H., Black, D., Anthony, P., *et al.* (1991). Randomised controlled trial of day and in-patient psychiatric treatment. 2: Comparison of two hospitals. *British Journal of Psychiatry*, **158**, 183–9.

Creed, F. H., Mbaya, P., Williams, B., Lancashire, S. & Tomenson, B. (1995). *Modified Cost-benefit Comparison of Day and In-patient Psychiatric Treatment*. Final Report to Department of Health.

Department of Health and Social Security (1975). *Better Services for the Mentally Ill*. Comnd 6233. London, HMSO.

Dick, P., Cameron, L., Cohen, D., *et al.* (1985a). Day and full-time psychiatric treatment: a controlled comparison. *British Journal of Psychiatry*, **147**, 246–50.

Dick, P., Ince, A. & Barlow, M. (1985b). Day treatment: suitability and referral procedure. *British Journal of Psychiatry*, **147**, 250–3.

Fenton, F. R., Tessier, L. & Struening, E. L. (1979). A comparative trial of home and hospital psychiatric care. *Archives of General Psychiatry*, **36**, 1073–9.

Fink, E. B., Longabaugh, R. & Stout, R. (1978). The paradoxical underutilization of partial hospitalization. *American Journal of Psychiatry*, **135**, 713–16.

Gudeman, J. E., Shore, M. F. & Dickey, B. (1983). Day hospitalisation and an inn instead of inpatient care for psychiatric patients. *New England Journal of Medicine*, **308**, 749–53.

Herz, M. I., Endicott, J., Spitzer, R. L., *et al.* (1971). Day versus inpatient hospitalisation, a controlled study. *American Journal of Psychiatry*, **127**, 1371–81.

Herz, M. I., Endicott, J., Spitzer, R. L. (1975). Brief hospitalization of patients with families: initial results. *American Journal of Psychiatry*, **132**, 413–17.

Hirsch, S. R., Platt, S., Knights, A. & Weyman, A. (1979). Shortening hospital stay for psychiatric care: effect on patients and their families. *British Medical Journal*, **1**, 442–6.

Hogarty, G. E., Dennis, H., Guy, W., *et al.* (1968). 'Who goes there?' – a critical evaluation of admissions to a psychiatric day hospital. *American Journal of Psychiatry*, **124**, 934–1003.

Kluiter, H., Giel, R., Nienhuis, F., Ruphan, M. & Wiersma, D. (1992). Predicting feasibility of day treatment for unselected patients referred for in-patient psychiatric treatment: results of a randomized trial. *American Journal of Psychiatry*, **149**, 1192–205.

Knapp, M. & Beecham, J. (1993). Reduced list costings: examination of an informed short cut in mental health research. *Health Economics*, **2**, 313–22.
Knights, A., Hirsch, S. R. & Platt, S. D. (1980) Clinical change as a function of brief admission to hospital in a controlled study using the present state examination. *British Journal of Psychiatry*, **137**, 170–80.
Lancet (1985). Day hospital for psychiatric care. *Lancet*, 2, 1106–7.
Lipius, S. H. (1973). Judgements of alternatives to hospitalization. *American Journal of Psychiatry*, **130**, 892–6.
Mbaya, P., Creed, F. H. & Tomenson, B. (1995). Different uses of psychiatric day hospitals. (Unpublished research paper)
McGrath, G. & Tantam, D. (1987). Long-stay patients in a psychiatric day hospital. *British Journal of Psychiatry*, **150**, 836–93.
Meltzer, D., Hale, A. S., Malik, S. J., Hogman, G. A. & Wood, S. (1991). Community care for patients with schizophrenia one year after hospital discharge. *British Medical Journal*, **303**, 1023–6.
Muijen, M., Marks, I., Connolly, J. & Audini, B. (1992). Home-based care and standard hospital care for patients with severe mental illness: a randomised controlled trial. *British Medical Journal*, **304**, 749–54.
Netten, A. & Smart, S. (1993). *Unit Costs of Community care.* Personal Social Services Research Unit, University of Kent.
Penk, W. E., Charles, H. L. & Van Hoose, T. A. (1978). Comparative effectiveness of day hospital and inpatient psychiatric treatment. *Journal of Consulting and Clinical Psychology*, **46**, 94–101.
Platt, S., Knights, A. C. & Hirsch, S. R. (1980). Caution and conservatism in the use of a psychiatric day hospital: evidence from a research project that failed. *Psychiatric Research*, **3**, 123–32.
Pryce, I. G. (1982). An expanding 'Stage Army' of long-stay psychiatric day-patients. *British Journal of Psychiatry*, **141**, 595–601.
Rosie, J. S. (1987). Partial hospitalization: a review of recent literature. *Hospital and Community Psychiatry*, **38**, 1291–9.
Schene, A. H., van Lieshout, P. A. H. & Mastboom, J. C. M. (1988). Different types of partial hospitalization programs: results of a nationwide survey in the Netherlands. *Acta Psychiatrica Scandinavica*, **78**, 515–22.
Schene, A. H., van Wijngaarden, B., Poelijoe, N. W. & Gersons, B. P. R. (1993). The Utrecht comparative study on psychiatric day treatment and inpatient treatment. *Acta Psychiatrica Scandanavica*, **87**, 427–36.
Tyrer, P. & Creed, F. H. (1995). *Community Psychiatry in Action.* Cambridge, Cambridge University Press.
Vaughan, P. J. (1983). The disordered development of day care in psychiatry. *Health Trends*, **15**, 91–4.
Vaughan, P. J. (1985). Developments in psychiatric day care. *British Journal of Psychiatry*, **147**, 1–4.
Washburn, S., Vannicelli, M. & Scheff, B. (1976). Irrational determinants of the place of psychiatric treatment. *Hospital and Community Psychiatry*, **27**, 179–82.
Wilder, J. F., Levin, G. & Zwerling, I. (1966). A two-year follow up evaluation of acute psychotic patients treated in a day hospital. *American*

Journal of Psychiatry, **122**, 1095–101.
Wilkinson, G. (1984). Day care for patients with psychiatric disorders. *British Medical Journal*, **288**, 1710–11.
Wykes, T. & Sturt, E. (1986). The measurement of social behaviour in psychiatric patients: an assessment of the reliability and validity of the SBS schedule. *British Journal of Psychiatry*, **148**, 1–11.
Zwerling, I. & Wilder, J. F. (1964). An evaluation of the applicability of the day hospital in treatment of acutely disturbed patients. *Israel Journal of Psychiatry and Related Disciplines*, **2**, 162–85.

16

Acute in-patient wards

Tom Sensky and Jan Scott

This chapter will outline the general aims of in-patient admission within an emergency mental health service, and consider aspects of the in-patient management of some particular clinical problems or patient groups. Resources required for in-patient units will be reviewed. The chapter ends with a brief description of one innovative model of in-patient care.

Recent decades have seen a dramatic shift in the focus of psychiatric care from mental hospitals to the community. The overall psychiatric in-patient population has dropped markedly, but this is accounted for largely by the rehabilitation and resettlement in the community of long-stay in-patients. The number of psychiatric patients in hospital for less than one year has changed very little. Alternatives to hospitalisation have been developed, including intensive community (Burti and Tansella, chapter 14) or day hospital provision (Creed, chapter 15). While pilot studies have demonstrated that such innovative approaches are viable and may have numerous advantages, there are many practical reasons why they cannot be easily implemented more widely in Britain and in other countries. Similarly, the impetus for the development of community mental health resource centres and crisis intervention teams was to reduce the need for in-patient admissions. For crisis intervention, a recent World Health Organization report (Katschnig, chapter 1) has concluded that, while crisis intervention may reduce the duration of in-patient admissions, its impact on the number of admissions remains unproven. Thus, although modern psychiatric services no longer have the in-patient unit as their main focus, the need for in-patient facilities remains as part of any comprehensive mental health care provision.

Aims of in-patient admission

Every admission should be managed as part of the patient's overall treatment plan. Whenever possible, planning for the patient's care after discharge should begin at the time of admission, or even before. One of the prime objectives should be to minimise the patient's length of stay in hospital.

Each admission should have specific indications and aims. Approximately 8% of admissions in England and Wales are involuntary, and here the indications for admission include those covered by the 1983 Mental Health Act. The patient must be suffering from a mental disorder as defined by the Act. Admission is considered necessary to prevent a deterioration of the patient's health, or in the interests of his or her safety or for the protection of others. There should be no appropriate alternative management available, and the patient must be unwilling or unable to accept voluntary admission. In addition to these obligatory indications, the Code of Practice emphasises the need to consider the context of the patient's assessment and the plan to admit – to attempt to understand the patient's view, and those of family, carers and others involved. In general, similar indications apply to voluntary admissions, except that these are arranged with the patient's informed consent, and often at his or her request.

In practice, common reasons for admission include the need for closer supervision of the patient's medical management (particularly the drug regime), to prevent harm to the patient or others as a result of the patient's disorder, or to respond to handicaps secondary to the disorder such as progressive self-neglect. Implicit in each of these indications is an end-point that can determine when in-patient care is no longer required. Another common indication for admission, particularly for patients with first episodes of major psychiatric disorder, is to observe the patient's behaviour and mental state more intensively than would be possible if the patient remained at home. In some instances, (particularly where the patient has some supports in the community) this aim can be met equally well by admission to a day hospital.

Good clinical practice should require that the patient's admission records state the expected aims of the admission. This is implicit in the treatment plan which should be formulated on admission, either by the multidisciplinary team or by each of the staff contributing to the initial assessment. Like the treatment plan, the aims of admission act as an initial point of reference, and can be updated or revised as the assessment continues.

The decision to admit

There is a considerable literature, particularly from the United States, of factors influencing the decision to admit to hospital patients who present as emergencies (Marson *et al.*, 1988). Most studies demonstrate the importance in decisions to admit of the severity of the patient's psychiatric symptoms, and perceived dangerousness. In some studies, the working diagnosis is important – patients diagnosed as having either a schizophreniform psychosis or mania are more likely to be admitted than others. In some studies, patients with substance misuse as their main diagnosis were also overrepresented among admissions (Oyewumi *et al.*, 1992).

Many conclusions drawn from such studies cannot easily be generalised, for two main reasons. Firstly, much of the earlier research in particular was probably carried out in settings where hospital and community-based psychiatric services were separately developed and the services they offered not co-ordinated. Few of the published studies have described the context of their emergency service. Where account **has** been taken of the resources available, these have influenced the decision to admit (Feigelson *et al*, 1978; Slagg, 1993). The second problem in extrapolating from results in North America is that the results are likely to be different where there exists a well established primary care system, as in Britain and many countries of Europe. In Britain, the majority of referrals for specialist psychiatric management come from general practitioners (GPs) or other doctors (Gater & Goldberg, 1991), but this pattern does not necessarily apply to other countries even where primary care is available (Gater *et al.*, 1991).

Despite such reservations, some of the conclusions from this work on decision-making in psychiatric emergencies warrants further consideration. For example, the influence of social support appears complex. While the decision to admit is commonly associated with poor social supports, this has not been a universal finding. In one study of four emergency services in a single Canadian city, those with good social supports were almost twice as likely to be admitted as those without (Oyewumi *et al.*, 1992). This apparently paradoxical result can be attributed to the possible impact of advocacy. Where patients present for help with family or friends, the latter can assist the assessment by providing further details of the patient's current difficulties, and also press for admission. If assertive advocacy does influence decisions to admit, this has important implications for training. Another finding that has similar implications is the observation that admission rates vary even when the services available are similar. Feigelson and colleagues (1978) demonstrated that admission rates were lower where the emergency assessments were carried out by more experienced psychiatrists.

Special clinical considerations

Suicidal intent

Where suicidal intent or behaviour occurs in the context of a clear depressive or schizophrenic disorder, the decision to admit is often straightforward. With depression in particular, the expectation is to reduce the risk of suicide by effective management of the affective disorder. However, in the absence of any evidence of a formal psychiatric diagnosis, it is always important to question whether in-patient admission is in the best interests of the patient and others who might be involved. In such instances, the need to have clear aims for the admission is especially important. Is it likely that the factors considered to give rise to the threat of suicide will be altered in any way by admission? Such decisions are particularly difficult when the patient is intoxicated at presentation. Under some circumstances, admission might even prove damaging to the patient's future care (see below).

Violence

The patient's potential dangerousness must be part of every emergency assessment. This is sometimes extremely difficult to assess accurately when the patient first presents. For example, the presence of police who assisted in bringing a patient to the casualty department (accident and emergency department in the UK; emergency room in the United States) can help to contain the patient and in some instances assist in making the patient feel safe, while in other instances the same circumstances can exacerbate the patient's violent behaviour. Because of such difficulties, it should be good practice to expect to admit all patients to the same admission ward for a preliminary assessment period (lasting some hours at least), unless there are clear indications that the patient's potential violence is unlikely to be contained without substantial risk to the patient or others (including other patients and staff). Moving all patients who **might** be violent to distant locked facilities may be unnecessary, disrupts the continuity of care, and also carries the risk of deskilling the admission ward staff in their management of violence. Intensive care facilities of some form should be provided in local in-patient units, but this carries resource implications (see below).

Among in-patients, as in the community, the prediction of violence remains difficult and imprecise, even allowing for systematic errors by clinicians (Monahan, 1981). Among patient factors related to violence, the best predictor is a past history of violence (McNiel *et al.*, 1988). The combination at admission of aggressive behaviour and the absence of anxiety can also be a useful predictor of later violence (Blomhoff *et al.*, 1990). A diagnosis of schizophrenia, and/or the presence of active hallucinations or delusions, are common among those patients involved in volent incidents (Noble & Rodger, 1989). However, these factors are not particularly helpful as predictors, because they apply equally to in-patients not involved in aggressive behaviour (James *et al.*, 1990). Similarly, other factors have been described which correlate with violence in some studies but not others. These include male gender and ethnic group. The ward setting is also important. There is clear evidence that patient violence escalates in situations of high staff turnover and increased reliance on a temporary workforce (James *et al.*, 1990). In this study, changes in staffing patterns accounted for 39% of the variance in violence. In a recent study, higher levels of violence against other people were found on an acute admission ward than an intensive care ward (Kho *et al.*, 1995). One explanation for this apparently paradoxical finding is that patients were accommodated in dormitories in the acute ward, but had their own rooms in the intensive care unit, and therefore had somewhere to withdraw to when tensions rose.

Offenders who might be suffering from mental disorder

In England and Wales, Section 136 of the 1983 Mental Health Act empowers a police constable to take to a **place of safety** a person in a public place whom the policeman suspects may be suffering from a mental illness, and in need of immediate care or control in the interests of the person or of others. In most instances, the preferred place of safety is a hospital. The aim of this provision is to allow prompt specialist mental health assessment of people who **may** be mentally ill. A proportion of those brought for assessment under Section 136 will have committed offences. In most localities, the police will have received little if any training in the nature or recognition of mental disorders. Early research demonstrated that despite this, a higher proportion than expected by chance of people brought to hospital under Section 136 were likely to remain in-patients following full mental health assessment. Similar findings have been reported from the United States (McNiel *et al.*, 1991). However, particular problems arise with people who show equivocal evidence of mental illness but might be very disturbed and require some form of restraint before assessment can be completed. Especially in such cases, effective liaison is essential between local police, psychiatric and social services. The use of Section 136 appears to depend on local relationships between these services (Szmuckler, 1981).

Special provision needs to be made for the rapid assessment and in-patient admission, when indicated, of people with mental disorder who appear before the courts. If an offender is remanded in custody, there may be considerable delays in arranging a psychiatric assessment, during which time the person may not receive adequate psychiatric care. In response to such problems, court diversion schemes have been recommended (Department of Health and Home Office, 1992) and developed (Blumenthal & Wessely, 1992; Joseph & Potter, 1993a,b), which allow for the rapid assessment of offenders before their initial court appearance, often by having psychiatrists or specially trained psychiatric nurses regularly available to assess people at the court. However, such schemes depend heavily on the assessing service having ready access to in-patient facilities with a range of security provisions, including local intensive care units with high staff–patient ratios (see below). Because the demand for such beds is variable, but when required, access often needs to be immediate, occupancy rates have to be relatively low for such facilities to continue to function effectively. At the same time, high staffing ratios also contribute to make such resources expensive relative to standard in-patient facilities.

Involuntary treatment

The grounds for involuntary commitment, and the legal and clinical processes involved, vary considerably among European countries (Segal, 1989; Whitney *et al.*, 1994), as they do among the states of the United States. In the United States, there is often the option of out-patient commitment for those patients unwilling to accept treatment voluntarily but not otherwise in need of in-patient admission (Task Force on Involuntary Outpatient Commitment, 1987). In the UK, this option does not formally exist, although there is evidence that such a facility could reduce in-patient admission rates and have other benefits for patients (Sensky *et al.*, 1991). In England and Wales, patients who require compulsory treatment can only receive this as in-patients and must, according to the law, be **liable to detention** in hospital, that is, their psychiatric disorder and mental state must warrant hospitalisation. A new **supervised discharge** provision has been proposed, to allow recall into hospital of patients previously subject to compulsory in-patient treatment. It remains to be seen how effective this provision will be.

Alcohol and substance misuse

Patients who present having taken alcohol or illicit drugs may be extremely difficult to assess accurately. Policies and procedures must be developed, based on resources available locally, for the management of such patients. Some hospitals have an informal policy of turning drunk patients away or insisting that they should be sober before they can be assessed. For such patients, there is a considerable advantage in having access to a brief admission ward or holding area attached to the casualty department.

Those who abuse alcohol or drugs are particularly prone to physical illness, which may be missed in casualty because of the way the patient presents. They must always have a thorough physical examination. Where this reveals abnormalities, the psychiatrist may have a vital role to play advocating the patient's needs to his physician colleagues, with whom a joint management plan should be agreed.

Patients who are physically ill

Patients who present with acute organic brain syndromes are especially difficult to manage on conventional psychiatric wards. Facilities are often inadequate for regular physical monitoring and for simple procedures like continuous intravenous infusion. Many psychiatric units are not designed to allow patients to be nursed in bed. On the other hand, patients who show disturbed behaviour may be difficult to manage in non-psychiatric settings. Similar considerations apply to patients who require admission after drug overdose. These problems are even worse where the psychiatric and medical wards are apart on separate sites. Then, providing a rapid and flexible response to the patient's changing needs can be particularly difficult.

A simple response to the admission of those with physical illness is to operate a policy whereby a patient will be admitted to the psychiatric unit only if considered **physically** fit for discharge. However, such a policy is not always practicable. Some suggest that such patients are best served by units with combined psychiatric and medical facilities (Hoffman, 1984), although others disagree (Fogel *et al.*, 1985). In the absence of such specialist resources, it is usually more feasible to provide psychiatric care for an in-patient in a medical unit than to provide adequate medical care in a psychiatric ward. It has even been suggested that all acute psychiatric emergencies can be effectively managed in medical admission wards (Reding & Maguire, 1973).

Ethnic minorities

A greater than expected compulsory admission rate among Afro-Caribbeans in Britain has been a consistent finding (Owens *et al.*, 1991). Amongst other ethnic groups, notably people originating from the Indian subcontinent, admission rates have been less consistent. Such inconsistencies are probably not attributable to differences in methodology between studies, but rather underline the complex effects of culture and ethnicity on the presentation of psychiatric disorder, on help-seeking and on acceptance of psychiatric care. Despite having similar ancestors, and possibly even the same mother tongue, a Sikh who comes to Britain from India for an arranged marriage may have little in common with another forced to leave East Africa as a refugee. An analysis of Mental Health Act admissions to one psychiatric unit in West London revealed an overall excess of Indian men, but closer scrutiny of these data revealed that the excess was accounted for by those who had migrated from East Africa; compulsory admission rates among immigrants from India were similar to those of matched UK-born patients.

With different cultural groups, it is particularly important to examine in-patient admission and treatment in the context of the overall psychiatric service. It is clear that the customary pathways to psychiatric care differ between cultural groups (Gater *et al.*, 1991). Bhui *et al.* (1993) reported that Asian patients reached one particular psychiatric service more often than expected via the casualty department or domiciliary visits, and relatively infrequently through their GPs, despite having an Asian GP in many instances.

Each psychiatric service clearly needs to learn from the local community which it aims to serve how best to meet the needs of its diverse ethnic and cultural groups. In doing so, the service is likely to become more receptive and responsive to the individual needs of all its patients. Particular barriers to adequate assessment for in-patient admission include language difficulties and other communication problems, and different idiomatic expressions of distress. Relatives sometimes face a conflict of interests when they are the only available translators while at the same time having their own needs, and often wishing to act as the patient's advocate. Once admitted, problems can arise explaining to the patient what he or she can expect to happen. The use of information sheets in different languages offers only a partial solution to this, because (particularly for older Asian people) patients who cannot speak English often cannot read in their mother tongue. It is probably uncommon for staff of in-patient units to be given specific guidance on the cultural practices of the minorities admitted to their unit, such as specific aspects of diet or worship.

Resources

Any discussion about in-patient facilities must clearly address the estimation of bed requirements, the nature of the in-patient environment, its specific and non-specific benefits and staffing issues.

Changing patterns of service delivery are affecting all these areas. In addition, few publications offer guidance on optimal staffing levels and multidisciplinary mix, and there is a need for more systematic evaluations in this area in the future.

In-patient beds

The level of in-patient resources provided for a given population has often been determined in a pragmatic way (from historic patterns of care in that area, or from the consequences of hospital closures) rather than through systematic planning. In recent years, the desire to develop a more coherent strategy has lead to an increased emphasis on two approaches (Thornicroft, 1991). The **top-down** model uses normative data, for example. The **bottom-up** model makes use, for example, of local survey data or individual needs assessment information. The combination of these two approaches allows more accurate planning, provided that other local resource and policy factors are also taken into account, such as alternative service provision, local policy on resettlement, social support networks and health beliefs of the community.

Estimates of bed requirements are summarised in Table 16.1. The median bed requirement for acute adult admissions has been estimated as 0.43 beds per 1000 population (Hirsch, 1988). In 1990, the mean number of acute beds was 0.54 per 1000 population (see Table 16.2), with considerable local variation (0.38 in Oxford; 0.76 in Mersey) (Wing, 1995). There is a 50% greater provision in Scotland, but available beds in Britain as a whole are generally lower than in other parts of Europe (Hirsch, 1988). Goldberg (1990) argues that the occupancy rate for such beds should be about 85%. Higher levels of short lengths of stay combined with high readmission rates may indicate insufficient bed provision to run the service effectively.

A number of sociodemographic factors correlate highly with bed usage and may therefore influence admission rates. The Jarman underprivileged area score (the most commonly quoted deprivation index in the UK) shows a significant positive association (correlation coefficient [r] = 0.6–0.8) with psychiatric admission rates (Jarman *et al.*, 1992). However, the Jarman index only explains 34% of the variation in admission rates between districts standardised for age, gender and marital status. Goldberg (1990) reported that three variables showed a strong (but not causal) association with admission

Table 16.1. *Estimated requirements for adult in-patients beds in England (per 250,000 population)*

Type	Number
Acute adult beds	108
New long stay beds	70
Special care beds	5–10
Secure unit beds	1–10

Table 16.2. *Mean adult in-patients beds in England (per 250,000 population)*

Type	Number
Acute	135
New long stay (1–5 yrs)	93
Old long stay (>5 yrs)	70
Total	298

(From Wing, 1995.)

rates (r=0.87). These were the percentage of illegitimate births, number of first notifications for drug dependency and the standardised mortality ratio for the area in question. Other factors which may be associated with admission rates in a given community include greater mobility of the population (r=0.73), greater ethnic minority representation (r=0.67) and poorer quality of the housing stock (r=0.84) (Thornicroft, 1991). Kammerling and O'Connor (1993) reported that the most powerful single indicator of serious mental illness that would need hospitalisation was the unemployment rate in people aged under 65 years. This factor explained 93% of the variance in admission rates (for the whole population, not just unemployed people). It was also demonstrated that there was a seven-fold difference in admission rates across the catchment areas investigated with a significant negative correlation between average length of stay and readmission rates (r= −0.64).

Individuals requiring in-patient treatment represent the tip of the psychiatric morbidity pyramid. In Britain, only about four admissions will occur for every 250 psychiatric 'cases' in the community (Goldberg, 1990). However, in-patient funding dominates the cost structure and the money spent on providing such hospital care in

England in 1987 (£1,200 million) represented 84% of the gross revenue expenditure on mental health (Office of Health Economics, 1989). As the number of in-patients continues to fall, the **per capita** cost of admissions is rising. This creates significant problems as, without bridging funds, it means that only limited monies have been available in many areas for the development of community-based service initiatives as alternatives to in-patient admission (Office of Health Economics, 1989).

In-patient environment and staffing

A further effect of the changing patterns of admissions is that in-patient units are increasingly faced with looking after the most severely disabled individuals who are often potentially dangerous to themselves or others. This creates a further tension within the system as the need to transfer monies and resources to the community where the majority (about 80%) of severely mentally ill people are treated has to be balanced against the need to provide adequate staffing levels to cope with the individuals most disturbed by their illness who have been admitted to hospital, and to ensure their safety and that of staff. Partly as a consequence of the changing nature of the in-patient environment, there has been a move away from mixed-gender acute psychiatric wards (as provided in other medical settings). Increasing fears for the safety of female patients who have reported physical and sexual harassment have led to public campaigns supporting moves to re-introduce single gender in-patient wards, or to develop smaller admission units (such as the nine-bedded 'Grange', described further below), which provide a more domestic 'normalising' environment and have single bedrooms. Preliminary reports suggest that such units may reduce the frequency of problems of harrassment, and avert the need to separate male and female in-patients (Scott *et al.*, 1992).

Other factors may influence the nature and safety of the in-patient environment. Staffing levels, staff training and experience must be adequate. The largest professional subgroup within mental health services is nursing (80,000 nurses were employed in such services in Britain in 1987). Unfortunately, the morale of this group of staff has suffered because the prestige of in-patient facilities has fallen whilst the nature of the work has become more demanding. This has resulted in greater staff turnover, often with the most skilled staff moving on. This adversely affects the in-patient environment, for example with regard to violent incidents, as already noted.

Estimates of required staffing levels and skills mix have been approximate at best. In the 1970s, Britain used the 'Aberdeen' and then the 'Cumbria' formulae. These approaches shared the characteristic that the nursing staff to patient ratio (and the ratio of qualified to unqualified staff) should be calculated from the dependency level. The latter was a function of the level of need of the patients admitted, and the rate of turnover (admissions and discharges) within the unit. Staff frequently suggested that these minimum levels meant that they operated merely as custodians (ensuring safety) rather than as therapists to the in-patients and that this may adversely affect outcome and discharge rates (Hargreaves & Shumway, 1990), but few more sophisticated methods have been documented. Indeed, in recent years, **local** policies on staffing have been the strongest determinant of nursing numbers.

Most in-patient units appear to operate what Maxmen *et al.* (1974) described as the **reactive environment** treatment model, in which the staff attempt to respond to the individual needs of each patient (Wright & Davis, 1993). Acute units that follow a specific theoretical or therapeutic model appear to be the exception rather than the rule. Most practise a pragmatic, broad based approach to therapy which Moline (1976) termed **rational eclecticism**. Such units show considerable variations in post-discharge outcome, as do those run according to the reactive environment model. However, predictors of good outcome may be identifiable (Hargreaves & Shumway, 1990). In a study of 191 treatment and environment factors that may predict post-discharge functioning in 22,000 in-patients (Ellsworth *et al.*, 1979; Collins *et al.*, 1985), a number of characteristics were shared by effective programmes even when patient and staff variables were taken into account. Patients who demonstrated the best post-discharge adjustment tended be treated in settings that had stable staffing, discouraged social isolation, had high levels of staff–patient interaction and used optimal medication. Multidisciplinary treatment programmes with clear roles and aims (including discharge plans) were also likely to improve outcome at follow-up (Hargreaves & Shumway, 1990). Interestingly, the most effective units also provided care for people with both acute and chronic disorders rather than targeting narrowly defined subgroups.

The future role of admission facilities in community services: one model

The recent shift towards home treatment for individuals suffering from mental illness has polarised the views of many of those involved in developing services (users, carers, purchasers and providers) who have tended to see the service options as **either** hospital **or** community. This is unfortunate as a truly integrated and effective service does not avoid the use of beds, but rather identifies the appropriate place of admission within the spectrum of services provided. This will be highlighted by describing a community-based mental health service to a deprived part of the Northeast of England.

The service was begun in 1988 and is now provided to 50,000 people in North Tyneside (ranking 58th out of 198 on the Jarman indices) extending from deprived inner city wards to more rural ex-mining communities. The area comprises predominantly social housing (80%), has a 20% male unemployment rate, but has a low ethnic minority population (1%). At the present time the mental health team comprises a senior lecturer and consultant psychiatrist, 0.5 senior psychiatric trainee, 3.5 community psychiatric nurses (CPNs), 2 occupational therapists (OTs), one junior doctor, a social worker (SW) dedicated to the team and administrative support. The admission unit is based in the community and has an establishment of 12.5 nurses for the 9 in-patient beds and the partial hospitalisation programme (Scott *et al.*, 1992).

The service has drawn on the Madison model (Stein & Test, 1980) and primarily aims to prove an assertive outreach programme for those with long-term and severe difficulties, with a secondary goal of providing a home-based early intervention service for new referrals (with early return to the primary care team when possible). The early intervention service aims to see emergency referrals within 24 hours, urgent referrals within 72 hours and routine referrals within 7 days. These targets are met for 75% of cases overall, but for all emergency and 90% of urgent referrals (Scott *et al.*, 1993). The co-existence of the assertive outreach programme and the early intervention service appears to allow the service to run safely with relatively low bed numbers provided in a 'domestic' environment. Eighty percent of the patients are treated at home. The community and in-patient staff are well integrated, and in-patient staff may also become involved in providing assertive outreach if they are seen as the most appropriate case manager for a given individual. All staff have admission rights to the unit but referring agencies do not. They may request assessment but the mental health team operate as gatekeepers to the unit.

The service currently receives between 430 and 520 referrals per year. A recent audit demonstrated that 66% of clients had psychotic or affective disorders, that those with the lowest global levels of functioning were receiving the most intensive input and that 80% of the CPN and 90% of the medical case load comprised the treatment of those individuals with long-term and severe disorders (Spear *et al.*, 1995). Thirty percent of newly referred patients have enduring forms of mental illness and are still in regular contact with the service one year after referral (Scott *et al.*, 1993). Over the course of a year, the in-patient unit treated 76 patients in the full and/or partial hospitalisation programmes (Scott, 1995).

For the full hospitalisation programme, the beds in this unit are used for three key purposes: to treat those in severe acute crisis, to provide an alternative setting when family or social networks are unable to cope and to offer 'asylum' to those in need of brief respite. The beds are less often used for assessment purposes alone as most of the individuals requiring this approach are managed in the partial hospitalisation programme. The latter is run from the in-patient facility and has three main aims (similar to those described by Klar *et al.*, 1982). Firstly, it allows intensive treatment of those in acute crisis who require flexible access to input but who refuse hospitalisation and cannot be admitted involuntarily. Secondly, it offers flexible and accessible aftercare (choice of seven days per week and variable hours of the day) by known staff for those recovering from an acute illness episode. Thirdly, it provides long-term psychosocial support for those with enduring illnesses who benefit from open access to staff who are known to them and willing to listen. The unit staff also offer telephone support to individuals known to them who make contact in crisis.

A breakdown of the recent use of the service over a 12-month period demonstrated that 31 new patients received a combination of full and partial hospitalisation whilst 18 received partial hospitalisation as an alternative to admission. Sixteen long-term service users regularly attended the partial hospitalisation programme without recourse to admission, and a further 11 long-term users attending the partial hospitalisation programme required at least one admission over the course of the year. The median costs of the full and partial hospitalisation programme showed that the use of partial as opposed to full hospitalisation reduced treatment costs for new referrals by 37%. Compared to a traditional district general hospital psychiatric unit service run in a catchment area of similar size and demography, the model of brief admission with intensive aftercare and partial hospitalisation saved an average of 400 patient bed-days per annum (Scott *et al.*, 1995). This confirms previous reports that brief admissions with intensive aftercare has clinical and cost-benefits for service users (for a review see Hargreaves & Shumway, 1990).

For many of the long-term service users, the previous model of treatment had comprised in-patient treatment and community follow-up with admission to the special care facility at the mental hospital at times of great distress. The new model of treatment (combining partial hospitalisation with intermittent brief admissions) did not have any detrimental effect on observer- or self-rated levels of functioning, but the median cost of treatment per patient per annum dropped by about 25% (range 13–61%) from £10,700 to £7900. In addition, patient and carer satisfaction ratings demonstrated that this approach was acceptable (Scott *et al.*, 1995). A further advantage of the partial hospitalisation service is that patients can establish relationships with the staff who care for them during their admissions. Although it may be argued that day hospitals can provide an equivalent service, the literature from the United States highlights that successful partial hospitalisation programmes benefit from geographic and philosophical proximity to the admission unit (Pang, 1985). The transitions between community, partial and full hospitalisation status may not always be as easily achieved by service users if they have to overcome additional inter-unit boundaries between different staff teams working in different settings (Hoge *et al.*, 1992). The model described represents a seam-free service where the treatment programme is tailored to the individual and they move easily across all components with little opportunity to fall through any 'gaps'.

As well as gains for service users, the above integrated model appears to have many benefits to mental health professionals working at the admission facility. Through the partial hospitalisation programme, staff get the opportunity to see a spectrum of disorders rather than dealing only with a narrow range of cases. The opportunity to extend their role into the community as case managers for a small number of patients on the assertive outreach programme also improves morale and provides variety in day to day working patterns.

Conclusions

Acute in-patient facilities have multiple functions. There is a need for continued access to beds for a significant minority of patients with severe mental illness. Particularly with the development of new service models, it is important to monitor and evaluate the quality and nature of in-patient provision for each service, and to ensure that the service can adequately manage those patients with special needs. There is a need to shift resources more rapidly to settings where the majority of service users are treated. However services develop, it is vital that the staff feel valued, that the units remain an integral part of the service, and that flexibility of functioning is preserved. This applies particularly to the use of brief admissions, with carefully planned discharges and intensive follow-up (to try to avert the 'revolving door' syndrome). By reducing the need for, or length of, some admissions, partial hospitalisation has potential benefits for service users and the service itself, and should be considered as one component of a comprehensive management programme for those with severe mental illness. However, we should also remember, as Tantam (1985) has commented, that in many instances 'it is not hospitalisation that is bad, but traditional aftercare that could be improved.'

References

Bhui, K., Strathdee, G. & Sufraz, R. (1993). Asian inpatients in a district psychiatric unit: an examination of presenting features and routes into care. *International Journal of Social Psychiatry*, **39**, 208–20.

Blomhoff, S., Seim, S. & Friis, S. (1990). Can prediction of violence among psychiatric inpatients be improved? *Hospital and Community Psychiatry*, **41**, 771–852.

Blumenthal, S. & Wessely, S. (1992). National survey of current arrangements for diversion from custody in England and Wales. *British Medical Journal*, **305**, 1322–5.

Collins, J., Ellsworth, R., Casey, N., Hyer, L., Hickey, R., Schoonover, R., Twemlow, S. & Nesselroade, J. (1985). Treatment characteristics of psychiatric programs that correlate with patient community adjustment. *Journal of Clinical Psychology*, **41**, 299–308.

Department of Health and Home Office (1992). *Review of Health and Social Services for Mentally Disordered Offenders and Others Requiring Similar Services (the Reed Report)*. London, HMSO.

Ellsworth, R., Collins, J., Casey, N., Schoonover, R., Hickey, R., Hyer, L., Twemlow, S. & Nesselroade, J. (1979). Some characteristics of effective psychiatric treatment programs. *Journal of Consulting and Clinical Psychology*, **47**, 799–817.

Feigelson, E. B., Davis, E. B., Mackinnon, R., Shands, H. C. & Schwartz, C. C. (1978). The decision to hospitalize. *American Journal of Psychiatry*, **135**, 354–7.

Fogel, B. S., Stroudemire, A. & Houpt, J. L. (1985). Contrasting models of combined medical and psychiatric inpatient treatment. *American Journal of Psychiatry*, **142**, 1085–9.

Gater, R., De Almedia e Souza, B., Barrientos, G., Caraveo, J., Chandrashekar, C. R., Dhadphale, M., Goldberg, D., Al Kathiri, A. H., Mubbashar, M., Silhan, K., Thong, D., Torres-Gonzales, F. & Sartorius, N. (1991). The pathways to psychiatric care: a cross-cultural study. *Psychological Medicine*, **21**, 761–74.

Gater, R. & Goldberg, D. (1991). Pathways to psychiatric care in South Manchester. *British Journal of Psychiatry*, **159**, 90–5.

Goldberg, D. (1990). Filters to care: a model. In *Indicators for Mental Health in the Population*, ed. R. Jenkins & S. Griffiths, London, HMSO.

Hargreaves, W. & Shumway, M. (1990). Effectiveness of mental health services for the severely mentally ill. In *New Directions for Mental Health Services*, ed. C. Taube, D. Mechanic & A. Hohmann, pp. 253–84. London, Hemisphere Publishing.

Hirsch, S. (1988). *Psychiatric Beds and Resources: Factors Influencing Bed Usage and Service Planning*. London, Gaskell.

Hoge, M. A., Davidson, L., Hill, W. L., Turner, V. E. & Ameli, R. (1992). The promise of partial hospitalisation: a reassessment. *Hospital and Community Psychiatry*, **43**, 345–54.

Hoffman, R. S. (1984). Operation of a medical-psychiatric unit in a general hospital setting. *General Hospital Psychiatry*, **6**, 93–9.

James, D., Fineberg, N., Shah, A. & Priest, R. (1990). An increase in violence on an acute psychiatric ward: a study of associated factors. *British Journal of Psychiatry*, **156**, 846–52.

Jarman, B., Hirsch, S., White, P. & Driscoll, R. (1992). Predicting psychiatric admission rates. *British Medical Journal*, **304**, 1146–52.

Joseph, P. L. & Potter, M. (1993a). Diversion from custody. I: Psychiatric assessment at the magistrates' court. *British Journal of Psychiatry*, **162**, 325–30.

Joseph, P. L. & Potter, M. (1993b). Diversion from custody. II: Effect on hospital and prison resources. *British Journal of Psychiatry*, **162**, 330–4.

Kammerling, R. & O'Connor, S. (1993). Unemployment rate as a predictor of rate of psychiatric admission. *British Medical Journal*, **307**,

1536–9.
Kho, K., Corcos, C., Mortimer, A. & Sensky, T. (1995). A prospective investigation of factors associated with incidents of aggression on psychiatric inpatient wards. (In press.)
Klar, H., Frances, A. & Clarkin, J. (1982). Selection criteria for partial hospitalisation. *Hospital and Community Psychiatry*, **33**, 929–33.
Marson, D. C., McGovern, M. P. & Pomp, H. C. (1988). Psychiatric decision making in the emergency room: a research overview. *American Journal of Psychiatry*, **145**, 918–25.
Maxmen, J., Tucker, G. & LeBow, M. (1974). *Rational Hospital Psychiatry*. New York, Brunner Mazel.
McNiel, D. E., Binder, R. L. & Greenfield, T. K. (1988). Predictors of violence in civilly committed acute psychiatric patients. *American Journal of Psychiatry*, **145**, 965–70.
McNiel, D. E., Hatcher, C., Zeiner, H., Wolfe, H. L. & Myers, R. S. (1991). Characteristics of persons referred by police to the psychiatric emergency room. *Hospital and Community Psychiatry*, **42**, 425–7.
Moline, R. (1976). Hospital psychiatry in transition: from therapeutic community to rational eclecticism. *Archives of General Psychiatry*, **33**, 1234–8.
Monahan, J. (1981). *Predicting Violent Behaviour: An Assessment of Clinical Techniques*. Beverley Hills, Sage.
Noble, P. & Rodger, S. (1989). Violence by psychiatric inpatients. *British Journal of Psychiatry*, **155**, 384–90.
Office of Health Economics (1989). *Mental Health in the 1990s: From Custody to Care*. London, OHE.
Owens, D., Harrison, G. & Boot, D. (1991). Ethnic factors in voluntary and compulsory admissions. *Psychological Medicine*, **21**, 185–96.
Oyewumi, L. K., Odejide, O. & Kazartian, S. S. (1992). Psychiatric emergency services in a Canadian city: II. Clinical characteristics and patients' disposition. *Canadian Journal of Psychiatry*, **37**, 96–9.
Pang, J. (1985). Partial hospitalisation: an alternative to inpatient care. *Psychiatric Clinics of North America*, **8**, 587–95.
Reding, G. R. & Maguire, B. (1973). Nonsegregated acute psychiatric admissions to general hospitals – continuity of care within the community hospital. *New England Journal of Medicine*, **289**, 185–9.
Scott, J. (1995). A 12-month evaluation of a partial hospitalisation programme. *International Journal of Mental Health*. (In press.)
Scott, J., McCluskey, S. & Smith, L. (1993). Three months in the life of a community mental health team. *Psychiatric Bulletin*, **18**, 615–17.
Scott, J., Normanton, M. & McKenna, J. (1992). Developing a community-orientated mental health service. *Psychiatric Bulletin*, **16**, 150–2.
Scott, J., Spear, J. & Joseph, S. (1995). A comparison of the equity, efficacy and effectiveness of community-based and hospital-based mental health services. (In press.)
Segal, S. P. (1989). Civil commitment standards and patient mix in

England/Wales, Italy and the United States. *American Journal of Psychiatry*, **146**, 187–93.

Sensky, T., Hughes, T. & Hirsch, S. (1991). Compulsory psychiatric treatment in the community: I. A controlled study of treatment with 'extended leave under the Mental Health Act: special characteristics of patients and impact of treatment. *British Journal of Psychiatry*, **158**, 792–9.

Slagg, N. B. (1993). Characteristics of emergency room patients that predict hospitalization or disposition to alternative treatments. *Hospital and Community Psychiatry*, **44**, 252–6.

Spear, J., Cole, A. & Scott, J. (1995). A cross-sectional evaluation of a community-orientated mental health service. *Psychiatric Bulletin*, **19**, 151–4.

Stein, L. & Test, M. (1980). Alternatives to mental hospital treatment: conceptual model, treatment program and clinical evaluation. *Archives of General Psychiatry*, **37**, 392–7.

Szmuckler, G. I. (1981). Compulsory admissions in a London borough: II. Circumstances surrounding admission: service implications. *Psychological Medicine*, **11**, 825–38.

Tantam, D. (1985). Annotation: alternatives to psychiatric hospitalisation. *British Journal of Psychiatry*, **146**, 1–4.

Task Force on Involuntary Outpatient Commitment (1987). *Involuntary Commitment to Outpatient Treatment.* Washington DC, American Psychiatric Association.

Thornicroft, G. (1991). *Mental health: the changing pattern of treatment and care.* South East Thames Regional Health Authority Seminar Report.

Whitney, L., Ruiz, P. & Langenbach, M. (1994). Detaining psychiatric patients: a European perspective. In *Psychiatry in Europe: Directions and Developments*, ed. T. Sensky, C. Katona, & S. Montgomery, pp. 137–42. London, Gaskell Press.

Wing, J. K. (1995). *Epidemiologically-Based Mental Health Needs Assessments.* London, HMSO. (In press.)

Wright, J. & Davis, M. (1993). Hospital psychiatry. In *Cognitive Therapy with Inpatients*, ed. J. Wright, M. Thase, A. T. Beck & J. Ludgate, pp. 35–60. New York, Guilford Press.

17

The future of mental health emergency services

MICHAEL PHELAN, GERALDINE STRATHDEE AND GRAHAM THORNICROFT

The contributors to this book have provided us with a wide overview of the current development of mental health emergency services in the 1990s. The different approaches and philosophies of care described reflect the current state of flux in service provision. However, there is a broad consensus on two major aspects of service provision. Firstly, many of the contributors have emphasised that a crisis service cannot stand alone, but must be viewed as an essential and integrated component of a comprehensive mental health system. No service can be complete without an adequate crisis service, but equally a crisis service cannot function without back-up and support. Secondly, it is clear that the development of a successful service is dependent on detailed strategic planning. Every area must assess the needs of the local population and plan services on this basis. There can never be a universal model to apply everywhere. Although many of the specific types of service described in this book can be widely adopted, the proportion of resources allocated to different aspects of the service, and the pattern of integration and communication must be decided locally.

In this chapter we will attempt to summarise the main themes which have emerged by briefly discussing the roles of different key groups and by suggesting priority action plans for the future.

Purchasers

In Britain, and elsewhere, purchasers of health care have an increasingly influential role in shaping the future development of services. Their fundamental task is to establish the needs of their local population and to ensure that as many of these needs as possible are met as efficiently as possible. To do this, purchasers require specific expertise in mental health as well as expertise in public health medicine. Contracts with provider units should therefore make specific mention of emergency care, and incorporate national policy guidelines, as well as any specific needs of the local population. Provider units need to be encouraged to be flexible and innovative in their approaches. Locally agreed minimum quality standards for the provision of emergency mental health care should be established. Failure to meet these standards should be investigated, and efforts by provider units to improve standards should be supported. Gradual improvement in services should be expected, and adequate resources provided for this.

Action plan for purchasers

- Identity emergency mental health care as a specific and high priority area.
- Establish local needs.
- Investigate current service utilisation, including data on diagnostic mix.
- Set locally agreed minimum standards of care, which incorporate national policy and guidance.
- Encourage flexible and innovative services.
- Ensure audit and monitoring of services.
- Provide adequate resources for staff training and supervision.
- Provide transitional funding for major service changes.

Clinicians

Any service can only be as effective as the clinicians who work in it. Staff have a responsibility to improve and broaden their skills, and to accept new ways of working. Crisis services have lagged behind rehabilitation services in providing multidisciplinary assessment and management of patients. Staff need to break through traditional professional barriers and have a greater understanding and respect for different professional skills. They need to listen to, and act on, criticism from service users and carers. Innovative work patterns will allow the flexible services that users demand. Clinical staff will always have the clearest and most immediate picture of any given service. They therefore have a responsibility to point out to purchasers deficiencies of care and to voice their concerns when resources are inadequate for them to provide a proper service.

Action plan for clinicians

- Understand the shortcomings of current care provision.
- Learn to work with change.
- Conduct routine evaluation.
- Make use of new technology.
- Be prepared to experiment.
- Break down professional barriers.
- Accept more flexible working patterns.
- Experienced staff to work at the front line.

Researchers

This book has demonstrated the important role that researchers have played during the last 30 years in establishing the feasibility, acceptability and effectiveness of many different innovative models of emergency care. In order that future service developments are guided by research findings it is essential that findings are clearly disseminated to policy makers and managers, as well as to clinicians. It is sometimes argued that many research findings cannot be generalised, and that results are distorted by the setting up of short lived experimental teams, with highly motivated staff. For this reason there is a constant need for further research to confirm previous findings in different settings, and to evaluate the effectiveness of different models of care. Randomised controlled trails (RCTs) are the most scientifically valid approach to comparing different types of care, and are routine in many types of medical research. However where RCTs are not clinically feasible there remains a need for other forms of controlled research. Currently much evaluative research is hampered by a lack of standardised and psychometrically robust instruments for measuring individual and service outcomes. Instruments which are short enough to be used on a routine basis by busy clinical staff need to be developed, so as to encourage evaluation of all services, and to allow direct comparison between different services.

Action plan for researchers

- Support routine evaluation.
- Conduct large detailed randomised controlled trials.
- Develop effective instruments for measuring patient outcome.
- Investigate the effects of service change on staff, carers and the wider community.
- Be sensitive to the needs of clinicians, carers and patients.
- Allow research to be guided by clinicians and others involved with services.
- Disseminate findings.

Managers

The development of more community based emergency services requires skilled management. In helping clinical staff provide the best possible service within the resources available, managers have a number of roles. They have a direct responsibility to provide the necessary infrastructure for the clinical service to function effectively. They need to introduce more flexible working patterns, but at the same time be sensitive to the needs of staff; for instance staff with children may have difficulty working in the evenings. With services moving away from centralised bases there is an increasing need for communication and safety equipment, and staff may need to be provided with cars. The establishment of crisis houses and community bases will involve negotiating with local authority planning departments, and ensuring that health and safety standards are met. Changes must be carefully discussed with local residents to help alleviate their concerns. In addition, managers need to liaise with the health purchasers and negotiate contracts which are workable, and acceptable to the clinical staff. They also have an important role in developing close links with a range of community agencies, such as social services, local housing associations, other provider units and the police.

Action plan for managers

- Collect and disseminate data.
- Encourage complaints and suggestions.
- Publicise available services.

- Financial support – costing of services.
- Shift resources.
- Provide communication aids/infrastructure/safety.
- Liaise with other providers.
- Highlight special needs to purchasers.

Voluntary organisations

There will always be a vital role for voluntary organisations alongside statutory services. They will often be perceived as less threatening than formal mental health services. Their flexibility can allow them to provide additional services, which are not necessarily provided by local services, such as specialist supported housing, and to respond quickly to changing local need. As independent bodies they have a role as a powerful national and local lobby, and advocate for people with severe mental illness. On a local level, voluntary organisations should establish close relationships with the statutory agencies, and take an active part in the planning of service changes. Staff working for statutory emergency services need to be aware of what local voluntary organisations can offer, so that they can make appropriate referrals.

Action plan for voluntary organisations

- Be aware of local service changes.
- Develop strong working relationships with statutory services.
- Provide alternatives/additions to statutory services, e.g. counselling services.
- Advocacy (individual and organisational).
- Ensure that staff receive mental health training.
- Encourage clients/residents to establish and maintain contact with primary and specialist mental health teams.
- Be aware of clients'/residents' signs of relapse and care plan.

Users

Users of mental health services are, at last, beginning to be listened to, and their views are a powerful force in the development of future services. Users have repeatedly emphasised the importance of being able to get urgent help when needed, and acute services have frequently been the subject of their sharpest criticism. On a national level user groups must continue to influence decisions about mental health legislation and policy changes. On a local level user groups need to encourage participation from a wide and representative sample of service users. Frequent contact with user representatives will raise staff awareness of different perceptions of the service they provide, and help them to question their current work practices. Dialogue with service providers should be on a regular and formal basis. As well as highlighting shortcomings in current provision, representatives should propose constructive ideas for service changes.

Action plan for users

- Continue to influence future service development.
- Canvas views from wide range of service users.
- Establish stable and regular communication with service purchasers and providers.
- Individual advocacy.
- Highlight examples of good, as well as bad, practice.

Carers

Service changes can have a profound impact on carers, and at times they will be affected more than anyone. Mental health services would very quickly collapse if it were not for their support. They must recognise their importance and feel comfortable in making their demands known. They will often be the first to know when their relative is beginning to relapse, and it is essential that they know how to contact local services. If their relative is not known to staff, the carer has a vital role in providing information and explaining what has helped in similar situations in the past. Carers should work closely with key workers in negotiating care plans and deciding on strategies for future relapse prevention. Carers must look after themselves, accept their limitations and be prepared to accept extra help when they need it.

Action plan for carers

- Recognise their own rights for help and support.
- Express opinions about service provision.
- Know how to contact services.
- Work closely with mental health staff.
- Seek help when it is needed.

Policy makers

Policy makers need to recognise the clear limitations of current emergency mental health provision, and the growing consensus, supported by research evidence, about how services should be changed. The challenge for the next 10 years is to ensure geographically widespread changes, not just in a few exceptional areas. They need to demand relevant and high quality research to guide future policy. Policy must be prepared in collaboration with people who have current, or recent, experience of working in clinical settings. When specific guidance is given it should be practical and clearly explained. It should reflect long-term strategies, rather than being a pragmatic response to recent events. If required, fresh legislation should be introduced to support changing work practices before introducing greater professional powers and further reductions in individual patient rights. However, alternative forms of care and treatment should be sought. Changes in policy and legislation should be carefully monitored, and reviewed regularly. Policy that cannot be implemented should be discarded when justified.

Action plan for policy makers

- Collect high quality national and regional data on service use.
- Canvas views of wide range of interested parties.
- Provide principled and co-ordinated policy and legislation.
- Provide clear guidance for clinicians and managers.
- Establish agreed national minimum standards of care.
- Ensure adequate and secure finance for services.
- Monitor adherence and effect of policy changes.
- Conduct detailed inquiries on individual cases which highlight deficiencies in current care arrangements.

Future challenges

The aims of this book are to inform the debate about the provision of emergency mental health services and to encourage the introduction of more flexible and community-based emergency services. Progress has been made in identifying the limitations of current services, and establishing models of alternative care, but in many areas the emergency mental health services which currently exist are not those which we would wish to use for our families. One touchstone for the future adequacy of these services is whether we could honestly say that we would use them ourselves.

Index